EATING TO EXTINCTION

EATING TO
EXTINCTION

THE WORLD'S
RAREST FOODS AND
WHY WE NEED
TO SAVE THEM

DAN SALADINO

FARRAR, STRAUS AND GIROUX

NEW YORK

Farrar, Straus and Giroux
120 Broadway, New York 10271

Copyright © 2021 by Dan Saladino
All rights reserved
Printed in the United States of America
Originally published in 2021 by Jonathan Cape, Great Britain
Published in the United States by Farrar, Straus and Giroux
First American edition, 2022

Library of Congress Cataloging-in-Publication Data
Names: Saladino, Dan, 1970– author.
Title: Eating to extinction : the world's rarest foods and why we need to
    save them / Dan Saladino.
Description: First American edition. | New York : Farrar, Straus and
    Giroux, 2022. | "Originally published in 2021 by Jonathan Cape,
    Great Britain." | Includes bibliographical references and index.
Identifiers: LCCN 2021041139 | ISBN 9780374605322 (hardcover)
Subjects: LCSH: Food—History. | Food supply—History. | Agrobiodiversity.
    Agrobiodiversity conservation. | Food industry and trade—Environmental
    aspects.
Classification: LCC TX357 .S23 2022 | DDC 641.3009—dc23
LC record available at https://lccn.loc.gov/2021041139

Our books may be purchased in bulk for promotional, educational, or business
    use. Please contact your local bookseller or the Macmillan Corporate and
    Premium Sales Department at 1-800-221-7945, extension 5442, or by
    email at MacmillanSpecialMarkets@macmillan.com.

www.fsgbooks.com
www.twitter.com/fsgbooks • www.facebook.com/fsgbooks

1   3   5   7   9   10   8   6   4   2

To Annabel, Harry and Charlie – my fellow travellers on the ark of taste

Nature has introduced great variety into the landscape, but man has displayed a passion for simplifying it.

Rachel Carson, *Silent Spring*

Tradition is not the worship of ashes, but the preservation of fire.

attributed to Gustav Mahler

Contents

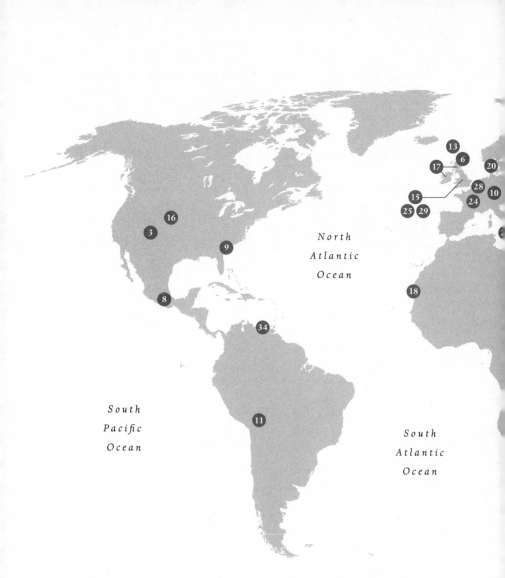

North
Atlantic
Ocean

South
Pacific
Ocean

South
Atlantic
Ocean

1 Hadza Honey (Lake Eyasi, Tanzania)
2 Murnong (Southern Australia)
3 Bear Root (Colorado, USA)
4 Memang Narang (Garo Hills, India)
5 Kavılca Wheat (Büyük Çatma, Anatolia)
6 Bere Barley (Orkney, Scotland)
7 Red Mouth Glutinous Rice (Sichuan, China)
8 Olotón Maize (Oaxaca, Mexico)
9 Geechee Red Pea (Sapelo Island, Georgia, USA)

10 Alb Lentil (Swabia, Germany)
11 Oca (Andes, Bolivia)
12 O-Higu Soybean (Okinawa, Japan)
13 Skerpikjøt (Faroe Islands)
14 Black Ogye Chicken (Yeonsan, South Korea)
15 Middle White Pig (Wye Valley, England)
16 Bison (Great Plains, USA)
17 Wild Atlantic Salmon (Ireland and Scotland)
18 Imraguen Butarikh (Banc D'Arguin, Mauritania)

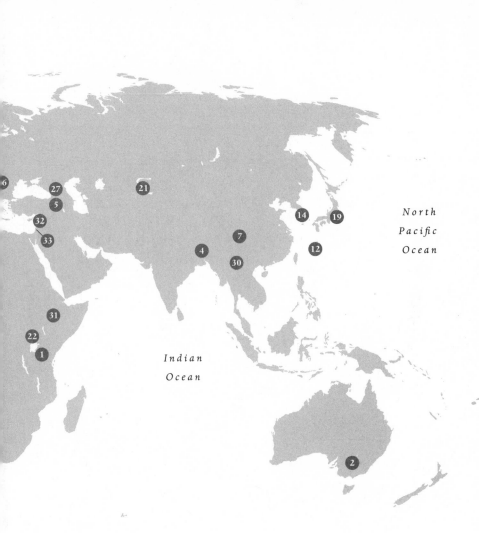

Introduction

In eastern Turkey, in a golden field overshadowed by grey mountains, I reached out and touched an endangered species. Its ancestors had evolved over millions of years and migrated here long ago. It had been indispensable to life in the villages across this plateau, but its time was running out. 'Just a few fields left,' the farmer said. 'Extinction will come easily.' This endangered species wasn't a rare bird or an elusive wild animal, it was food, a type of wheat: a less familiar character in the extinction story now playing out around the world, but one we all need to know.

The tall crop, heavy with grains, was ready to harvest. A whisper of a breeze made its surface swirl like a sea. To most of us, one field of wheat might look much like any other, but this crop was extraordinary. Kavilca (pronounced Kav-all-jah) had turned eastern Anatolian landscapes the colour of honey for four hundred generations (around 10,000 years). It was one of the world's earliest cultivated foods, and now one of the rarest.

How could this be possible? Wheat is an ubiquitous grass that covers more farmland than any other crop, grown on every continent except Antarctica. How can a food be close to extinction and yet at the same time appear to be everywhere? The answer is that one type of wheat is different to another. Each has a unique story to tell, and many varieties are at risk, including ones with important characteristics we need to combat crop diseases or climate change. Kavilca's rarity is emblematic of the mass extinction taking place in our food. We are losing diversity in all the crops that feed the world. Yet diversity was the rule for millennia; thousands of different types of wheat have been recorded, each one distinctive in the way it looked, grew and tasted. Few of these varieties have survived into the twenty-first century. Instead, all over the world, from Punjab to Iowa, the Western Cape to East Anglia, wheat fields have been cloaked in a blanket of uniformity, and the same is happening to all our food, at a faster and faster pace.

Many aspects of our lives are becoming more homogeneous. We can shop from identical outlets, see the same brands and buy into the same fashions around the world. The same is true of our diet. In a short space of time it has become possible for us to eat the same food wherever we are, creating an edible form of uniformity. 'But hang on,' you might say, 'I eat a greater variety of foods than my parents or grandparents ever did.' And on one level, that is true. Whether you're in London, Los Angeles or Lima, you can eat sushi, curry, or McDonald's; bite into an avocado, banana or mango; sip a Coke, a Budweiser or a branded bottle of water – and all in a single day. What we're being offered appears at first to be diverse, until you realise it is the same kind of 'diversity' that is spreading around the globe in identical fashion; what the world buys and eats is becoming more and more the same.

Consider these facts: the source of much of the world's food – seeds – is mostly in the control of just four corporations; half of all the world's cheeses are produced with bacteria or enzymes manufactured by a single company; one in four beers drunk around the world is the product of one brewer; from the USA to China, most global pork production is based around the genetics of a single breed of pig; and, perhaps most famously, although there are more than 1,500 different varieties of banana, global trade is dominated by just one, the Cavendish, a cloned fruit grown in monocultures so vast their scale can only be comprehended from the view of an aeroplane or by satellite.

This level of uniformity, from the genetics of the world's most widely consumed crops, wheat, rice and maize, right through to the meals they become, has never been experienced before. The human diet has undergone more change in the last 150 years (roughly six generations) than in the entire previous one million years (around 40,000 generations). And in the last half a century, trade, technology and corporate power have extended these dietary changes right across the world. We are living and eating our way through one big unparalleled experiment.

For most of our evolution as a species, as hunter-gatherers and then as farmers, human diets were enormously varied. Our food was the product of a place and crops were adapted to a particular environment, shaped by the knowledge and the preferences of the people who lived there as well as the climate, soil, water and even altitude. This diversity was stored and passed on in the seeds farmers saved, in the flavours of the fruits and vegetables people grew, the breeds of animals they reared, the bread they baked, the cheeses they produced and the drinks they made.

Kavilca wheat is one of the survivors of disappearing diversity, but only just. Like all the endangered foods in this book, it has a distinctive history and a connection to a specific part of the world and its people. I came across it in a village called Büyük Çatma, north of the part of Turkey where the very first farmers began cultivating wheat 12,000 years ago. From the time when prehistoric tribes farmed this land and on through Roman, Ottoman, Soviet and then Turkish rule, Kavilca was the most important food source here. It is only during our lifetimes that this singular grain, perfectly adapted to its environment and with a taste like no other, has become endangered and pushed to the brink of extinction. The same is true of many thousands of other crops and foods. We should all know their stories and the reasons for their decline, not just as an exercise in food history or to satisfy culinary curiosity but also, as we'll see, because our survival depends on it.

Under the big open sky of eastern Anatolia, I watched the farmer as he worked until dusk, harvesting the last of the Kavilca wheat from his field. 'I want to plant Kavilca again next year,' the farmer said. 'But my neighbours? I'm not so sure.' I was witnessing the closing chapter of a story that had begun thousands of years before. It felt like a privilege but also a tragedy.

I reported on food stories for BBC radio for almost a decade before I realised the extent of the extinction process taking place. I had stumbled into food journalism, but for me, food soon became the perfect lens through which I could understand the inner workings of the world. Food shows us where real power lies; it can explain conflicts and wars; showcase human creativity and invention; account for the rise and fall of empires; and expose the causes and consequences of disasters. Food stories are perhaps the most essential stories of all.

My entry into food journalism took place during a crisis. It was 2008, and while the world was mostly focusing on the financial turmoil ripping through the banking system, a momentous food story was also unfolding. Wheat, rice and maize prices were spiralling to record highs, tripling on global markets at their peak. This pushed tens of millions of the poorest people on Earth towards hunger and also fuelled the tensions that later exploded into the Arab Spring. Riots and protests toppled governments in Tunisia and Egypt and helped trigger the conflict in Syria. For the first time in decades, people were asking serious questions about the future of our food. With 7.5 billion people on Earth and a projected 10 billion by 2050, crop scientists began telling the world that global harvests needed to increase by 70 per cent. Faced with these forecasts, the disappearance of one type of wheat like Kavilca might have seemed an irrelevance. Surely what the planet needed was more food? Calling for greater diversity seemed like an indulgence. But now we're starting to realise that diversity is essential for our future.

Evidence of this shift in thinking came in September 2019 at the Climate Action Summit held at the United Nations headquarters in New York. Emmanuel Faber, who was then CEO of the dairy giant Danone, told the business leaders and politicians present that the food system the world had created over the last century was at a dead end. 'We thought with science we could change the cycle of life and its rules,' he said, that we could feed ourselves with monocultures and base most of the world's food supply on a handful of plants. This approach was now bankrupt, Faber explained. 'We've been killing life and now we need to restore it.'

Faber was making a pledge to save diversity backed by twenty global food businesses, including Unilever, Nestlé, Mars and Kellogg – companies with combined food sales in a hundred countries of about $500 billion. He said the world urgently needed to save the crops and 'the traditional seeds that are dying', and that agricultural biodiversity needed to be restored. At the event, Faber expressed concern that in parts of the dairy industry 99 per cent of the cows are a single breed, the Holstein. 'It's over-simplistic now,' he said of the global food system. 'We have a complete loss of diversity.'

If the businesses that helped create and spread homogeneity in our food are now voicing concerns over lost diversity, then we should all take notice. The enormity of what we're losing is only now dawning on us; but if we act now, we can save it.

The endangered foods in this book are part of the bigger crisis unfolding across the planet: the loss of all kinds of biodiversity. Just as we are losing diversity in jungles and rainforests, we're losing it in fields and farms. But what exactly does 'biodiversity' mean when applied to food? Part of the answer lies at the end of a tunnel cut 135 metres deep into a mountain on the remote Arctic island of Svalbard. This is the most secure place scientists could find to build the world's largest seed vault, home of a collection of more than one million seeds, a living record of thousands of years of farming history. These seeds were sent to Svalbard for safekeeping, usually by governments but also by indigenous people looking to preserve their most precious and often endangered traditional foods. The collection represents one form of diversity being lost from our food: genetic diversity, or, put another way, the variation created since the dawn of agriculture by farmers all over the world. There are varieties of more than 1,000 different crops inside the vault, including 170,000 unique samples of rice, 39,000 samples of maize, 21,000 samples of potato and 35,000 samples of millet (there are also the wild relatives of all of these crops). And tucked away in one of the boxes of seed (all kept at –18°C) is a handful of Kavilca grains, just one of the 213,000 different samples of wheat being safeguarded. Diversity stored in a vault isn't the same as that tended by farmers growing crops we can eat, but it's a recognition of the importance of diversity and a way of keeping our options open.

In addition to the seeds at Svalbard, in other parts of the world collections of living diversity are managed by universities and other institutions. For example, at Brogdale in Kent, home of the UK's National Fruit Collection, there are 2,000 varieties of apple while at the University of California Riverside more than 1,000 different varieties of citrus are being conserved. Across the planet there are 8,000 livestock breeds (of cows, sheep, pigs and so on) being saved, mostly on small farms, many at risk of extinction. Much of our food supply has been narrowed down to a tiny fraction of this diverse array of plants and animals, and in some cases we are dependent on just one variety or a handful of breeds.

The rich profusion of diversity, provided by nature and guided by human hands, is not just one of the most beautiful features of our food and farming history. We nurtured diversity because we needed it and, in the creation of cuisines and the evolution of cultures, we have celebrated it. In the village of Büyük Çatma in eastern Turkey, farmers grew Kavilca for millennia because in the harshest, wettest, coldest winters, no other crop produced as much food. What's more, countless cooks experimented with the grain and used its distinctive textures and tastes to craft recipes, creating what we might refer to today as a food culture. Wherever you look in human history, all communities had their own versions of Kavilca, life-giving foods that forged identities or inspired rituals and religions, such as gods made of maize in Central America and oranges believed to repel spirits in South Asia. Whether plants or animals, these were unique genetic resources, all adapted to their place in the world. You can multiply Kavilca's story a million times, for each and every seed stored inside Svalbard, for all the ancient breeds of farm animals that still exist, and for every traditional style of cheese and bread made around the world. Each one of these foods is a piece of human history.

The decline in the diversity of our food, and the fact that so many foods have become endangered, didn't happen by accident: it is an entirely human-made process. The biggest loss of crop diversity came in the decades that followed the Second World War when, in an attempt to save millions from starvation, crop scientists found ways to produce grains such as rice and wheat on a phenomenal scale. To grow the extra food the world desperately needed diversity was sacrificed, as thousands of traditional varieties were replaced by a small number of new super-productive ones. These plants were designed to grow quickly and produce lots more grain. The strategy that ensured this – more agrochemicals, more irrigation, plus new genetics – came to be known as the 'Green Revolution'. And it worked spectacularly well, at least to begin with.

Because of it, grain production tripled, and between 1970 and 2020 the human population more than doubled. Leaving the environmental, dietary and social legacy of that strategy to one side (we will get there), the danger of creating more uniform crops is that, like a stock portfolio with just a few holdings, they become vulnerable to catastrophes. A global food system that depends on just a narrow selection of plants – and only a very small number of varieties of these – is at greater risk of succumbing to diseases, pests and climate extremes.

Quite *how* vulnerable can be understood when you look across a field of Kavilca. As an older form of wheat, it stands taller than the modern varieties you're likely to see today. There are good evolutionary reasons for this; as they grow, longer stalks put distance between the ears of wheat and the soil, which is where most plant diseases live. One of these diseases is caused by a ruinous (and incredibly sneaky) fungus called *Fusarium graminearum*, which is spreading through Europe, Asia and the Americas. After tricking its way inside the wheat, it leaves behind a worthless crop and tonnes of grain made toxic to humans and animals. Once the fungus is in a field, it is impossible to remove.

The disease it causes (Fusarium head blight) creates billions of dollars of damage a year and presents a serious risk to future food security. The genetics of modern wheat makes it more susceptible to head blight than older varieties. Like most crop diseases spreading around the world, the problem is getting worse too. Climate change, particularly warmer, wetter weather, is accelerating the fungus's spread. Although the Green Revolution was based on ingenious science, it attempted to oversimplify nature, and this is starting to backfire on us. In creating fields of identical wheat, we abandoned thousands of highly adapted and resilient varieties. Far too often their valuable traits were lost forever. We're starting to see our mistake – there was wisdom in what went before.

Kavilca is just one endangered food, but it illustrates, as do all of the foods in this book, the interconnectedness of farming, food, environment, diet and health. The physicist Albert-László Barabási, an expert in unravelling complex networks both human-made and natural, argues that the driving force of science during the twentieth century was a relentless kind of reductionism; convinced by our own cleverness, we believed we were capable of deciphering nature in all its complexity and then overriding it. And yes, we have been brilliant at fathoming the constituent parts, but we have too often failed to understand nature as a whole. Like a child taking apart a favourite toy, Barabási says, we have no idea how to put it back together again. In riding reductionism, 'we run into the hard wall of complexity'.

The endangered foods in this book represent a time before that scientific reductionism took hold. These foods offered much more than a supply of calories delivered in ever greater quantities, they helped us work more in harmony with nature. Take, for example, a humble legume called the Swabian lentil, once grown widely in the Alps of southern Germany. Beloved for its flavour, the *Alb-linse* fed the people in this mountainous region because it was able to nourish the otherwise ungenerous soil. Or consider a rare variety of maize found high up in a village in Oaxaca, Mexico, that oozes a self-fertilising mucus which scientists believe could help reduce agriculture's dependence on fossil fuels. Many of the world's endangered foods are so complex that scientists are only just beginning to unlock their secrets.

Of the 6,000 plant species humans have eaten over time, the world now mostly eats just nine, of which just three – rice, wheat and maize – provide 50 per cent of all calories. Add potato, barley, palm oil, soy and sugar (beet and cane) and you have 75 per cent of all the calories that fuel our species. Since the Green Revolution, we eat more refined grains, vegetable oils, sugar and meat, and we depend on foods produced further and further away from the places we live. As thousands of foods have become endangered and extinct, a small number have risen to dominance. Often this has happened without us really noticing. Take soy, domesticated in China thousands of years ago, a bean relatively obscure outside Asia until the 1970s and now one of the world's most traded agricultural commodities. Used in feed for pigs, chickens, cattle and farmed fish, which in turn feed us, soy plays a starring role in an increasingly homogeneous diet eaten by billions of people. Seen in the context of 2 million years of human evolution, these dietary shifts taking place at a global level, all pointing towards uniformity, are unprecedented. This is happening as we're just beginning to understand the importance of diversity to our own health. The richer our gut microbiomes (the trillions of bacteria, fungi and other microbes we all host) the better for us. And the more diverse our diets, the richer our gut microbiomes become.

What an individual human diet looked like even a few thousand years ago isn't easy to untangle from the archaeological record, let alone further back in our evolution, but we do know it was far richer in diversity than the one most of us eat today. In the Jutland Peninsula of western Denmark in 1950, peat diggers discovered the intact body of a man who had been executed (or possibly sacrificed) 2,500 years ago. The body had been so well protected in the wet, boggy conditions it was first thought to be the victim of a recent murder. Inside the man's stomach was a porridge made with barley, flax and the seeds of forty different plants, some of them gathered from the wild. In present-day East Africa, the Hadza, who are among the last of the world's hunter-gatherers, eat from a potential wild menu that consists of more than eight hundred plant and animal species, including numerous types of tubers, berries, leaves, small mammals, large game, birds and types of honey. The Hadza are a surviving link back to early-human diets. We can't replicate their diets in the industrialised world but we can learn from them nonetheless.

On top of the nutritional loss and genetic loss taking place, there is a cultural one. Over millennia, humans discovered myriad ways of cooking, crafting, baking, fermenting, smoking, drying and distilling their foods and drinks. The number of people in possession of many of the world's traditional food skills, and much of the world's ancient knowledge, is dwindling, from methods of cheese-making to techniques for preserving cuts of meat. These are essential parts of our heritage and are being lost. We look to paintings, sculptures, cathedrals and temples for the greatest examples of human creativity and vision, but we should also look to the endangered foods in this book, whether a cultivated red grain of rice from south-western China, a rare cheese from the Accursed Mountains of Albania, or a piece of cake baked in western Syria; each of these foods is the product of invention and imagination and the wisdom of generations of unknown cooks and farmers.

This book is definitely not a call to return to some kind of halcyon past. But it is a plea to consider what the past can teach us about how to inhabit the world now and in the future. Our current food system is contributing to the destruction of the planet: one million plant and animal species are now threatened with extinction; we clear swathes of forests to plant immense monocultures and then burn through millions of barrels of oil a day to make fertilisers to feed them. Out at sea, we have significantly altered 90 per cent of the oceans; marine wilderness is disappearing. And while we destroy biodiversity, we extract tremendous quantities of water from rivers and aquifers to irrigate Green Revolution crops in a loan that cannot be repaid. Our food is both the cause and a victim of all of this harm. The productivity of a quarter of the land surface of the Earth has been seriously compromised, hampering our ability to grow food. We are farming on borrowed time.

I can't claim that the foods in this book will provide answers to all of these problems, but I believe they should be part of the solution. Bere barley, for example, is a food so perfectly adapted to the harsh environment of Orkney that no fertilisers or other chemicals are needed for it to grow. *Skerpikjøt*, a fermented hunk of sheep meat from the Faroe Islands, shows us how far our relationship with animals has changed – and needs to change again. And murnong, a juicy, nutritious and once abundant root from southern Australia, is proof that the world has much to learn from indigenous peoples about eating more in harmony with nature.

Many argue that the only serious answer to our food problems lies not in returning to a more diverse food system, but in launching a second Green Revolution, one based around biotechnology, such as transgenics and gene editing. But even that approach will depend on saving endangered foods. Crop breeders and other food scientists have joined in the race to save disappearing diversity because endangered plants and animals – including many featured in this book – are seen as possessing the genetic toolkit we need to tackle drought and disease, to contend with climate change and to improve the quality of our diets. Whichever path we take, we can't afford to let these foods go extinct.

The concept of being *endangered* and *at risk of extinction* is usually reserved for wildlife. Since the 1960s, the Red List, compiled by the International Union for Conservation of Nature, has catalogued vulnerable plant and animal species (around 105,000 at the time of writing), highlighting those at risk of extinction (nearly 30,000). It's only if you know something is about to disappear, the thinking goes, that you can galvanise action to save it.

A version of the Red List dedicated solely to food was created in the mid-1990s, in the small Piedmontese town of Bra, in northern Italy, when a group of friends realised that crops, animal breeds and traditional dishes were disappearing from their region. They created an online catalogue for endangered foods and named it the Ark of Taste. Led by the journalist Carlo Petrini, the group had already set up the Slow Food organisation, which called on people 'to defend themselves against the universal madness of "the fast life" ... escape the tediousness of "fast-food" [and] rediscover the rich varieties and aromas of local cuisines'. They saw that when a food, a local product or crop became endangered, so too did a way of life, knowledge and skill, a local economy and an ecosystem. Their call to respect diversity captured the imaginations of farmers, cooks and campaigners from around the world, who started to add their own endangered foods to the Ark.

The Ark of Taste inspired this book. As I write, it contains 5,312 foods from 130 countries, with 762 products on a waiting list ready to be assessed. Here, we will meet people saving endangered foods, including the farmer who showed me the rare field of Kavilca wheat and others like him. There are likely to be other champions in your own part of the world. These foods represent much more than sustenance. They are history, identity, pleasure, culture, geography, genetics, science, creativity and craft. And our future.

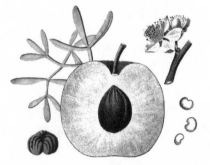

Food:
A Very Brief History

[Biodiversity] is the assembly of life that took a billion
years to evolve. It has eaten the storms – folded them
into its genes – and created the world that created us.
It holds the world steady.

E.O. Wilson, *The Diversity of Life*

To grasp the scale of the decline in the diversity of the world's food, we need to comprehend the almost incomprehensible amount of time it took for biodiversity to evolve. So huge is the timeline involved here, I'm going to call on the help of Kavilca wheat once more, to provide some useful points of reference.

Four and a half billion years before the first farmers planted Kavilca seeds, there was nothing on the menu. Earth was a fiery landscape with burning lava spouting from volcanoes and its surface bombarded by meteors. Geologists call this hellish time the Hadean period, after the Greek god of the underworld. One billion years later, the first microscopic organisms appeared, followed a further billion years later by forms of bacteria capable of using energy from the sun and water to produce nutrients. These first acts of photosynthesis produced oxygen and made it possible for more complex life forms to evolve. Fast-forward another one and a half billion years and multicellular life forms show up on Earth, and a mere 100 million after that, sponges and tiny, plate-like creatures called Placozoa evolved, perhaps the last common ancestors of all animals. But there was still nothing on Earth you and I would recognise as food.

Things started to become a little more interesting (at least from our point of view) 530 million years ago; the continents were dividing and different life forms proliferated in the oceans following the Cambrian Explosion, evolution's 'Big Bang'. This was the beginning of biodiversity as we know it. Shelled creatures resembling clams and snails appeared in the oceans, along with oyster-like bivalves, eel-like conodonts and *Nectocaris pteryx*, a kite-shaped, stalk-eyed, carnivorous ancestor of squid, octopus and cuttlefish. By the time the Earth entered its next geological age, the Ordovician, less than 500 million years ago, most of the ancestors of all the major life forms that populate our world today had arrived. Plants made their big move from sea to land to begin a long, co-evolutionary journey with another life form, insects.

The first plants on land were mosses and ferns, which released spores into the air to reproduce. They also helped to break apart Earth's rocky surface, turning it into a substrate, which slowly developed into soil. Four hundred million years ago Earth's environment went from being moist and tropical to drier and (for most plants) more hostile. In response plants evolved preservation chambers that could provide an embryo protection as well as a store of food: seeds. Around 250 million years ago, some plants came up with the added evolutionary advantage of growing spectacular flowers and seductive fruits to attract the greatest number of insects and mammals to disperse grains of pollen and seeds. Grasses evolved 60 million years ago, a big moment in terms of our food history. Dinosaurs missed out on this food source by around 6 million years, but mammals, including humans, were waiting in the wings to reap the benefits; from these grasses came rice, maize, barley and wheat (at last, Kavilca is on its way!).

Six million years ago, ape-like hominids appeared, among them *Sahelanthropus tchadensis* (Sahel Man), a species that spent most of its time foraging among forest canopies, eating leaves, nuts, seeds, roots, fruits and insects. In Ethiopia 4 million years ago, a human ancestor called *Ardipithecus ramidus* (nicknamed Ardi) also climbed trees but spent a little more of its time finding food by walking on two feet. Then, 2 million years ago, Earth's climate changed and brought humans down from the trees and onto the ground. The wetlands of East Africa had become savannah and to survive our ancestors scavenged meat and hunted animals. In the Olduvai Gorge in northern Tanzania, early humans left behind stone tools used to strip flesh off carcasses and (perhaps more importantly) break into bones to gain access to the nutrient rich marrow. The human body changed again during this period; toes and forearms became shorter and legs longer as we turned into the long-distance runners of the animal kingdom, capable of tracking and killing larger creatures. Partly thanks to meat eating our teeth became smaller and our brains became bigger (three times larger than the brains of apes). The human gut also shrank in size, but within it a complex ecosystem of trillions of microbes evolved, helping us adapt to more diverse diets.

Between 800,000 and 300,000 years ago, the use of fire and cooking expanded the human diet, turning inedible plants into food and making meat easier to digest. Sophisticated weapons made human hunters more lethal; half a million years ago, spears were being used to kill land animals. Later, lethal barbs crafted from bones helped our ancestors to haul giant catfish out of lakes. Seventy thousand years ago, our species *Homo sapiens* spread out of East Africa and began to establish its dominance over the planet. Sixty-five thousand years ago, a group of hunter-gatherers reached Australia, where they devised fish traps along rivers (and used lakes to practise aquaculture).

Containers made from animal skins were being used to move food around 30,000 years ago, and later, baskets woven from plant fibres. In China, 20,000 years ago, long before the birth of agriculture, new cooking technology was in use: pots for boiling and steaming wild rice. By then groups of humans had made the long trek from north-east Asia to the Americas, taking much of this know-how with them.

Then came one of the most momentous events in the history of *Homo sapiens*: the birth of agriculture. In the Black Desert, in present-day Jordan, Natufian hunter-gatherers had long ground up the seeds of wild grasses into rough flour, and mixed in pulverised plant roots to make a dough which they cooked over fire. Scientists in the twenty-first century who recreated this early form of flatbread described the taste as 'nutty and a little bitter'. This mixture of different ingredients is the earliest evidence of a cuisine. The Natufians who made that bread 13,000 years ago are the transitional link between millions of years of human hunter-gatherers and agriculture. In the Fertile Crescent, an arc of land that sweeps across Iraq, south-eastern Turkey, Syria, Lebanon, Israel and Jordan, the necessary wild plants, climate and imagination led humans to become settled farmers. Over the next few thousand years, through unconscious decisions, accidental discoveries and luck, some humans transformed the plants they found around them, selecting the biggest seeds and the grains easiest to harvest, domesticating and taming them. During this time human biology changed yet again as our saliva and our gut microbiomes evolved to break down the greater amounts of starch produced by agriculture.

Early in this transition from foraging to farming came emmer, a type of wheat that would go on to be prized by ancient Egyptians. One of the few surviving varieties of this early form of wheat is Kavilca.

Wheat was not domesticated alone of course. In the Fertile Crescent, the Neolithic food package also included chickpeas and lentils, followed by figs and dates. Hunter-gatherers in other parts of the world domesticated the wild plants that grew in their ecosystems: rice and millets along the Yangtze and Yellow River basins in China; corn, squash and beans in south-eastern Mexico; potatoes and quinoa around Lake Titicaca in the Andes; mung beans and millets in India; sorghum and cowpeas in sub-Saharan Africa; and bananas and sugar cane in Papua New Guinea. The transformation of wild plants into cultivated crops took thousands of years and involved more than 150 generations of farmers. Alongside plants, these early farmers domesticated all of the animal species kept as livestock today: cows, sheep, pigs and goats, as well as camels, llamas and yaks. This resulted in another biological change, the ability of adult humans in some parts of the world to digest milk more easily.

Around 3,500 years ago, the remarkable transition from humans being dependent on wild foods to mostly cultivated ones neared completion. No new plants or animals of significance to human diets have been domesticated since. Why? Partly because by then the plants most suited to farming had been encountered. Domestication was also a slow and arduous task. Why go to the trouble when trade and migration were opening up access to new plants transformed by other civilisations? Globalisation in the ancient world helped bring an end to the domestication effort.

As the suite of domesticated plants and animals spread all over the world, moved around by farmers from one region to another, they evolved and adapted in new environments. To paraphrase the botanist E.O. Wilson, they 'ate the storms', adjusted to the soils, the climate, the altitude (and human inclinations) and 'folded them into their genes'. This is how the world ended up with so many varieties of corn, rice and wheat and all the other food crops.

Through innovation and experimentation, humans transformed their food in more intricate ways. People in central Europe started preserving milk by reducing its water content and concentrating the fats and proteins, so making cheese; in the Caucasus, grapes were crushed and converted into wine; in China, cooks deployed a wondrous process that turned inedible soybeans into white, silky blocks of tofu; in the Amazon, forest dwellers co-opted bacteria and yeasts to ferment a toxic tuber, cassava, into a safe and delicious food; and farmers in southern Mexico added toxic mineral lime to corn, to extract more nutrients from the grain and make a soft dough for tortillas.

Over millennia, food, cooking and eating became the most powerful expression of the human imagination. So, when a food becomes endangered, another seed lost, another skill forgotten, it is worth remembering the epic story of how they got here.

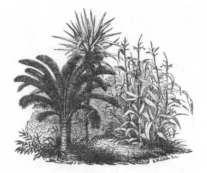

Part One
Wild

The question must be raised. Why farm? Hunter gatherers paint pictures, recite poetry, play musical instruments ... they do everything farmers do ... but they don't work as hard.

Jack Harlan, *Crops and Man*

We were born to eat wild. For most of our history, human survival meant foraging for plants, collecting nuts and seeds, and tracking and killing animals. By any measure, hunting and gathering has been our most successful lifestyle to date. In the late 1960s, the anthropologists Richard Lee and Irven DeVore estimated that of the 85,000 million people who had ever lived, 90 per cent were hunters and gatherers and only about 6 per cent lived as farmers. The barely significant number that remained were experimenting with life in the industrialised world. Our physiology, psychology, fears, hopes *and* dietary preferences have been shaped by our evolution as hunters and gatherers. Our bodies haven't changed that much but our way of life and our diets have, profoundly and at speed.

Of the 7.8 billion of us on the planet today, just a few thousand people continue to source most of their calories from the wild. Colonialism has historically played its part in this decline, and other forces are at work today. The farms, plantations and industries that feed most of us are destroying the habitats of many traditional societies. Manufactured and branded products from the industrialised world make it into the furthest reaches of the Amazon forest and the African savannah, in a form of neocolonialism through food. If the last of the hunter-gatherers ceased to exist – which could happen within our lifetimes – the world would lose valuable knowledge amassed over countless generations, and a link to the way of life that formed us. It would be a tragic end to a 2-million-year-long story.

But look more closely and it becomes clear that 'wild' food isn't just the preserve of the few remaining hunter-gatherers. Indigenous farming communities all over the world also still rely heavily on wild food. The Mbuti people in the Congo eat more than three hundred different species of animals and plants in addition to the cassava and plantains they cultivate. Across India, 1,400 wild plant species feature in rural diets, including 650 different fruits. And whereas many indigenous people get the bulk of their calories from wheat, corn, rice and millet, most of their micronutrients (the vitamins and minerals) still come from wild food. Rice farmers in north-eastern Thailand, for instance, forage for a wild spinach found around the edges of their paddies, a food which complements the starchy grain they grow. The choice between the cultivated and uncultivated is not a binary one – it is more of a sliding scale. It has always been this way. The first farmers to sow seeds would have starved if they hadn't continued to hunt and forage for wild food, as would the hundreds of generations of farmers who followed. In more modern times all human societies which have experienced scarcity have looked to the wild for sustenance. At the beginning of the twentieth-century Sicilians who went hungry after poor harvests searched for snails to eat; Americans in the depression era turned to wild blackberries and dandelions; people in wartime Britain gathered nettles; and in China during the Great Famine of the 1950s, people looked to bitter grasses for survival.

Today, one billion people source at least a portion of their diet from the wild, whether for sustenance or pleasure (the figure is 3.3 billion if you include fish). In Oaxaca in southern Mexico, city dwellers queue at markets to satisfy cravings for toasted flying ants. In Maputo, Mozambique, affluent eaters pay top dollar for cuts of wild 'bush' meat. And on the outskirts of Moscow, New York, Tokyo and London, you can find urban foragers venturing into woodlands to find berries and mushrooms when they are in season. But even though the call of the wild remains strong, the practice and the knowledge of how to find and eat wild foods are disappearing. So too, of course, are the wild plants, animals and their habitats. By the time you get to the next full stop, the world will have lost the equivalent of a football pitch of primary forest. Deforestation to make way for monocultures of soy, palm oil and cattle has contributed to thousands of the world's wild food species becoming endangered or threatened with extinction. One source of hope is the world's indigenous people who make up less than 5 per cent of the total human population but inhabit 25 per cent of the world's land surface. In the twenty-first century they are among the most important stewards of the natural world and defenders of biodiversity. The wild foods they protect are crucial for all of our future food security, including the 'crop wild relatives' that may hold the genetic keys to problems such as drought and disease resistance.

Wild foods are also becoming endangered at a time when we are struggling to understand what our diets should look like. We look to incomplete science for answers but ignore lessons already learned. Although wild foods provide less than 1 per cent of all of the calories consumed around the world today, they account for a much higher proportion of nutrients. Among hunter-gatherers such as the Hadza, rates of obesity, type 2 diabetes, heart disease and cancer are so low that cases are hard to find. This is partly because of the rich diversity of foods they eat and the high levels of fibre they consume (five times more than people in the industrialised world). Bitterness and sourness, both associated with wild foods, are often signals of health-giving properties. In the Peruvian Amazon, people gather camu camu (*Myrciaria dubia*), a fruit which resembles a cherry and contains twenty times more vitamin C than an orange.

The foods we are about to meet in this part all help to explain why wild foods matter. The answers to the mess we're in, environmentally and physically, will not, of course, include a return to the wild, but they can be informed by the knowledge that has carried our species this far, over millennia. We might not be able to imitate the hunter-gatherers that remain, but we can and should be inspired by the people who continue to venture into the wild.

I

Hadza Honey

Lake Eyasi, Tanzania

It was April, the rainy season. Short downpours had brought pockets of colour to the greens and browns of the East African savannah as small delicate flowers bloomed. Nectar was becoming abundant and, with it, honey. I was with a group of Hadza hunters, a scattered population of just over one thousand people. The tribe has lived in the dry bush of northern Tanzania, near the shore of Lake Eyasi, for tens of thousands of years, perhaps hundreds of thousands of years. Now, fewer than two hundred Hadza live fully as hunter-gatherers, making them the last people in Africa to practise no form of agriculture. The group I was with had walked far away from the camp and deep into the bush, led by a young man named Sigwazi. As he walked, he whistled.

This wasn't a melodious tune, more a series of angular ups and downs on a musical scale, each passage finished with a high-pitched twirl. To my ears there was no obvious musical pattern to follow but something in the bush was paying close attention to this whistle. Noticing movement above the trees, Sigwazi broke into a sprint, weaving through the scrub and around baobab trees as he continued the whistle. A wordless conversation was under way, an exchange between a human and a bird. Sigwazi looked towards the flutter of activity in the canopy, and there perched on a branch was an olive-grey bird the size of a starling.

Barring a few flashes of white on its tail, the bird looked plain and unassuming, but after a few more whistles from the hunter, it revealed itself to be exceptional. 'Ach-ech-ech-ech' came its reply to Sigwazi's whistle, signalling that a deal was on. The bird had agreed to lead the hunter to honey hidden among the branches of the giant baobabs. These trees are as wide as they are tall, living for up to a thousand years, fed by a root system so deep that they can access water in periods of extreme drought. Finding a bees' nest concealed among the baobab's tall branches can take a hunter-gatherer several hours as they need to inspect tree after tree; with the assistance of a honeyguide, it takes a fraction of that time. The bird's scientific name captures its talent perfectly: *Indicator indicator*.

Somehow, over hundreds of thousands of years, the two species, humans and honeyguides, found a way of sharing their different skills. The bird can find the bees' nests but can't get to the wax it wants to eat without being stung to death. Humans, meanwhile, struggle to find the nests, but armed with smoke can pacify the bees. Theirs is the most complex and productive of any partnership between humans and wild animals.

To reach the most isolated Hadza camps from Dar es Salaam, Tanzania's largest city, involves an eighteen-hour drive by jeep. Their home is set among a patchwork of shrubs, rocks, trees and dust, a landscape occupied by humans for at least 2 million years. Looking out across the horizon of Hadza country, it's possible to see human history in microcosm. Just a few miles north is Laetoli, the site where a group of our distant ancestors walked through wet volcanic ash and left behind the earliest known human footprints. Even closer is the Olduvai Gorge, the place where some of the oldest stone tools and hand axes have been discovered. Within walking distance is the salt-water expanse of Lake Eyasi, where human skeletons, 130,000 years old, have been excavated.

The Hadza are no proxy for our Stone Age relatives; they are thoroughly modern humans. But their foraging way of life is the closest we have to that of early *Homo sapiens*, and the Hadza diet offers the best insight into the foods that fuelled our evolution. I watched the Hadza follow trails that were impossible for me to see, and read the earth as if it was a much-loved book, knowing exactly where golden Congolobe berries were ripest and Panjuako tubers were at their thickest, where long-snouted bush pigs were likely to feed and when the squirrel-like hyrax might gather. They picked up on sounds I didn't notice and paused to feel changes in the gentlest of breezes so they could approach animals undetected. It was still a month until the dry season, when the large game congregate around water, making them easier to find. For now, the easiest way of finding meat was to dig it out from underground, which is why earlier Sigwazi had lured a porcupine from its den beneath a baobab tree. The offal (the heart, liver and kidney) were eaten on the spot, cooked for moments on a makeshift fire, but the carcass was carried back to camp, and shared among the rest of the group. Meat, however, isn't the Hadza's favourite food. Honey is, which is why the conversation with the honeyguide is so valuable.

The collaboration between human and bird was chronicled by Portuguese missionaries in the 1500s, but it took until 2016 for outsiders to understand the conversation more fully. When a team of scientists walked through the savannah playing loops of different recordings, they discovered that the attention of the honeyguide wasn't caught by just any human sound: the birds were listening out for specific phrases. In the case of the Yao people of Mozambique, this was 'brrr-hm … ', whereas in northern Tanzania the birds responded to the twists and twirls of the Hadza's whistles. These calls are passed down from one generation of hunter to another and, in each case, the researchers found, repeating the traditional phrases not only doubled the chance of being guided by a bird, but also tripled the chance of finding a bees' nest and honey.

What makes this even more remarkable is that the honeyguide is a brood parasite; it lays its eggs in other birds' nests. More brutal than the cuckoo, the chicks use their sharp-hooked bills to dispatch their rivals as they hatch. How the bird learns the skill of conversing with the Hadza we still don't know. One theory is that, just like the hunters, they are social learners; they watch and listen to their more experienced peers. It's possible this inter-species conversation predates the arrival of *Homo sapiens* and reaches back a million years or more to our ancestors' first use of fire and smoke. This idea is part of a compelling argument that it was honey and bee larvae, as much as meat, that made the human brain larger and helped us to outcompete all other species. Meat eating gets all the glory, the argument goes, because stone tools used in hunting turn up in the archaeological record, while evidence of eating honey does not. But there are plenty of other clues. Our closest relatives in the animal kingdom – chimpanzees, bonobos, gorillas and orangutans – all eagerly gorge on honey and bee larvae, nature's most energy-dense food. And in the earliest rock art discovered, inside caves in Spain, India, Australia and South Africa, there are depictions of honey collecting dating back at least 40,000 years.

But perhaps the most persuasive evidence of honey's importance to human evolution is the diets of the world's few remaining hunter-gatherers, including that of the Hadza. One-fifth of all of their calories across a year comes from honey, around half of which is the result of help from the honeyguide bird. The other half the Hadza can find themselves, as it comes from various species of bee that nest closer to the ground. Some are tiny, gnat-like and stingless, and produce a type of honey that is highly perfumed and delicately tangy. The Hadza find these nests by inspecting trees for the needle-sized tubes used by the bees to get inside the trunk. This type of honey, called *kanowa* or *mulangeko* in Hadzane (the Hadza's language), comes in modest, snack-like portions, and is gathered by chopping into the colonised section of tree. But on this occasion Sigwazi and the honeyguide wanted more. Together they were going to find the honey and wax of the larger (and more aggressive) *Apis mellifera scutellata*, the African honeybee.

Sigwazi watched as the bird he had attracted with his whistle hovered above one of the baobabs. This signalled there was honey; now it was time for Sigwazi to start climbing. He was short (five feet tall at most), wiry and slim. I figured his physique was the reason he was the member of the group chosen to climb the tree, but I came to realise it was more a question of bravery. Sigwazi was the one least concerned about disturbing a bees' nest, being stung or, worse still, falling thirty feet to the ground. He handed his bow and arrow to a fellow hunter, stripped off his ripped T-shirt and frayed shorts and removed the string of red and yellow beads from around his neck. By now almost naked, he started to chop up fallen branches with an axe and sharpen them into thin sticks. Baobabs are so soft and sponge-like that hunters can drive these pegs into their trunks with ease to create a makeshift ladder up towards the canopy. Swinging back and forth, Sigwazi made his way up the baobab, forcing a new peg in above his head as he climbed, clinging on, balancing and hammering all at once. As he neared the top of the tree another hunter climbed up behind and handed him a bunch of smouldering leaves. With these, Sigwazi closed in on the nest and immediately launched into a mid-air dance punctuated with high-pitched yelps. Bees were swarming around the honey thief and stinging as he scooped his hand into the nest and pulled out chunks of honeycomb. These rained down on the other Hadza hunters as

Sigwazi tossed them below. They cupped their hands to their mouths and started to feast, spitting out pieces of wax as they ate, leaving behind warm melting liquid that tasted both sweet and sour, bright and acidic like citrus. As I joined them I could feel writhing larvae inside my mouth and the crunch of dead bees. The honeyguide bird perched silently nearby, waiting for its share of the raid once the crowd of hunters had gone.

When the rest of the honey was taken back to the camp, women gathered armfuls of baobab pods, each one the size of two cupped hands. With bare feet, they brought their heels down to open the pods with a crunch. Inside were clusters of kidney-shaped seeds coated in a white powdery pulp which tasted like effervescent vitamin C tablets. The seeds, pulp, water and a little honey were placed into a bucket and stirred into a whirlpool with a stick. When everything settled, it looked like a thick creamy soup. Each sip fizzed in the mouth. This, I was told, is a food Hadza babies are weaned on.

Someone who had watched this exact scene long before me, as a 23-year-old Cambridge student, was James Woodburn. In 1957, to complete his PhD, he travelled to Tanzania in search of Africa's last hunter-gatherers. He followed two Italian ivory hunters tracking an elephant herd. Near Lake Eyasi, after the animals were killed and the tusks removed, Woodburn watched as Hadza hunters appeared out of the scrubland and into the clearing to take away the mountain of meat (elephants are the only big game that Hadza don't hunt – they say their poison is not strong enough to kill them). Woodburn followed the hunters back to their camp and spent the next two years living alongside them. To survive Hadza country without Hadza skills, he brought in supplies of rice and lentils to add to the small amounts of wild food he managed to forage for himself.

Woodburn learned to speak Hadzane (his language skills had been honed as a military interpreter), and gained new insights that brought the Hadza to wider attention in the 1960s. This included work carried out with paediatricians, which showed how exceptionally well nourished Hadza children were compared with their contemporaries in nearby farming communities. During the six decades that have followed, Woodburn has returned to Hadza country on a regular basis, staying with the tribe, studying their way of life and recording how it has changed over time. Luckily for me, my visit to Hadza country coincided with one of his.

'They have stayed as hunter-gatherers because it is a life that makes sense to them,' Woodburn said as we sat by a campfire, the last of Sigwazi's porcupine crackling as it cooked, 'they regard it as a wonderful life.' It's a way of life that's endured, he believes, largely because of the autonomy it brings; no Hadza has control over another, a fact made possible because of the abundance of wild food around them. Apart from the very young and the very old, everyone in the camp is self-sufficient, each skilled enough to feed themselves, even children as young as six. 'Once this way of life stops making sense to them,' Woodburn said, 'it finally comes to an end.'

When Woodburn first met the Hadza, the outside world had stood at a distance. The foragers still didn't know which country they lived in and their knowledge of what lay beyond Hadza country came largely from encounters with neighbouring tribes – the Iraqw, the Datoga and the Isanzu. With these pastoralists and farmers, the Hadza traded meat, skins and honey for millet, maize, marijuana and metal (to make axes and arrowheads). Other things they knew about the outside world had been passed down the generations, including stories of abductions of their forebears. Tanzania was at the centre of the East African slave trade until the middle of the nineteenth century, which was why the Hadza, until recently, always ran from strangers who appeared in the bush. But in the mid-1960s, there was no avoiding the world outside. Following independence from Britain, the Tanzanian government, encouraged by American missionaries, attempted to settle the Hadza in villages by force. Hunter-gatherers from remote bush camps were taken away in trucks to purpose-built villages, escorted by armed guards. Many became ill from infections and died. Within two years, most of those who had survived returned to their camps and to foraging. Efforts to settle and convert the Hadza, not only to Christianity but also to agriculture, have continued. And yet, against the odds, their hunter-gatherer way of life – the life that makes sense to them – has persisted. Now, though, a new set of forces is bearing down on the Hadza. Agriculture is spilling over into their land and products made by the global food industry have reached the camps. Woodburn said he hadn't forseen the scale of these pressures on the Hadza. No one had.

*

One-third of the Earth's land surface is now dedicated to food production – a quarter of this for crops, three-quarters for grazing animals – and farming's expansion into the wild is continuing (nearly 4 million hectares of tropical rainforest are lost each year). Agriculture is reaching into parts of the world once thought impossible to be farmed. Among them, Hadza country. At the beginning of the twenty-first century, tens of thousands of hectares of land used by the Hadza was converted by outsiders into pasture for livestock or to grow crops each year. Along with it went some of the Hadza's access to wild foods, including giant baobab trees that take hundreds of years to grow. Supplies of nutritious baobab pods were depleted, and so were sources of honey. In 2012, after years of campaigning, the Hadza were awarded rights of occupancy over 150,000 hectares of land, but this still didn't stop the problem. Neighbouring tribes faced with water shortages caused by irrigation and climate change moved cattle closer to the Hadza's camps and waterholes. The cattle ate the vegetation that brought in game and disrupted migration routes which meant there was less for the Hadza to hunt. Across the whole of Africa, two-thirds of the continent's productive land is now at risk of becoming degraded, half of this severe enough to lead to desertification. The biggest cause is overgrazing of livestock.

The Hadza are ill-equipped to stop this encroachment; they have no possessions, no money and no leaders. They're skilled hunters but they avoid conflict. Instead of confronting tribes arriving on their land, they move deeper into the bush. But even here, farmers edge ever closer, expanding pasture and planting sorghum and corn, though there's barely enough water to irrigate crops. The Hadza have to contend with the effects of climate change too; they see its impact in the lack of water, disappearance of edible plants and decline in nectar and therefore quantity of honey they find. To survive, many rely on food from NGOs and missionaries. The last hunter-gatherers in Africa are being pinched from all sides.

A thirty-minute drive from Sigwazi's honey hunting, we reached a crossing point where different tribes gather to take water from a newly installed pump. Here, they also visit a small mudbrick hut lit by a single light bulb that hangs from the corrugated roof. Inside, from floor to ceiling, are shelves stacked with cans of sugary sodas and packets of biscuits. We were hours from the nearest city, an enormous wilderness lay between us and the nearest road, and yet some of the biggest food and drink brands in the world had made it this far.

In the place where our ancestors first evolved, sugar in plastic bottles is replacing the sweetness of the food that helped to make us human, honey. Scientists who monitor birdlife in the savannah describe melancholy scenes of birds swooping down, calling 'ach-ech-ech-ech' in the hope of a reply, as their interaction with humans becomes rarer. The conversation between the two species, thousands, possibly millions of years in the making, may soon fall silent.

Encircling the mudbrick hut were newly planted fields of corn. I felt I could have been watching a film in which hundreds of thousands of years of human history was being played on fast-forward, from wild to farmed and from foraged to processed, bottled and branded.

2

Murnong

For as long as anyone could remember, there were only a couple of places left where foragers were guaranteed to find murnong, a radish-like root with a crisp bite and the taste of sweet coconut. One was a cemetery on Forge Creek Road in the town of Bairnsdale, Victoria, where the plant's bright yellow flowers could be seen clustered around gravestones; the other was along a nearby railway track, where a line of tall fences protected the bullet-sized root and its shoots from grazing animals. Before European invaders arrived in the eighteenth century, the grasslands and rocky hillsides of Victoria had been covered in these plants, a crop that grew so thick that from a distance it seemed to form a blanket of yellow.

The first humans to make the journey from the Afro-Asian land mass to Australia did so more than 60,000 years ago, and when they arrived, the plants and animals they found would have been alien to them. But just as the Hadza do today, these hunter-gatherers knew that, armed with digging sticks, a guaranteed supply of food could be found underground. Seeds, fruits and honey are seasonal, but roots and tubers are available all year round, and as the storage organs of plants, they're energy-rich. In south-eastern Australia, the most important of these subterranean foods was murnong. For the tribes who lived here over tens of thousands of years, including the Wurundjeri, the Wathaurong, Gunditjmara and Jaara, the importance of this one root is hard to overstate. Without murnong, life in south-eastern Australia would have been precarious, perhaps impossible. But by the 1860s the food was as good as extinct, making its retreat into cemeteries and sidings, places where either the dead were resting or the living kept away, and knowledge of the plant was lost to generations of Aboriginal people.

In 1985, a botanist in her sixties, Beth Gott, marked out a plot of land at Monash University in Melbourne. It was to be a garden dedicated to Aboriginal wild plants. Gott had become interested in indigenous foods and medicines during fieldwork in the Americas and Asia, and on her return to Australia she embarked on the most thorough study of Aboriginal plant knowledge ever conducted. From her base at Monash, she catalogued more than a thousand different species, including sleep-inducing dune thistles and silver cones picked from woorike trees used to make sweet-tasting drinks. After years of study, she concluded that one indigenous food in particular had been crucial to pre-colonial life in Australia. Some Aboriginal people called it the yam daisy, but most referred to it as murnong. Gott set out to find the plant in the wild, and grow it in her garden, but finding murnong wasn't easy and uncovering its history was just as hard. So much knowledge had been lost, much of it through violence.

In the deserts of southern Australia, between 1953 and 1957, the British government exploded nuclear bombs, part of a series of missile tests that continued well into the 1960s. Clearing the area for these explosions involved patrols rounding up the remaining 10,000 or so Aboriginal hunter-gatherers who roamed the Western Desert. As a result, the last of Australia's self-sufficient foragers were forced off their land and into the industrialised world. In other parts of the country, Aboriginal people had been moved off their land long before and confined to reservations. This latest clearance destroyed most of what was left of the living knowledge accumulated and practised over 60,000 years. In the 1980s, Gott set out to see if any of this knowledge had survived and to record it. If she could find some of the wild foods and medicinal plants, she would try to save those too.

Her source material, perhaps ironically, included the journals of the early colonists. The first reports sent back to Britain in 1770 by Captain James Cook and botanist Joseph Banks gave no information about the food eaten by the Aboriginal people or about anything that resembled a food culture, save for 'small fires and fresh mussels broiling upon them' and 'vast heaps of the largest oyster shells I ever saw'. The impression Cook and Banks gave was that 'the natives' were few in number, nomadic and basically savages. But a few decades later, another Englishman told a different story. William Buckley was transported to Australia as a convict but escaped from Sullivan Bay in Victoria and ended up living with members of the Wathaurong tribe for thirty years. This so-called 'wild white man' told of surviving on a diet of wild meat and murnong and how 'a man may live on the root for weeks'. In 1837, another settler described the tribe's diet consisting of the 'meat of the country when they can kill it, but chiefly roots'.

As she uncovered more documents, Beth Gott built up a picture of murnong's presence in the open spaces and woodlands of southern Australia, where it grew in the 'millions'. In 1841, George Augustus Robinson wrote how murnong was picked by women 'spread over the plain as far as I could see them ... each had a load as much as she could carry'. Edward Curr, a Yorkshireman who settled in Australia in the 1820s, described the 'yams as so abundant and so easily procured that one might have collected in an hour, with a pointed stick, as many as would have served a family for the day'.

There are images too. In the State Library of Victoria are hundreds of sketches made by a nineteen-year-old settler called Henry Godfrey, who arrived in Australia in 1843. *Women gathering murnong* shows two central figures against the backdrop of a forest canopy. Long cloaks and small sacks hang from their shoulders. One of the foragers is holding a hatchet which is about to be sunk into the ground to break the earth. The other has a stick in hand ready to dig. It's a joyful scene; children are playing with dogs as others sit around relaxing among the trees, arms raised, animated as they talk and gather food.

Murnong grows up to 40cm tall. At the tip of its leafless stalk are buds heavy enough to make the plant tilt over into the shape of a shepherd's hook. In the spring these open out into a spray of petals, so that the plant takes on the look of a big dandelion, as brightly coloured as a child's drawing of the sun. Below ground, the swollen tubers can grow as round as radishes or as thin as tapering carrots. When broken, every part of the plant exudes a milky liquid that leaves fingers stained. Left untouched, the tubers grow in tight clumps, but disturbed by digging, they're easily separated and scattered. This, Gott realised, was what had made the food so abundant. The actions of Aboriginal gatherers over thousands of years had spread murnong across the landscape. From the journals and diaries, it was clear

Aboriginal people were aware of this, which is why some argue they should be considered the world's earliest farmers.

Fire also played a role. The plant needs direct sunlight, and so in the dry season Aboriginal people would set the bush alight. They did this with precision, knowing exactly when and where to start a fire, and where the fire would end. This cleared away dead vegetation, but left murnong, with its tubers underground, unharmed. Harvesting was also easier in this open ground, and the ash left from the fire fertilised the soil. With this technique, a patchwork of murnong was created across south-eastern Australia. Beth Gott was ridiculed in the 1980s for researching Aboriginal fire techniques, but by January 2020, the world had caught up with her. Vast tracts of Australia burned in the worst bush fires in living memory, 11 million hectares of land scorched, thousands of homes destroyed, and tens of people killed. In the Aboriginal communities, in which people knew how to fight fire with fire, the damage was less severe; lighting hundreds of small fires during the year had tamed the undergrowth and prevented bigger fires from taking hold.

Murnong can be eaten raw, but Aboriginal cooks also made earth ovens in the ground in which hot stones were used to bake the tubers covered in layers of grass. In the journals, Gott found descriptions of communal feasts in which reed baskets filled with murnong, stacked three feet high, were cooked over fire. These sweet, nutritious roots were eaten with seeds, shellfish and possum. The only time of year when this didn't happen was winter, when the tubers were less succulent and often tasted bitter. But across the year, Gott calculated, Aboriginal people consumed an average of 2kg of murnong each per day at least. The supply of this food must have seemed never-ending.

From the arrival of the first colonists in 1788, when livestock was offloaded from ships, sheep began eating their way through the landscape. Before the gold rush of the 1850s, a 'grass rush' had taken hold across southern Australia. The region had some of the greatest expanses of grasslands in the world but, unlike the Serengeti and the American Plains, there were no migrating animals roaming free and no wildlife to plunder the murnong fields. In the first decades of European settlement, farmers introduced millions of sheep, their numbers doubling every two or three years. Awaiting the sheep were thousands of square miles of pristine grass and vegetation, and the animals loved murnong. The soil was also light and soft, so they could nose their way right through to the roots. They cropped the plants with their teeth and, along with cattle, their hard hooves compacted the soil.

In 1839, just five years after the founding of Melbourne, James Dredge, a Methodist preacher who had spent a year with the Tonge-worong people living in a bark hut, recorded in his diary a conversation with an Aboriginal man named Moonin. 'Too many jumbuck [sheep] and bulgana [cattle],' Moonin said, 'plenty eat it myrnyong, all gone the murnong.' A year later, Edward Curr added in his journal that 'several thousand sheep not only learnt to root up these vegetables with their noses, but they for the most part lived on them for the first year', after which murnong became scarce.

The state-appointed 'Chief Protectors of the Aborigines', the colonists on the ground and in a position to see how quickly things were changing in the Aboriginal territories, were aware of what was happening to murnong. One alerted his superiors to scenes of starvation. In the eyes of most of the Europeans, however, murnong was little more than a weed, and so the indigenous people were left looking on as more livestock arrived and swept through the landscape, eating up their supplies of food. A missionary, Francis Tuckfield, wrote that 'the Aborigines' ... murnong and other valuable roots are eaten by the white man's sheep, and their deprivations, abuses and miseries are daily increasing'. The colonists introduced other invasive species which made the situation worse, including grasses that outcompeted murnong and encouraged yet more grazing and trampling by sheep and cattle. Then, in 1859, rabbits were brought to Australia. If there had been any wild murnong left, the herbivores finished it off.

At this time, Aboriginal people were also the target of organised massacres and forced settlement. At Myall Creek in 1838, as a reprisal for disturbing cattle (a cause of murnong's decline), twenty-eight unarmed men, women and children were rounded up and killed. Other settlers talked of there being 'no more harm in shooting a native, than in shooting a dog'. Disease also played a role, but violence was the chief cause in the decline in the indigenous population, the worst of which was in Victoria. As soon as the British made it through the hills, they just kept pushing along the river network, where most

Aboriginal settlements were. It was the most rapid and brutal land-grab in Australian history. Because of Beth Gott's research we know that as well as attacks, many Aboriginal people must have died because their food supplies were destroyed. Prior to first contact, the indigenous population was estimated to have been between 750,000 and 1.5 million. By 1901, that number was more like 100,000. From an estimated seven hundred Aboriginal groups in the early 1800s, by the end of the nineteenth century just seventeen groups were left. In place of the murnong and the other foods that were lost, the Aboriginal people were issued supplies of flour and sugar (as well as blankets) by the colonists: this was the start of a policy of food rationing for Aboriginal communities that continued into the 1960s. When the invaders arrived, the Aboriginal people were fitter and healthier than most Europeans. Today, Aboriginal people can expect to die a decade earlier than Australia's non-indigenous population. Lack of access to affordable and healthy food is one factor in this.

As Beth Gott started growing Aboriginal plants in her garden at Monash in the early 1980s, an expert in public health based in Western Australia named Kerin O'Dea started taking indigenous people back to the wild. Her hunch was that Western foods were contributing to obesity and type 2 diabetes among the Aboriginal population. In a simple but radical experiment, she took ten middle-aged, overweight, diabetic and pre-diabetic Aboriginal people from cities to spend seven weeks in a remote part of the bush and live as hunters and gatherers, including digging up tubers. Even after this short period, all had lost weight and had seen the symptoms of their diabetes reversed. O'Dea concluded that it wasn't necessary to revert to a traditional lifestyle to tackle diabetes, but incorporating features of that lifestyle, including dietary ones, could bring great benefits. By then, however, many indigenous ingredients, along with murnong, had become endangered.

But things are changing. Murnong is making a slow return back to Australian consciousness and cooking. Aboriginal community gardens now have plots dedicated to the plant and harvest celebrations featuring digging sticks and ceremonial dances are being revived after two hundred years. After learning about the plant from the Aboriginal writer and farmer Bruce Pascoe, one of Australia's most celebrated chefs, Ben Shewry, sourced some seeds and started to grow murnong in his garden. 'It's the most important ingredient I serve,' he says, explaining that his customers are blown away by how delicious the plant tastes and moved by its story. Some of the seeds now used to grow murnong came from places where it had sprung up in the wild, including Bairnsdale's railway sidings and cemetery. Others were sourced from Beth Gott's Aboriginal garden, and so murnong's future now lies elsewhere: in the hands of growers and gardeners spread right across Victoria, and inside their kitchens as well.

3

Bear Root

Colorado, USA

From a distance you can see how Sleeping Ute Mountain got its name. Native people in southwestern Colorado say that its long shape was formed by a warrior god who, injured in battle, fell into a deep sleep as he rested on the ground. He has stayed there ever since, his arms folded across his chest forming one peak, his head, knees and toes making up the others. The mountain was sacred when it was given its name and it remains sacred today. In early summer, Sun Dancers from the Ute Mountain tribe gather on one of the peaks called Horse Mountain (which appears to form the warrior god's ribcage). Below the mountain is the town of Towaoc, home to around a thousand people, mostly Native Americans. And it was here that I watched a meal being cooked inside the town's community centre, overseen by Karlos Baca, a former chef, now teacher. His students had travelled from reservations in Texas, New Mexico and Colorado (Apache, Navajo and Pueblo). 'Most are places where there are more gas stations than grocery stores,' Baca told me. 'Here I'm teaching them how to survive the American food system.' Baca is on the front line of a food war, one being waged against indigenous people. The way he sees it, the first casualty is their health. 'That's why we need to decolonise our diets,' he says.

Laid out on the steel kitchen worktops were elk hunted from nearby forests and jars of flour made from acorns that Baca had soaked for weeks to leach out their bitter tannins. 'No wheat, no pork, no chicken,' Baca told the ten women and men who had gathered around him, some in their twenties, others their sixties. 'This is pre-colonial food.'

I watched as the group made cookies with amaranth seeds, turned maize into flatbreads and slow-cooked the elk into a stew. Above the sound of the kitchen clatter, Baca coached his students. Tall and heavily built, his black hair plaited and his arms covered in intertwined tattoos, he spoke quietly and with purpose. 'Come on, keep cooking,' he urged the team. 'This food shaped who we are, food that sustained our ancestors.' He explained later that he believed there is within each of us a kind of biological memory, a connection with food that exists on a cellular level. All he was doing, he said, was teaching people to tap into that memory through cooking. 'Think about it. These ingredients were part of our diets for thousands of years, how can that not have been passed on in some physical way?'

During the class, he took a handful of blue maize flour and mixed in some water, turning the grey-white powder into a deep purple porridge. To this, he added a pinch of burnt wood ash that made the colour of the maize more intense. With a small blade, he sliced tiny slivers from what looked like a gnarled and blackened piece of wood. 'I can tell you my life story through this one bowl,' Baca said, 'and this food can also show you what happened to my people.'

Baca, who is in his mid-forties, had turned his back on a career cooking in high-end restaurants to focus his energy on rescuing the food knowledge and skills of his ancestors, the Tewa, Diné and Ute tribes. He was born in a former mining town, Durango, in south-west Colorado, and after his parents' divorce when he was three, moved with his mother to Cortez, a town north of Towaoc, close to Ute Mountain reservation. There he remembers opening up boxes sent to reservations by the United States Department of Agriculture, food rations distributed to Native American families. Inside the boxes were cans of processed pork, bags of white flour and bottles of juice concentrate. 'None of that food was healthy,' he says, 'just junk that tricked your body into thinking you were full.' Summertime was different because then he went to live on the Southern Ute reservation with his grandparents, Fanny and Manuel Baca. His grandfather had survived one of the most brutal clashes of the Second World War, the Battle of Ryukyu on Okinawa. When he returned home, he opted for a life away from towns and cities, and spent time hunting, fishing and foraging, keeping hold of some of the old food ways. In the summer he took his grandson on these adventures and so Baca got to follow elk trails and pick wild sumac.

As a chef, Baca worked in all kinds of restaurants: Creole, barbecue, Italian, even Japanese sushi. But wherever he went and whichever kitchen he worked in, there was one food he says he never cooked, 'the food of my people'. The more he learned about his Native American roots, the more he realised America's first food culture had not only been written out of cookbooks, but out of history books as well.

By the time he had worked his way up to the position of executive chef at an exclusive retreat in the Colorado Mountains, on a six-figure salary, serving meals to rich tourists, he was disillusioned. One day, he walked away from it all, sold his car, put everything he owned into storage and, for two years, hitchhiked around the four corners of America, talking to the elders on reservations and reading every book he could lay his hands on about America's indigenous food. 'I wanted to find out what that food had been and if I could bring back some of our lost knowledge.'

Small details from his childhood took on a new significance. 'My grandfather always dressed exactly the same – heavy boots, blue jeans, a plaid shirt and a gambler style hat,' says Baca. 'And in his shirt pocket he always carried chiltepin chilli peppers and a gnarly piece of root.' At the first sign of a cold, Baca's grandfather would dip into his pocket, produce these two ingredients and make a tonic – 'He was like a walking medicine cabinet.' In the kitchen, his grandmother made a porridge of blue cornmeal, a warm, comforting mush that everyone on the reservation used to eat. 'It was the first food you'd be fed as a baby and the last you ate before you died,' says Baca. The food, bowls of blue cornmeal and that gnarly black root, made a big impact on him. Some indigenous people called the root osha, others chuchupate. To Baca, in the language of the Ute tribe, it was kwiyag'atu tukapi.

From the Ute community centre, we drove into the forest of the La Plata Mountain in the southernmost Rockies. We climbed past tall oak trees and silver-trunked aspens thick with leaves turning autumnal orange and red. Above the tree line were miles of valleys and mountain peaks stretching far into the distance, rising and falling across 13,000 feet. Deep in the forest and away from the path, Baca led us to a thick, green plant, with parsley-like leaves and small, snowflake-like flowers. He dug his hands into the earth and gently brushed away the soil to reveal a tangle of roots with a chocolate-brown surface. 'This one's young, maybe three years old,' he said, 'too young to be disturbed,' and he patted it back into place. Instead, he passed me a piece of leaf to eat. It tasted of crisp celery and fresh carrot with the added heat of pepper and the numbing sensation of a chest rub. The osha plant can take a decade to mature, at which point indigenous people will harvest only some of its roots, allowing the plant to carry on growing, unharmed. Its leaves can be added to soups or cooked with meat but, as with murnong, the real treasure lies beneath the soil. For thousands of years, the plant's dark brown, twig-like roots have been used not only as a spice to flavour food but also as a potent medicine. There are stories of animals much larger than humans digging up this plant, chewing its roots and rubbing it into their fur. Which is why it goes by the name 'bear root'.

Legends shared by Native Americans of bears interacting with the root were first put to the test in the late 1970s. A young Harvard student, Shawn Sigstedt (now a professor of biology at Colorado University), had gone to live with a Navajo community in Arizona to study traditional medicine. There, he came across bear root, or osha as they called it. Navajo healers told him how, long ago, hunters learned of the plant's powers by watching bears wake from hibernation and seek out the plant, dig up the roots and chew them up into a paste which they then rubbed over their bodies with their paws.

Intrigued by the story, Sigstedt took his research to a zoo in Colorado Springs and started to feed pieces of osha to two captive black bears. Their reaction to the root astonished him; the animals did exactly as the Navajo described. But as well as chewing the plant and rubbing the puréed root with their paws, they shook their heads and sprayed the osha from their mouths, creating what Sigstedt described as an aerosol effect. Sigstedt spent years studying bear behaviour and analysing the root which had antibacterial, antiviral and antifungal properties. It also contained painkilling chemicals and a powerful insecticide. What Stigstedt had been told by the Navajo in the 1970s weren't legends, they were scientifically accurate observations. Even a sniff of the tiniest flake of bear root has a distinctly medicinal smell. It packs a menthol punch which leaves you with a sharp, cleansing sensation.

Osha is a powerful plant, and it is also a highly regional one, found mostly around the southern end of the Rocky Mountains in the forests of south-western Colorado (it is also called Colorado cough root). One theory is the plant lives in symbiosis with microbes found only in the high altitude of the Rockies and Mexico's Sierra Nevada, which is why people have so far found it impossible to cultivate. And so indigenous people with access to bear root traded it far and wide, and each tribe who adopted it used it in a slightly different way. The Navajo, Zuni, Southern Ute and Lakota used osha to treat stomach pains and toothache; the Lakota smoked the root to relieve headaches; the Tarahumara of north-eastern Mexico, who are legendary long-distance runners, ate bear root to increase stamina and ease joint pain. Further south, Pueblo tribes used it in a con-coction they sprinkled across their maize fields to keep pests away; Comanche elders in Oklahoma tied pieces of the root around their ankles to repel snakes, and if they were bitten, they would chew the root into a pulp to treat the wound. The Chiricahua and Mescelero Apache, meanwhile, added the root to stews to spice up the flavour of meat.

To some indigenous people, bear root was a sacred plant and the places where it grew were often kept secret. Even mentioning its name was sometimes forbidden in the presence of outsiders. But they couldn't keep it secret forever. Its scientific name is *Ligusticum porteri*, named after a nineteenth-century preacher turned botanist, Thomas Conrad Porter, who was an early Western convert to the plant's medicinal powers. Bear root joined echinacea, goldenseal and American ginseng as a plant used by indigenous people and com-mercialised by colonists. Part of Porter's legacy is that bear root is a highly sought-after product in the multi-billion dollar herbal medi-cine trade, marketed as a remedy for chest infections, sore throats and arthritis. Becoming a lucrative wild medicinal plant has helped it become a species at risk.

'In the mountains it's foraged on an industrial scale,' Baca told me. 'The Forest Service caught one guy with hundreds of pounds of root in the trunk of his car.'

Indigenous knowledge of wild plants such as bear root is something Baca is teaching fellow Native Americans. Knowing these ingredients provides a gateway to traditional ways of cooking and much healthier diets; it can also help dispel some myths. There are a few foods Americans think of as traditional native staples, the most famous being frybread, dough pancakes that puff up as they're cooked in corn oil on hot skillets. It's still cooked in homes on reservations in Arizona and New Mexico where it has a strong association with Navajo culture and is sold as an indigenous street food, often described as an 'American Indian food'. But 'Navajo frybread' was never a traditional food – it was created 150 years ago out of desperation. Deep in the winter of 1864, the US Army forced 8,500 Navajo men, women and children off their land in north-eastern Arizona and onto the Bosque Redondo reservation, an internment camp that was three hundred miles away in New Mexico. Getting there involved a trek that is now known as the 'Long Walk'. Along the way, hundreds of Navajo died of exposure and starvation. They had not only lost their homes, but also been made to abandon their crops, seeds and food stores. To reduce the numbers dying of starvation, the government sent food parcels, rations that included white flour, sugar and lard. This was how frybread came to be. 'I go into neighbourhoods and still see people cooking up frybread,' says Baca. 'I don't want to embarrass them, but I make sure they know the history of that food.'

Baca isn't alone in his mission to decolonise indigenous diets. In the twenty-first century, a movement of Native American activists and cooks has grown up, people who are reclaiming their identity through food. Some of this work is being recorded by Elizabeth Hoover, an Associate Professor at the University of California, Berkeley, who has Mohawk, Mi'kmaq, French-Canadian and Irish ancestry. In a road trip over twenty thousand miles she visited forty different Native American communities to learn how they were using garden projects to grow traditional foods. Like Baca, she realised that the modern food system was killing indigenous people. The highest rates of type 2 diabetes in America are found on reservations; the disease is twice as prevalent among Native Americans as it is in the white population. Typically, these communities are located in food deserts, where access to healthy food is most limited. The irony is that a hundred years before, if their ancestors had stepped into a real desert, they would have known exactly how to find good food. And yet in many places Hoover saw that this bleak situation was changing.

In Arizona, she spent time with people returning to the desert to revive the tradition of harvesting cactus fruit. In Rhode Island, she met Narragansett people who had combed through seed banks in search of a rare white maize once grown by their great-great-grandparents. In the south-west, members of the Zuni tribe had rediscovered an amber-coloured bean last harvested a century ago. These were fragments of an ancient food system that had barely made it into the nineteenth century. With the first wave of European colonists came smallpox and other diseases that killed millions of indigenous people. Then, in the 1800s, as the settlers pushed their way further west, yet more native tribes were dispossessed and displaced, each one a sovereign nation in its own right, with its own distinct food and farming culture.

The 'Indian Removal Act' of 1830 sanctioned the expulsion of indigenous people from the southern United States. Many took seeds with them to reservations in parts of Oklahoma, where the soil was thin and water scarce, and their traditional crops failed. A century later, many of their descendants found themselves in the heart of the American dust bowl, where nothing grew. There were observers of this forced migration who realised something important was being lost. One was a seed trader called Oscar Wills, who visited reservations across the Dakotas collecting soon-to-be endangered varieties of corn, potatoes, beans and squash from the tribes. Wills's collection resulted in some indigenous plants being saved by curious backyard gardeners, leaving behind a seed trail for Elizabeth Hoover and other researchers to follow.

In recent years employment has provided another incentive for Native Americans to restore lost wild foods. In north-western Minnesota, on the White Earth Indian reservation, home of the Ojibwe people, the community worked out they were spending $7 million a year on food that was mostly being bought in from thousands of miles away. In search of an alternative, they looked at what their ancestors had once eaten, and this led them to the region's lakes and a unique species of wild rice. These green, yellow and brown grains, unrelated to Asian rice, grow on forty lakes in the area and had been the Ojibwe's most important food source for a thousand years. The grains have a dark, earthy flavour. 'A wild taste, a taste of the lakes,' says the

environmentalist Winona LaDuke, who is half-Ojibwe and has led
efforts to bring the rice-harvesting skills back.

At the end of the summer, the rice harvesters look out for the Wild
Rice Moon (called Manoominike-Giizis), which signals that the rice
has ripened and that it's time for the Ojibwe to head out to the lakes
in their canoes. At the rear, one harvester pushes a long pole to direct
the vessel, while another in the front holds two pieces of wood that
look like drumsticks, one to fold the tall grass across the canoe and
the other to knock it down. This creates a rhythmic sound of a swish
followed by the noise of rice grains hitting the bottom of the boat.
Back on the reservation, the rice is parched over fires and then laid
on the ground. 'To take the hulls off, our people used to dance all
night long over the rice,' says LaDuke. 'Today, we use machines, but
we still like to dance.'

Like bear root, the rice is sacred food and a medicine, but it has
also been a lifeline for the community. Long-term unemployment is
common on the White Earth reservation, and poverty can cut across
several generations. Many of the ricers are young; their average age
is around twenty-five. 'It's not an old dying thing,' LaDuke says. 'It's
a living tradition, a real source of income and a way of telling the
world who we are.' Around a third of the families on the 12,000-strong
reservation generate part of their income from harvesting wild rice.
'And during the pandemic when the food system looked less secure,'
she says, 'the rice was something we could depend on.'

Inside Baca's house in Durango, one of the bedrooms has been converted into a larder to store the ingredients he's discovered during the
years he's been foraging in forests and travelling around the US. It's
a repository of endangered knowledge, rare plants and seeds. There
are jars of beans, bags of corn, squashes on tables and dried chillis in
plastic bags. In a two-metre-long blue box, filled to the brim with
ingredients, are wild onion husks, sumac, white pine needles, fireweed,
nettles, parsley flowers, wild mint, purslane, porcini powder, juniper
berries, smoked trout roe, amaranth seeds and Navajo tea. Everything
has been gathered by hand. And that's just the top layer. After digging
deeper, Baca pulls out a small bag containing a dark brown, gnarly
piece of bear root, the smallest of pieces carefully taken from a mature

wild plant. 'We're standing at the edge of a cliff,' he says. 'This knowledge and all these ingredients are being lost.'

He cooked up a pan of blue maize and bear root. One mouthful took me back into the forest. There was the cosy warmth of the porridge followed by the pungent burst of the root. Baca picked up a spoon and tasted. 'My grandfather has just come alive. I see him standing in his boots, jeans and his big broad hat. Memories and history in a bowl.'

4

Memang Narang

Garo Hills, India

Unlike bear root, which only grows in a particular place, many of the plants we depend on have spread far and wide and are now cultivated right around the globe. Knowing where these crops originated is increasingly important for the future of our food. Saving a wild citrus, for instance, that grows in the Garo Hills of India may prove to be vital for the future of citrus everywhere.

Across the planet, there are around one billion citrus trees in cultivation, growing in countries ranging from Italy to Haiti and Vietnam to Senegal. Oranges, lemons, limes and grapefruits are among the world's most popular fruits. Less well known is the fact that they have an extremely complicated sex life, and a family tree that is complex and perplexing. In fact, you could say these fruits are the product of genetic chaos. The simple version is this: all of the world's commercial citrus fruits have three main ancestors: the mandarin (*Citrus reticulata*), the pomelo (*Citrus grandis*) and the citron (*Citrus medica*). These citrus ancestors were all happy to be fertilised by each other's pollen. And so, during the evolution of citrus, when these plants were swapping around their genes, it resulted in oranges (a hybrid of the mandarin and the pomelo), lemons (a hybrid of citrons and sour oranges), limes (a citron–mandarin cross), and the most recent, the grapefruit, the result of a hybridisation event that took place roughly three hundred years ago in Barbados, this time between a sweet orange and a pomelo.

Citrus also mutates easily. Explore some of the side branches of this family tree and you will see how a single chance seedling can go on to produce a new fruit. For example, a farmer in nineteenth-century Algeria spotted something a little different growing on one branch of a mandarin tree, the result of a gene mutation. This is how we got the clementine. Generations of farmers noticing these subtle changes and selecting desirable variations is the history of fruit breeding.

In 2018, the origins of citrus became a little clearer as scientists solved some more of the fruit's mysteries. They had sequenced the citrus genome and through some DNA detective work, pieced together millions of years of evolutionary history. This revealed ten older ancestors and, further back still, around 8 million years ago, a single wild fruit, the true ancient ancestor of all of the world's citrus. There are still gaps to fill in this story but one thing the researchers were confident of was that all the ancient citrus species, including the very first ancestor, evolved in north-eastern India and in the borderlands of south-western China and Myanmar.

This region is a biodiversity hotspot, where fragments of primitive fruit DNA show up in the archaeological record, including 8-million-year-old citrus leaves dug up in Yunnan, south-west China. That was a time of rapid climate change; the landscape became drier as violent monsoons started to ease and conditions became more conducive to plant life. This allowed the ancestor of citrus to spread across Asia and, as it did, it adapted to new environments and began to diversify. Different species then intermingled and hybridised, and spontaneous mutations created different shapes, sizes, colours, aromas and tastes. Millions of years later, humans selected some of these fruits from the wild and domesticated them, resulting in the citrus we have today.

The sexual compatibility of different citrus fruits, along with the tendency to mutate and create infinite possibilities for diversity, make citrus unusual. Yet out of thousands of potential varieties, we have ended up cultivating just a few and cloning these to make up the bulk of today's global crop. Valencia and Navel oranges, the Lisbon lemon and the Persian lime dominate the world's citrus groves and our fruit bowls. But there are indigenous people who still live among wild ancient relatives of citrus, perhaps even the oldest ancestor of all. And what they are protecting is precious.

In north-east India, close to the Himalayas and the border with Myanmar, Bangladesh and China, is the state of Meghalaya, home of the Khasi, a matrilineal tribe in which property and family names are passed down from mother to daughter. In this area of exceptional biodiversity there are orange-scented villages and forests of wild citrus which, until just a few decades ago, were cut off from the outside world. 'Diversity is the name of the game in this region,' says Phrang Roy, a renowned expert on Meghalaya's indigenous cultures and a member of the Khasi tribe. 'The people here speak more than 200 different languages, and nature offers even more variety. Two-thirds of India's biodiversity is in this one region.' Over thousands of years, people from across Asia moved into Meghalaya and settled, creating an extraordinarily rich cultural diversity. The food of the indigenous tribes includes crops such as millet and sweet potato which are farmed, but also foraged ingredients such as edible insects and honey. Wild citrus, however, holds a special kind of status; it is a medicine, a fruit to cook and preserve, and a sacred plant. In one Khasi community, when a baby is born, the umbilical cord is cut and placed in a bamboo basket, which is then hung from the branch of an orange tree. 'In their minds,' says Roy, 'it's as if the tree has become a godparent to the child, and the lives of the child and the plant have become intertwined, forever connected.'

Other tribes live in Meghalaya's densely forested Garo Hills. Surrounding the Garo tribes are forests of a wild citrus they call *memang narang* (scientific name: *Citrus indica*), which means 'the fruit of ghosts'. The name originates from the fruit's use in a death ritual in which the freshly picked oranges are placed over the body of a dying relative. This is seen as a way of absorbing the spirit, leaving the person to move on into the next world unencumbered by ghosts. Science can also explain this ritual, usually performed by the *ojha*, part medicine men, part priests, part botanists, as the wild fruit contains high levels of antimicrobial compounds which act as an insecticide. In hot and humid conditions, these chemicals help to keep bugs away from the bodies of the deceased.

As medicine, *memang narang* is used as a cure for ailments such as colds and stomach aches and even (the *ojha* believe) smallpox. Tonics made from citrus can be found across Asia, particularly where the fruit still grows wild and so has a long history (in Myanmar as well as north-east India, and south-west China). Beliefs in the fruit's medicinal powers travelled with it across the world; citrus features in ancient Greek medical texts and famously was used in the nineteenth century by the British Navy to combat scurvy. Today, all over the world, people feeling under the weather take citrus-flavoured vitamin C tablets and drink glasses of orange juice for their health.

The Khasi and Garo tribes also enjoy wild *memang narang* as food. The fruit is about 5cm in diameter and scarlet red when ripe, with a thin, soft skin. It looks like a mandarin but has the broad leaves of a citron, and to most of us, its taste would seem pretty extreme. 'There's an appreciation of sourness and bitterness in these communities the rest of the world has lost,' says Roy. In fact, we didn't just lose sourness and bitterness, it was methodically removed from our food. Plant breeders in the twentieth century, especially after the juice industry took off in the 1950s, focused on producing larger and sweeter oranges that could be transported around the world. The orange varieties selected had low levels of phenols, bitter-tasting (but also health-giving) compounds. This meant they appealed to the increasingly sweet global palate, but left the global crop more vulnerable to pests and diseases because the bitter chemicals present in wild citrus such as *memang narang* are a big part of the plant's natural defences. As we reduce these compounds in our quest for more sweetness, farmers have to compensate and protect the fruit with more chemical sprays.

Even if we never get to taste the bitterness of *memang narang*, we still make use of its linguistic legacy. References to the fruit can be found in Sanskrit and ancient Hindi literature, including the *Charaka Samhita*, a medical text thought to be a thousand years old. It's here the word narang or naranga first emerges, which along the Silk Road became the Persian *neranji*, and eventually *naranja* in Spain, *laranja* in Portugal, *arancia* in Italy and *orange* in France. In the 1590s, soon after the arrival of the fruit on British shores, Shakespeare included the reference 'orange tawny beard' in *A Midsummer Night's Dream*.

Much of the Garo Hills are still unexplored by botanists and seed collectors, and it's likely there are more citrus species here yet to be catalogued by outsiders. In the 1930s, plant explorers who reached the hills, and further north into Assam, described seeing immense landscapes of undisturbed wild citrus trees. In the 1950s, another generation of botanists started to catalogue this awe-inspiring diversity. But researchers on field trips in the twenty-first century no longer find the same level of diversity. Illegal logging, road building and agriculture have decimated vast areas where wild citrus grew.

This is a problem for the Khasi and Garo tribes, but it's also a worry for all of us (at least those of us who enjoy eating citrus). The genome of *Citrus indica* is yet to be sequenced by the team researching the origins and evolution of citrus. 'We know it's ancient and it could be a critical link in the citrus story,' says Fred Gmitter, a world authority on citrus at the University of Florida and a member of the team doing the genome work. 'It could even be the original ancestor of all citrus.' He doesn't know for sure because so little research has been carried out on the wild fruit. Scientists on the ground told him it hadn't been safe to work there for decades. In the 1990s and early 2000s, separatist rebels in Meghalaya used the Garo Hills as a hiding place, turning parts of the forest into no-go areas. This put the wild citrus at risk. 'For rebels hiding in the hills, everything was short term,' says Phrang Roy. 'Wild animals were killed for food and trees cut down for firewood.'

With one billion citrus trees around the world, could losing wild forests in India be a problem? Fred Gmitter says yes. 'Within those forests there could be ancestors of commercial citrus with unique genes resistant to diseases or capable of coping with climate change, genes we've lost because we've bred them out of the global crop.' Making the matter even more urgent is huanglongbing (usually referred to as citrus greening disease), a bacterial infection that's making its way around the world. 'It might well be the deadliest disease fruit growers have ever had to contend with,' he says. The disease has already ravaged Florida's $6.5 billion citrus industry, forcing some growers out of business. Farmers in other parts of the world have been looking on nervously as the disease spreads. When the University of Florida announced a breakthrough in the summer of 2020 – a molecule that could control the disease – it turned out it had been discovered in a relative of *memang narang*, another ancient wild species of citrus. 'The indigenous people protecting this wild fruit,' says Gmitter, 'are safeguarding the genes that could save a billion trees.'

Mapping the wild

A century before Fred Gmitter and his team sequenced the citrus genome (in fact, before we really understood what genes were), a Russian botanist was making the argument that to protect the future of our food we need to save biodiversity. Nikolai Vavilov was an adventurer and explorer and the first scientist to make the connection between the importance of plant diversity and food security. Today, his ideas are more important than ever.

Vavilov is best known for coining the term 'centres of origin', the idea that the crops that feed us today all began life somewhere in the world as wild plants and then, during the last 12,000 years, were selected and domesticated by humans. Where, when and how this had happened with each food was what Vavilov spent his life trying to understand, convinced that the future of the human race depended on finding answers to these questions. He argued that a plant's origin was where its diversity was greatest; this is where the most valuable genetic traits could be found – the ones with tolerance to drought or disease, resistance to parasites, or an ability to grow in poor soils.

Vavilov identified eight 'centres of origin'. They included the 'East Asian centre' in which he estimated 20 per cent of the world's cultivated flora had evolved (including soybeans and millet in northern China). Another was the 'Inter-Asiatic', which went from Iran and Syria eastwards on to north-western India, where wheat, rye and most of our fruit originated. The 'Central American centre', which covered the southernmost part of the USA and Mexico, was the home of corn, beans, pumpkins, cocoa and avocados. Later botanists refined his idea into 'centres of diversity': places where the greatest genetic variation of a species could be found.

Born into a merchant family in Moscow in 1887, Vavilov studied at the Moscow Agricultural Institute and later came to stress how dependent the world had become on a narrow range of plants for its food. He travelled for twenty-five years on 180 expeditions, spending much of the 1920s and 30s trekking on horseback through far-flung parts of the Soviet Union, Afghanistan, Iran, China and Korea, across Spain, Algeria and Eritrea, and on to Argentina, Bolivia, Peru, Brazil and Mexico. More than any other scientist before or since, he explained where our food comes from. Known for his relentless work ethic and his ability to survive on little sleep, Vavilov and his colleagues collected over 150,000 seed samples, which were housed in the institute in St Petersburg that now takes his name: the world's first seed bank.

As he travelled, Vavilov realised that many of the habitats in these centres of origin were changing, that industry, urbanisation and farming were eroding these precious genetic resources. Diversity was disappearing and with that came risks. Crop failures in Russia had resulted in famine and, just half a century before, in Ireland, there had been the Great Famine. The same genetically identical potato, the lumper, had been planted year after year in the same soil. A fungal disease had attacked these monocultures resulting in mass emigration and the loss of one million lives through starvation.

After decades of research and travel in his bid to help feed the world, in the late 1930s Vavilov found himself on the losing side of a bitter feud. The now discredited theories of Soviet biologist Trofim Lysenko were in the ascendancy. Inspired more by Marxist ideology than Mendelian genetics, they included the idea that plants could be 'educated' and crops improved by exposing them to extreme conditions. Vavilov fell out of favour with Stalin and was sent to a prison camp. During the war, his seed collection came close to being lost as the German Army blockaded Leningrad in a 28-month siege. The Soviets had plans in place to save works of art from the city's galleries but had done little to protect the seed bank. The Nazis, however, recognised its potential as a future food resource and saw the institute as an asset they needed to target. Fortunately, Vavilov had so inspired his fellow scientists that they moved hundreds of boxes of seeds to a basement and took shifts inside the dark building, in the sub-zero temperatures, to protect the collection. What happened next is well known to botanists, but it's a story we should all know.

Surrounded by seeds they could have eaten, the caretakers of the collection faced hunger rather than jeopardise the genetic resource. By the end of the 900-day siege, in the spring of 1944, nine of them had died of starvation, including the curator of the rice collection. He was found at his desk surrounded by bags of rice. 'We were students of Vavilov,' one survivor said, explaining their heroic efforts to protect the seeds. By then, Nikolai Vavilov was already dead. In 1943, at the age of fifty-five, he was claimed by the very thing he had spent his life working to prevent: starvation. He died in a Soviet prison and was buried in an unmarked grave.

This book includes foods thought to have gone extinct, but which have been brought 'back to life' and restored to farmers' fields because their seeds were collected by Vavilov and his colleagues and kept safe inside the institute. Nearly a century after his death, a new generation is following in Vavilov's footsteps.

Scientists at the Millennium Seed Bank in Sussex are today's 'students of Vavilov'. They travel around the world collecting endangered seeds which are then stored away for safekeeping. Inside Cold Room number 1, held at a steady −20°C, are floor-to-ceiling shelves filled with jars that contain every imaginable colour of seed, from black pumpkin-like seeds to purple flying-saucer-shaped legumes. Over one million wild seeds are held in this storeroom alone, including many from plants now extinct in the outside world. 'You are standing in the most biodiverse place on the planet,' reads a sign outside the vault.

The seed bank looks like the lair of a Bond villain. Its walls are made from half-metre-thick reinforced concrete, strong enough to withstand the impact of a plane crash (Gatwick Airport is nearby). If radiation is detected from a nuclear explosion, the bank's monitors will shut the air supply off to the vaults. The building is designed to last at least five hundred years.

'For too long, we've ignored the plants that Vavilov valued, the crop wild relatives,' says Chris Cockel of the Royal Botanic Gardens, Kew, which oversees the collection. For decades, these wild plants were regarded mostly as weeds; now we realise we need them to breed the crops of the future. Searching for the wild plants today are explorers from Kew, along with scientists in more than a hundred countries who send in boxes of seed samples. The cold rooms at the Millennium Seed Bank are part of a global backup plan.

A few months before I visited, the team had travelled to Laos to collect seeds of wild plants growing on the fringes of paddy fields. By the time they arrived, the plants were all gone. 'The farmers had been told to clear them away,' says Cockel. They had probably been growing there for thousands of years but were lost in a moment. We're at the eleventh hour; as Vavilov knew all too well, the more diversity we lose, the greater the risks we face. As we'll see in the next part of the book, we are taking huge risks with cereals – wheat, barley, rice and maize – the crops that feed most of the world. To produce more and more, diversity has been reduced down to a fraction of what existed before. Now the race is on to bring diversity back.

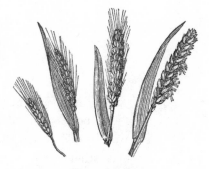

Part Two
Cereal

Sin maíz no hay país (Without maize there is no country)

Slogan used during food protests in Mexico in 2007

It could have been a weapon, spiky, shielded and hefty, but in fact I was holding an ear of wild wheat, perfectly evolved to protect the plant's future, its seeds. This cluster of golden grain had been gathered from the foot of a mountain in southern Turkey, part of the Fertile Crescent. It is now safely stored away in the laboratory of the Institute of Archaeology at University College London.

This is how wheat looked before it was redesigned and repurposed by four hundred generations of farmers. It had evolved in the wild to reproduce happily without any human assistance. After ripening in the sun, its brittle grains 'shatter', blown free of the plant by a light breeze or an animal brushing past, to be scattered across the ground. Each seed is equipped with two long bristles called awns. In the dry heat of the day, these bristles bend outwards, while at night, dampened by dew, they straighten. Over days, this movement (like a swimmer doing breaststroke) pushes the grain into the soil, the bristles acting as both an engine and a navigator. Once the grain has been driven down into the soil, the two bristles work like a drill. Powered by the air, they send the grain safely into the earth, ready to germinate. Our pre-agricultural ancestors gathered wild grains just like this one using beating sticks and baskets, crushed them with stones and turned them into porridges and flatbreads.

After they started to cultivate them, consciously or unconsciously they selected plants with a genetic mutation which meant their seeds didn't fall so easily to the ground. Plants with *non-shattering* grains, which stuck together, were easier to harvest and so more attractive. This phenomenon changed the course of human history. This mutant wheat was sown all around and its genes travelled far and wide. Humans got to harvest more food, while the plant benefitted by having its seeds dispersed. As the historian Jacob Bronowski puts it, 'the life of each, bread and man, depended on the other ... a true fairy tale of genetics'. Because the non-shattering wheat made it possible for humans to produce more food than was possible to gather as foragers, populations grew, settlements expanded, cities were created, foundations were laid for trade and civilisations flourished. And it all began with a selection of grasses from the Poaceae family.

There are around 11,000 different species of grass in this genus but in different parts of the world and at roughly the same time, humans started to focus on the seeds of just a handful. In the Fertile Crescent, it was wheat and barley; in Asia, rice and millet; and in Central America, corn. In each case, the farmer-led transformation followed the same pattern, from self-sufficient wild seeds to bigger, non-shattering ones that could be grown at greater densities; all were more dependent on human hands for propagation. This way, farmers, wherever they were in the world, had a steady supply of energy-dense grain that they could eat but also, crucially, store and replant. Thousands of years on, these cereals are still the most important foods in the human diet and supply half the world's calories.

In among thousands of other matchbox-sized containers at UCL are tiny cobs of ancient maize, no more than 5cm long, found preserved in caves in Mexico, 4,000 years old. And there are charred grains of rice excavated from fireplaces abandoned in the fifth century BCE. Each seed is a clue as to how, over 12,000 years, we changed wild plants, and how, in turn, those plants changed us.

But there's another characteristic of cereals that I want to explore, and that is their diversity. One reason these plants proved to be so valuable was their adaptability. When farmers migrated and traded, their crops travelled with them, evolving to meet the demands of each new location, so creating the enormous variation found inside the Vavilov Institute, the Svalbard Seed Vault or UCL's archaeobotany laboratory.

The diversity of the world's cereals is visible in their morphology – some maize cobs are long and thin, others fat and round; ears of wheat might have bristly awns, others appear 'naked'; rice varieties might be red, purple or black. Hidden from view, genetic diversity also includes the plant's physiology and those features we now know are priceless: the ability to resist disease, survive in cold temperatures, grow in deserts, thrive at high altitudes, flower under low levels of sunlight or tolerate saline soils. And of course they also have unique flavours and textures. All these factors determined why a community might save one variety of cereal and a different community another. The name given to a genetically diverse crop grown in a specific area whose seeds were kept and sown year after year and passed down through many generations, is a 'landrace'.

Over hundreds and possibly thousands of years, landraces of wheat, rice, maize and other cultivated grains continually evolved and adapted to their local environment, and were intimately linked to an ecosystem and to a population of people and their culture. This connection between plant and place also manifested itself in cooking styles and recipes, as a feedback loop took place between farmers in fields and cooks in kitchens. From a family of unlikely grasses, humans crafted an unfathomable number of distinctive foods: breads, dumplings, porridges, pilafs, pastas, puddings, noodles, tamales, tortillas, naans and chapatis.

To explore how this diversity came into being, how it was lost and why we need to save it, let's go in search of some of the world's most endangered, and most fascinating, grains.

5

Kavilca Wheat

Büyük Çatma, Anatolia

In the small Anatolian village of Büyük Çatma, families had risen at sunrise and then slaughtered sheep to whispered prayers. The festival of Eid had fallen in late August and husbands and wives worked together, hunched over tables, butchering the fresh carcasses. This produced a breakfast of hearts, kidneys and livers still warm from the slaughter, flash-fried and served in cubes of glistening fat and delicate slivers of muscle. The call to prayer from the nearby mosque broke the silence in the village outside.

Büyük Çatma lies on Turkey's eastern border; head north and you cross into Georgia, to the east lies Armenia and Iran, keep heading south and you'll reach Iraq. Over thousands of years, various cultures and empires have claimed this soil: prehistoric tribes, Hellenic warriors, Romans, Byzantines, Ottomans and Soviets. None settled longer than five hundred years. Throughout it all a rare source of continuity has been a particular type of grain, Kavilca, an emmer wheat, one of the first plants domesticated by Neolithic farmers. It still grows in the fields around the village.

White geese waddled between the houses, pecking at what looked like a wall built with black roof tiles stacked in a zigzag pattern. 'Fuel,' one of the farmers, Nejdet Dasdemir, explained. Manure had been moulded into cakes and stacked for the winter, ready to be used to warm homes and heat the clay ovens inside kitchens. People are mostly self-sufficient here; they have small herds of cattle and sheep, make cheese and butter, grow their own vegetables and keep beehives.

It was harvest time, and the last uncut field of golden-yellow Kavilca formed an oasis against the backdrop of the grey-green mountains. The mature ears of wheat were now so heavy they bowed down, their long, protective bristles waving in the wind. Dasdemir walked among the chest-high stalks, picked off an ear and broke it apart. The grains were encased in a tight-fitting, protective shell, a glume. He rubbed it between his fingers. 'Most wheat gives up its grains easily,' he said. 'Kavilca is stubborn.' Kavilca also produces lower yields than modern varieties. I was starting to wonder why it hadn't gone extinct long ago.

Resilience is part of the answer. The land around Büyük Çatma is high and harsh, a tough place to live, for people and plants. At an altitude of 1,500 metres, temperatures drop to below −30°C in the winter, and heavy snow can close the village off for weeks. During the spring it rains and the air is damp, an invitation for all kinds of diseases to attack crops. Few crops do well here. Kavilca is an exception; it evolved in this environment over thousands of years, adapted, survived and thrived. Dasdemir and the other farmers viewed Kavilca as an inheritance, handed down by their ancestors. 'We have an emotional connection with this food,' he said. 'We love the way the wheat looks in our fields, and the smell and taste of the grain when it's cooked.'

From the field, we went in search of the only local miller stubborn enough to still work with the stubborn wheat. Erdem Kaya looked tired when we arrived at his mill on the outskirts of the village. During harvest time, he finishes work at one o'clock in the morning and starts again at six. A beanpole of a man, dressed in a green overall, unshaven and melancholy-looking, he lives and works alone. His father had been a miller, he had been born in the mill and it was all he had ever known. The grey-stone mill stands beside the Kars Çayi River, the source of the power for the two large circular grinding stones inside. A sweet smell hung in the air like freshly baked cake. Kaya disappeared up a ladder and pulled a long wooden lever to start the flow of water. The whole room seemed to creak and then sigh as machinery juddered into life, a series of belts slapped into action and the giant stones began to turn.

Modern bread wheat is free-threshing which means its naked grains easily come loose from their ears, ready to be milled into flour. Because of their tough hulls, Kavilca grains have to be milled twice. The first step removes the husks. After these outer shells have been separated (winnowed away), a second round of grinding breaks the grains into tiny pieces, leaving it looking like fine shingle on a beach. It is the most difficult wheat Kaya works with, but also the most satisfying.

'When they cook with it in the village, I can smell it from the mill,' he said. 'That's not true with the other grains.' He handed us a sack of Kavilca and we left him to his work.

The aroma Kaya described wafts from a variety of traditional Anatolian dishes that feature Kavilca, one of which was cooked with the grains we had collected from the mill. Back in the village Erdal Göksu and his wife Filiz, also farmers, roasted a goose on top of the cracked wheat so that its fat dripped down and cooked the grains. Filiz moved around the kitchen, a white, embroidered scarf covering her head, and added bowl after bowl to the table: cream and soft cheeses, pickled cabbage, peppers stuffed with spiced lamb and, at the centre of it all, a large dish piled with Kavilca shaped into a ring, its brown grains glistening with the fat and juices from the goose, with flakes of tender, buttery meat in the centre. The grains tasted rich, nutty and satisfying. 'This is a taste we recognise deep within us,' Filiz said, 'we feel it in our bodies.'

Kavilca is now endangered, but as an emmer wheat its history goes back to the very beginnings of farming. Emmer wheat was one of the first wild grasses domesticated by Neolithic farmers; it was also the grain of ancient Egypt, of Mesopotamia and Greece, the food eaten by the people who built Stonehenge and the sailors who forged the maritime networks of Phoenicia. How did such an essential, world changing food end up on the brink of extinction?

Dasdemir had given me a handful of old desiccated Kavilca seeds, a souvenir to take back to Britain, a reminder of Büyük Çatma. These I showed to a farmer in Oxford, John Letts, an expert in ancient grains. In the early 1990s, Letts studied archaeobotany at UCL. This led him to Turkey in search of the history of wheat. Staying in rural villages there, he remembers waking to the thud-thud-thud of women pounding away with enormous pestles and mortars, removing the hulls from emmer and cracking the grains. Curious about Britain's wheat history, back home he started a search for ancient grains.

It wasn't an easy trail to follow but a breakthrough came in 1993. Workmen repairing the thatched roof of a medieval house in Buckinghamshire discovered at its base a smoke-blackened jumble of straw and weeds, untouched for six hundred years. This old thatch was stripped and about to be destroyed when the inspector overseeing work on the listed building recognised its importance and saved some of it in a shoebox. The box was stored at the Oxford Museum of Natural History until someone made the connection with Letts's research and sent him what was left of the medieval thatch. When he opened the box, he felt he had been handed gold. 'Inside were landrace wheats that hadn't been grown in England for centuries,' says Letts. 'It was treasure, biological treasure, a type of genetic diversity Britain had completely lost.' The discovery made it possible for him to recreate a medieval wheat field and, over the years, he added to the collection. Today, in fields around his farm, he grows some of the rarest and most ancient varieties of wheat in the world, including emmer. These he mills for bakers looking for older and less familiar flavours.

Selecting one of the ears of dried Kavilca with a pair of tweezers and peering through a magnifying glass, Letts looked intrigued and then excited. 'This seems different,' he said, 'smaller and darker than any emmer I know. I'm getting the same chill I felt when I opened up that shoebox all those years ago.' He twirled one of the spikes between his fingers and held it up to the light. 'I think I'm holding one of the oldest wheats in the world.'

The heart of the Fertile Crescent lies south of Büyük Çatma on the south-eastern edge of Turkey. Ecologically this is a remarkable place, a transition zone between desert and grassland with low rainfall on one side, lush mountainous steppe and oak woodlands on the other. Here, among scattered trees, our hunter-gatherer ancestors foraged from patches of tall grasses, including wild species of wheat and barley. They harvested grains using flint sickles with handles carved from wood and bone. Hard basalt rock served as their grinding stones. In prehistoric hearths, archaeologists have found charred remains of ancient flatbreads made from the seeds of wild grasses. Our ancestors were bakers long before they became farmers.

In the late 1960s, the American botanist Jack Harlan set out to experience something of this lost food history. In the Karacadag Mountains of south-eastern Turkey, one of the hotspots of domestication, he became a hunter-gatherer. First, without tools he hand-stripped ripe ears from the wild wheat that grew along the slopes, and then he tried harvesting the grains using a flint blade. Harlan concluded that one family harvesting around the Karacadag for three weeks, 'without even working very hard, could gather more grain than it could possibly consume in a year'.

Around 12,000 years ago, some hunter-gatherers across the Fertile Crescent started to cultivate patches of these wild grasses. Climate change had created drier conditions, and other foods, including meat, became harder to find, so the appeal of grains grew stronger. The early farmers focused on two different species of wild wheat: einkorn (*Triticum monococcum*), a small, tough and frugal plant (*einkorn* is German for 'one grain'), and emmer (*Triticum dicoccum*), which had twice the number of grains in each spikelet. Einkorn and emmer were domesticated separately, but eventually both spread throughout the Fertile Crescent. We know hunter-gatherers traded materials such as obsidian for tool making, and it's likely they also exchanged seeds. The non-shattering genetic mutation spread too, though it took at least 2,000 years for it to stabilise and become 'fixed' in these wheats.

To the east of the Fertile Crescent, by 6000 BCE, emmer and einkorn were growing in parts of today's Pakistan, arriving in Rajasthan and Haryana in north-west India by 3000 BCE; to the south, they spread through Palestine and Israel, and on to Egypt by around 4500 BCE; to the west, the two wheats went through Greece, the Balkans and along the Danube to southern Europe; and by 3000 BCE, einkorn and emmer were growing in Oman and Yemen and traded across the Red Sea into Ethiopia. Part of the success of both of these grains came down to the tight-fitting glumes (or husks) the miller of Büyük Çatma has to contend with. This protective coating not only has antimicrobial properties that keep fungal infections at bay, it also provides the grain with physical protection from cold, damp conditions and insects and birds, making it possible to store for long periods. Einkorn was hardier, but emmer, with double the number of grains, dominated, and went on to become the world's most widely grown wheat. This is how things stayed for thousands of years.

Meanwhile, evolving in the background was a weed that had appeared on the fringes of the emmer fields. This weed was an accidental hybrid of cultivated emmer and wild 'goat-faced' grass. We know that this hybrid was growing among einkorn and emmer by around 7000 BCE and started to be selected by Neolithic farmers. Today we call this 'weed' bread wheat, *Triticum aestivum*, and it makes up more than 95 per cent of the global wheat crop, a food for most of the people on Earth. In the ancient world, the plant didn't look too promising – its grains were small and lacked the tight protective glumes – and it was only with the building of more advanced granaries capable of offering man-made protection that bread wheat eventually displaced emmer. Its advantage was that its grains came away from the chaff easily, and its paper-thin coating meant its husk didn't need to be removed before milling. This 'naked' wheat was also chemically different; its gluten proteins were stickier, so the dough had greater elasticity, producing a lighter loaf of bread, and it was more versatile.

While bread wheat took over in most parts of the world, emmer and einkorn continued to be grown in remote and mountainous regions: in the Alps in Switzerland and Germany; in Italy's Apennine Mountains; in the Basque region of Spain; and in the Himalayas and the Nilgiri Mountains in India (though after the British arrived in the nineteenth century, Indian farmers were ordered to replace their ancient wheats with bread wheat, using seeds supplied from the Empire). In the 1920s, Nikolai Vavilov tracked down varieties of emmer just as they were becoming endangered in Asturias, in northern Spain, and in the mountains of western Georgia. By this time a marginal crop, emmer was typically boiled up and eaten by the poor or, more often than not, relegated to the status of animal feed. Morocco's western Rif is one of the last remaining places where einkorn is still grown, in the mountainous Jabala region, where it's used in the winter months to make flatbreads. In Ethiopia, specific varieties of emmer are used for brewing beer. And, of course, in Büyük Çatma the emmer they call Kavilca has continued to be cultivated through the grain's rise and fall.

One consistent feature of all wheat – einkorn, emmer and bread wheat – in this 12,000-year history, has been diversity. For a sense of scale, there are more than 560,000 different samples of wheat saved as seed in collections around the world. And these are only the wheat varieties crop experts have been able to collect. Many others will have already gone extinct. The greatest loss took place during the twentieth century following a series of scientific breakthroughs.

Charles Darwin's *On the Origin of Species* (1859) and Gregor Mendel's rules of inheritance gleaned from his famous pea experiments (1866) provided plant breeders with the foundations of an agricultural revolution. Experimental research programmes were launched in the late nineteenth century by the British and the United States Department of Agriculture (USDA), and also by scientists in Russia. The emerging science of crop genetics was quickly put into practice on wheat, then, as now, the world's most widely grown crop. At Cambridge University in the early 1900s, the first Professor of Agricultural Botany, Rowland Biffen, applied Mendelian genetics to breed new higher-yielding varieties; he identified attractive traits in wheats found across the British Empire and hybridised (crossed) them with other varieties.

Around the same time, inside a lab in a district of Berlin, the chemist Fritz Haber succeeded in 'fixing' nitrogen into liquid ammonia, creating the basis for synthetic fertiliser. Until this point, lack of nitrogen in soil had been the biggest brake on the industrialisation of crop production; but in a lab, using extreme temperatures and extraordinary pressures, Haber and his assistant Carl Bosch managed to synthesise nitrogen on a large scale. It was one of the most important discoveries in modern history. As the science writer Charles C. Mann puts it, 'More than 3 billion men, women and children – an incomprehensibly vast cloud of dreams, fears and explorations – owe their existence to two early-twentieth-century German chemists.' However, there was a drawback which needed to be overcome. When farmers applied the new chemical fertilisers to their fields, crops became so tall and their grains so heavy they fell over (or lodged), which either made harvesting too difficult or left food rotting away on the ground. This problem took decades to solve, and the solution was ingenious.

In occupied Japan in 1946, an American biologist, Cecil Salmon, came across a strange-looking wheat that grew just two feet tall instead of the usual four or five. The 'dwarf wheat', called 'Norin 10', was sent first to the USDA and later, in 1952, it caught the attention of a plant breeder working on a remote research station in Mexico. Norman Borlaug, originally from Iowa, had been developing disease-resistant varieties of wheat to help peasant farmers. He began working with Norin 10, crossing it with traditional Mexican varieties. By shrinking wheat plants, he figured, he could strengthen the stem and unleash the power of the new fertilisers. In search of improved wheat, working alone for months on end, he cross-pollinated thousands of plants by hand. He would sleep in a rat-infested research station with broken windows and no running water. In the absence of a tractor or a horse, he strapped a harness around his chest to pull a plough across fields.

After years of arduous experiments, Borlaug succeeded in creating new disease-resistant, higher-yielding varieties. By 1963, 95 per cent of Mexico's wheat was Borlaug's varieties, Lerma Rojo 64 and Sonora 64, which tripled the country's wheat harvest. They were soon adopted in India, Pakistan and Afghanistan, and within the space of a decade, right across the wheat-growing world. Famines that had been anticipated were averted, and in Cold War politics, the Green Revolution became a powerful tool to halt the spread of communism in developing countries. Borlaug became known as the man who saved a billion lives and in 1970 was awarded the Nobel Peace Prize.

But the Green Revolution had other consequences. Borlaug's dwarf wheats were part of a package: they needed lots of water through irrigation and huge amounts of fertiliser produced by the energy-hungry Haber–Bosch process. This food revolution was nourished by fossil fuels. Nearly half of all the crops consumed by humans today depend on nitrogen derived from synthetic fertiliser. And there was another essential feature of the Green Revolution package: uniformity.

In a single hectare of Kavilca there could be as many as 3 million individual plants and considerable genetic diversity. I saw this in Büyük Çatma. Some plants were taller than others, some grains dark brown, others the colour of amber. Landrace wheats evolve as mixed populations, and for good evolutionary reasons as variation in the crop bestows resilience; if some plants fail in a sun-scorched year, others with a different set of genetic traits will still produce. Having this larger and more diverse gene pool gives a field of landrace wheat the biological toolkit to deal with whatever the environment throws at it. Over time this diversity allows the landrace to adapt to longer-term changes in climate and growing conditions. Animals can run away from threats, but plants survive or die depending on their ability to adapt.

The Green Revolution created monocultures of genetically identical plants. The new science of breeding made it possible to select *against* diversity rather than embrace it. Each plant could be guaranteed to grow to an identical height and mature at the same time, making harvesting more efficient. The chemical composition of the grains could also be controlled to deliver the balance of proteins and starches demanded by an expanding global food industry.

Crop breeders might argue that modern wheat is extremely diverse, and it's true that in Europe alone, a farmer can select from the many hundreds of licensed varieties that appear each year on the European Union's 'approved list'. This list is decided by committees of seed companies and crop scientists. About one-fifth of the list gets refreshed each year as new varieties are added. But how diverse is it really? These so-called 'elite varieties' are slightly different versions of the same theme, all coming from the same narrow gene pool. Every single one (by law) is bred for yield and homogeneity. The nutritional value of the wheat (e.g. zinc, iron and fibre levels) is not considered, and neither is flavour. And most farmers don't even get to choose the wheat they grow as they often are in long-term contracts with the food industry, including the industrial bakers who supply bread to supermarkets. It's these companies that often decide which specific variety of wheat a farmer will grow that year. This way, consistency and uniformity can be maintained right through the process, from sowing seeds to the finished loaf. The entire system, the wheat-breeding programmes and the approved list, is also designed around one type of product: white bread made with refined flour for which most of the nutrients in the grain are removed in the milling process. Again, by law, these nutrients are then put back in through the process of 'fortification'. This isn't the fault of the plant breeders; they are paid to create what the current food system demands: cheap grain and a commodity that can turn a profit on global markets. After 12,000 years of farming such a rich variety of wheat, what a strange state of affairs we find ourselves in.

Unlike most revolutions, the Green one achieved exactly what it set out to do, which was to boost the supply of calories for the world. But the planet is now paying a heavy price. Borlaug said the Green Revolution was only buying us time, twenty to thirty years at most. He hadn't intended it to be a long-term fix for feeding the world but the world became locked into this intensive system. The land that was cleared, the fossil fuels used, and the water extracted – all are contributing not only to food diversity becoming endangered, but also, potentially, the endangerment of life on Earth. What's more, the original promise is stalling; in many parts of the world wheat yields have plateaued. In riding reductionism, we really did run into the hard wall of complexity.

In 2020, the Covid-19 pandemic showed us how a microscopic virus can threaten human life, destabilise economies and disrupt social norms. Microscopic diseases can also bring chaos to food security. I mentioned one example of a devastating crop disease at the beginning of this book, Fusarium head blight. I also described it as sneaky. It has a devious (yet strangely impressive) modus operandi: the fungus lies dormant in fields, but when it rains, droplets splash its spores upwards and onto the ears of wheat. From here, it penetrates deep inside the plant where, by secreting an arsenal of proteins, the fungus gives itself an invisibility cloak. This allows it to bypass the plant's defences and travel hidden between the cells, spreading out. Then the fungus delivers its *coup de grâce*: by releasing a chemical signal it effectively causes the plant to commit suicide. It then gets to fulfil its mission, which is to feast on all the nutrients the wheat had stored inside its seeds ready for its own reproduction.

What has made head blight even more successful in recent years, decimating crops at an alarming rate, is that the gene responsible for dwarfing the world's wheat had a hitchhiker, a section of DNA that made it even more susceptible to this disease. The more uniform wheat became, the more that gene spread and the easier it became for the head blight to attack fields full of food. It has turned millions of tonnes of wheat into shrivelled, grey, chalky grains at a global cost running into billions of dollars. So far, the most promising solution to this threat lies with the ancient wheats, einkorn and emmer, both of which have greater resistance to the fungus.

Even more devastating is a relatively new disease called wheat blast. Caused by the fungus *Magnaporthe oryzae* it reduced harvests in parts of Brazil and Bolivia by two-thirds before crossing the Pacific and arriving in South Asia on a shipment of grain. When it was discovered in Bangladesh in 2016, thousands of farmers were ordered by the government to set fire to their fields of unharvested wheat, to burn their crops and throw away any seeds they had saved from the previous year. This fungus infects spikes of wheat and turns the plant a pinkish colour, covering the grains in black spots. Soon after, the grains shrivel and deform, eventually destroying the crop. What makes wheat blast so remarkable is that it originated as a disease that only affected rice plantations. But a new high-yielding variety of wheat had been bred without a particular defensive gene, and this allowed the fungus to cross the species barrier and mutate to attack wheat. As with Fusarium head blight, scientists are now looking for a source of resistance within old landrace varieties of wheat.

This is history repeating itself. In the late 1940s, Jack Harlan came across 'a miserable looking wheat, tall and thin-stemmed', in a remote part of eastern Turkey. He picked a few samples and took them back with him to the USA, where they remained in a seed bank for nearly two decades. In the 1960s, when a disease called 'stripe rust' broke out across wheat fields in the American north-west, plant breeders experimented with Harlan's Turkish wheat. It turned out to have resistance not only to the outbreak but also to fourteen other diseases. Tonnes of food and millions of dollars were saved thanks to Harlan's chance find.

Today, the future potential of pre-Green Revolution wheats is being explored at Britain's world-renowned centre for plant science, the John Innes Centre in East Anglia. The centre hosts a collection of wheats assembled a century ago by a Cambridge University botanist named Arthur Watkins. While serving as an officer in the First World War in France, Watkins became infatuated with the crop. He noticed how each French village had fields of different-looking wheat. After the war, at the School of Agriculture in Cambridge, he corresponded with Nikolai Vavilov and realised the importance of the genetic diversity he'd seen in France. He then came up with an ingenious method for building his own collection. Using the Civil Service network, he contacted staff based in British consulates in the Middle East, Asia, Europe and the Americas to help 'collect as many wheat varieties as possible from around the world'. This, he told them, was for his own scientific curiosity and also for 'breeding improved varieties of wheat'. He asked them to find the oldest landrace wheats they could find because, he said, 'these are always a mixture of many distinct types'. Hundreds of consulate workers explored local markets and farms to buy seeds for Watkins and posted them off to him in Cambridge.

By the end of the 1930s, Watkins had collected 7,400 wheat samples – einkorn, emmer and bread wheats, including lots of different and rare varieties. He turned this into a living collection at the School of Agriculture, which was then the biggest of its kind in the world. Watkins died in obscurity but the collection he left behind is a unique and priceless snapshot of wheat diversity around the world before it was swept away by the Green Revolution. Researchers at John Innes are now searching through Watkins's collection for genes that could be transferred into modern varieties in order to improve their yield, hardiness or disease resistance.

What became of Kavilca in this story? Borlaug's Green Revolution wheat arrived in Turkey in the 1960s. Funded by the Rockefeller Foundation, farmers were handed free supplies of seeds, fertilisers and pesticides; agriculture in Turkey underwent more change in a single generation than it had in five hundred years. By the end of the decade, farms had become bigger, the number of farmers fewer and Turkey's rural population had dropped from around three-quarters of the national total to less than a quarter (all universal features of the Green Revolution, from Mexico to India). The people who stayed in the countryside stopped saving their traditional seeds. Landrace wheats became associated with ignorance and poverty.

The extent of Turkey's lost diversity is only known to us because of the work of a young botanist named Mirza Gökgöl. In 1929, inspired by Vavilov, he set out on horseback, travelling from village to village, collecting every type of wild and cultivated wheat he could find, assembling a collection of 18,000 varieties. He did this for more than a quarter of a century. 'He was a one-man army,' says Dr Alptekin Karagoz, a leading expert in Turkey's wheat diversity. 'What he found was priceless.'

Among the seeds Gökgöl collected was Kavilca, or *gernik* as he described it in old Anatolian Turkish. 'One of the oldest cultivated wheat species,' he wrote in the 1930s, 'in excavations in Babylonia and Egypt, this emmer has been unearthed. While the poor fed on barley, the high-ranking ate emmer.' In eastern Turkey, Gökgöl met farmers who valued emmer's ability to grow in the thin soils and cold damp temperatures of the high Anatolian plateau. He watched as villagers gathered together in a communal exercise of threshing the wheat and removing the hulls, and he studied the transformation of cracked wheat into nourishing dishes of pilafs and flatbreads. He saw how Kavilca wasn't just a crop – it supported a whole way of life.

But in Gökgöl's later travels, even in the most remote villages, he found that Kavilca was being replaced by what he described as 'soft and ordinary inferior wheats' and was 'doomed to go extinct'. By the end of the 1960s, Kavilca was remembered by only the oldest farmers and cooks. A decade later, that memory was close to becoming myth.

Picking up the baton from Gökgöl, Karagoz also spent years travelling across Turkey on seed-hunting expeditions for the Ankara Gene Bank. In 2004, he took Gökgöl's vast wheat encyclopedias with him on the road, and found that most of what Gökgöl had recorded was gone. By then, less than 5 per cent of wheat being grown in Turkey was a landrace variety. By 2016, it was estimated to be 1 per cent. Even the living wheat collection planted by Gökgöl was lost. His garden, holding some of Turkey's oldest wheat varieties, had been abandoned after his death in the 1980s.

That 1 per cent included the Kavilca grown in small family plots in Büyük Çatma. Lack of roads to the remote village meant the 'revolutionary' seeds and fertilisers hadn't made it here. Even if they had, the high altitude would have been too much for Borlaug's bread wheats, and the rain and moisture-loving fungal diseases would have overwhelmed them.

The Turkish farmers in Büyük Çatma had saved their precious landrace wheat, but Britain had lost its own. In the late summer of 2020, I walked among the wheat that was growing around John Letts's farm in Oxford, the legacy of the shoebox of medieval straw and weeds he had been given in the early 1990s. Letts was on a mission to restore what Britain had lost. He had scoured the contents of every seed bank and plant collection prepared to give him access and sowed every type of pre-Green Revolution wheat he could find. Hearing their names turned them into characters as rich and colourful as Kavilca: Red Lammas, Devon Orange Blue Rough Chaff, Blue Cone Rivet, Duck-bill and Golden Drop.

The crop was tall, twice the height of modern wheat and was growing well above my shoulders. There was also diversity in the field. Each plant looked subtly different to its neighbour; tiny variations in the colour, shape and size of the grains, just like the field of Kavilca I had stood in with Nejdet Dasdemir. Letts's landrace population will discover its own strengths and weaknesses and evolve in the years to come, its gene pool wide enough to give it options to adapt.

Another similarity to Kavilca was that Letts's wheat had a complex root system, much deeper than modern varieties, which have been bred to grow in just a few inches of fertilised soil. Landraces evolved without that luxury and send their roots far down in search of food; deeper roots mean greater access to minerals and nutrients. 'Try to imagine beneath our feet,' said Letts, 'how far those roots have travelled in search of nutrients.' Working out if one wheat produces more nutrient-rich food than another isn't easy; there are lots of variables at play: the type of soil, the method of farming, right through to how the grains have been milled, baked or cooked. But we do know for certain that levels of minerals such as zinc and iron are higher in older wheats than in modern ones.

After the harvest, we took some grains to a large wooden barn filled with different kinds of milling machines. One of these, about the size of a washing machine, could remove the hull from Kavilca in seconds, Letts told me. I wished the miller Erdem Kaya had been there to watch. 'Growing old varieties isn't about going back in time,' Letts said. 'With new technology we can now start to realise their full potential.'

In my hand were the dried Kavilca seeds and I thought about the millennia the wheat had survived through, all the empires that had come and gone, the countless people who had lived, loved and died, the thousands of harvests that had been reaped. Throughout all of this, the plant had toughed it out. Tried and tested, it had evolved and adapted. 'The people who selected that wheat thousands of years ago weren't stupid,' Letts said, 'and neither were the farmers in Turkey who saved it.'

6

Bere Barley

As John Letts set out to prove, everywhere has – or once had – its own version of Kavilca, a food ecologically, culturally and culinarily linked to that specific place. On the Orkney Islands, twenty miles north of the Scottish mainland, it was a type of barley. Early settlers arrived here 5,000 years ago, and the Neolithic package – the crops domesticated in the Fertile Crescent – reached these islands around 4,000 years ago, part of its westward sweep out of the Near East. In the seventh century, Celtic missionaries arrived on the islands, followed in the eighth by Vikings. Throughout all this, the people who came to be known as 'Orcadians' were sustained by barley. Tougher and more tolerant to a cold climate than wheat, this cereal made life possible in this exposed and weather-beaten place. And the type that grew best on Orkney and adapted to its challenging conditions was given the name bere (Anglo-Saxon for barley).

One advantage of bere is that it is fast-growing, so much so that it can be the last crop to be sown but the first ready for harvest, soaking up the light of the prolonged summer days in the northern hemisphere. 'From flag leaf – the last leaf to appear on a stalk – to harvest it's ninety days,' Rae Phillips of Orkney's Barony Mill told me. Even in harsher years, when winter winds and colder temperatures sweep in early, bere will have grown quickly enough to produce grain when other crops have failed. In good years, modern barley and even wheat fed by fertilisers and fungicides yield more than bere, but in a bad year those crops might give nothing at all.

When the weather is rough (and on Orkney it can get very rough), it's possible to watch bere's resilience in action. It grows five feet tall – higher than modern dwarf cereals – but when winds gust across it, it will bow over as if it's shielding its grains, hunkering down until things calm down and ready to rise again in time for the harvest. Thousands of years of adaptation have made bere Orkney-proof.

Milling was in Rae Phillips's blood. His grandfather and father worked Barony, a mill which dates back to the 1600s. Just like einkorn and emmer, bere has hulled grains, with tight-fitting glumes, so milling it involves skill, patience and three sets of stones (one more than Kavilca). At Barony Mill these are all powered by water from the nearby Boardhouse Loch. The first set, the shelling stones, crack the husk; then burr stones create a coarse powder; and the final set, the Orkney stones, turn the powder into a fine meal, soft brown-coloured flour with a deliciously nutty smell. This is placed in a kiln for six hours to drive out moisture. The whole process takes around three days. 'And you can't speed it up,' said Phillips, which is one reason why Barony is the only mill left on Orkney still working with bere. Another is that barley is no longer a major part of human diets.

Neolithic people in the Fertile Crescent domesticated wheat and barley at the same time. Barley was wheat's hardier cousin, able to grow in cooler, wetter weather and poorer soils. Combined, the two crops provided early farmers with more resilience: if neither einkorn nor emmer delivered, the chances were that barley would. Barley and wheat were more than likely grown together as a crop, along with, much later, oats and rye. These farmers had unconsciously selected in wild barley the same mutations that had been favoured in wheat: non-shattering ears that made them easier to gather. And as wheat radiated out from the Fertile Crescent, so too did barley. When early farmers in Britain were hit by a period of climate change and colder and wetter weather in around 3000 BCE, wheat struggled, but barley didn't. This tougher cereal became a mainstay of farming, particularly in Scotland's Northern Isles.

If you look at traditional baking cultures across Western and Northern Europe, you can see (and taste) how climate has shaped food. One general rule is that the further north you travel in Europe, the flatter bread becomes. In places with plenty of sun and long hot summers it's possible to grow cereals such as bread wheat, which have higher levels of the protein gluten. This chemical property adds so much elasticity to dough that, when baked, bubbles of trapped air can make it rise into a fluffy loaf. In colder northern climates, however, the lower levels of sunlight favour barley, rye and oats. These cereals have a different chemical structure and lower levels of gluten, and because of this, in the places where they've traditionally been grown, instead of loaves, you find flatbreads. Southern Sweden, for example, had more of a wheat culture and fluffy loaves, whereas bakers in northern Sweden, where barley grew, made flatbreads and *knäckebröd* (baked crackers). In Orkney, the textures and flavours of bere barley shaped traditional recipes and cooking. An important food here was bannocks – soft, round biscuity flatbreads cooked over fire.

This rich baking diversity across Europe started to decline towards the end of the nineteenth century. Until then, most grain was still milled by stone, a process that left the wheatgerm and its oils in the flour (this is the most nutritious part of the grain, and contains protein, vitamins and minerals). Unlike the flour we buy today, this was more like a fresh food, one that was best consumed within a few weeks of milling before the oils began to turn rancid and the flour went mouldy. This changed with the introduction of roller mills, which used steel cylinders to crush grains and made it possible to remove the germ. Although this took away the most nutritious part of the grain, the refined white flour that resulted could be stored for much longer and transported over longer distances. Later, after the Green Revolution and the introduction of modern wheats fed with fertiliser and chemicals, it became possible to cultivate wheat in places where only barley had traditionally grown. With these changes in crops and milling technology, most of what remained of Europe's flatbread culture disappeared, as did many landrace varieties of barley.

Of all the barley grown around the world today, only 2 per cent is eaten by humans. The majority, around 60 per cent, is used as animal feed, while the remainder is used to make malt (for brewing beer and distilling whisky) and a very small proportion is fermented to make soy sauce and miso. Like emmer and einkorn, barley tends to be eaten as food in more remote and inhospitable places. In the highlands of Ethiopia, barley water made with roasted grains survives as a traditional drink, and in Tibet, people still depend on *tsampa*, a mix of barley flour and tea as a high-altitude energy fix.

In Europe, by the 1960s, bere was fast disappearing from the parts of Scotland where it had grown for thousands of years. On the Outer

Hebrides, just six crofters were left growing the cereal, the bere mixed into fields with oats and rye and used mostly to feed livestock. On Shetland, sheep farming had replaced grain production and so bere was in the hands of just two farmers. It was only on Orkney that it had survived as a crop for human consumption. But as more processed food began to be imported onto the island, bere also started to disappear from Orkney's fields, bannocks pushed off household stoves by sliced white bread. In the 1990s, the doors of Barony Mill closed and Rae Phillips retired. The world had moved on, and his skills had become an anachronism.

In 2006, Peter Martin, an agronomist working on Orkney, started researching bere, part of a project launched by the Scottish government to protect the nation's disappearing landrace varieties. Bere not only had to contend with Orkney's extremes of wind and cold, but its sandy and alkaline soil, with low levels of copper, magnesium and zinc. Even if you add lots of nitrogen, modern crops still struggle in this soil. Yet, somehow, bere had thrived on the island for thousands of years.

Fortunately for Martin, small patches of bere could still be found on Orkney, including some left growing next to the old mill. He began an experiment and planted a small field of bere at Orkney's Agronomy Institute. Without fertiliser, the bere grew, whereas the modern barley planted alongside it for comparison completely failed. Martin found high levels of folate, iron, iodine and magnesium in the bere, all important in the human diet. Realising this was a crop too important to lose, he set about producing more seed to help bring the crop back. Inspired by the return of their landrace barley, a new generation of Orcadian farmers, bakers and brewers got involved, planting the barley and using it to bake bannocks and produce beer. Distilleries in the Highlands have also used bere to make whisky.

Rae Phillips came out of retirement to reopen Barony Mill. Without his skills (and patience) it would have been impossible to save bere. When we last spoke in 2018, he was in his mid-seventies and excited about working again. His voice was slow and steady and almost musical. 'We're milling more bere now than we did in the 1950s,' he said. A few months later, the news reached me that he had passed away. A new miller, trained by Phillips, Ali Harcus, stepped in to keep the flame and the bere alive. The mill he said was 'working sweetly' and the flour tasted good. Another precious grain had been saved by a few plots of land and rare knowledge passed from one miller to another.

7

Red Mouth Glutinous Rice

Sichuan, China

Sun Wenxiang grows rice on his farm in the far south of the province of Sichuan in south-west China. He lives with his wife near Dragon Rider Mountain, the peaks of which look like a human riding a mythical winged creature. When I arrived Sun was busy tending to his special home-brewed fertiliser. He applies this to his fields, but he also adds it to the feed he gives his pigs and uses it to clean his house, his teeth and his hair. Sun, who is in his late forties, looked incongruous in the farmyard, pigs grunting in a nearby pen as he stirred his elixir. He was wearing a black double-breasted jacket, mud-soiled and worn, part of the suit he said he reserved for visitors from outside the village. The liquid in the barrels, and its multiple uses, he explained, was all part of his approach to self-sufficiency.

We set off down a narrow, muddy path, with terraces of soybeans, chilli plants and some patches of wheat on either side. Ducks and chickens were busy along the edges of rice paddies, pecking away at insects and tugging at weeds. Sun pointed out the different rice varieties as we passed them. Some had black grains, some were suited for making porridge-like congee and others for making wine. None of Sun's landrace varieties needed artificial fertilisers or pesticides. 'The rice looks after itself,' he said, apart from a helping hand from his fermented tonic and the ducks and chickens who keep the insect numbers under control and add fertiliser to the soil. He pointed across the valley to the rows of rice fields and paddies belonging to his neighbours. These farms, he said, had replaced their old rice varieties in the 1970s with higher-yielding ones issued by the government. They now seemed to be engaged in an endless battle with pests and diseases. Sun's family had resisted and stuck with the landraces. This had left him with a heavy responsibility. 'If I give them up, they'll go extinct,' he said. The plants around our feet were now more endangered than the panda bears in China's nature reserves.

There are few solid records of how much rice diversity China has lost since the 1970s, but there is evidence of a massive reduction. In the 1950s, farmers in Hunan, east of Sichuan, grew more than 1,300 varieties; by 2014, the number had decreased to 84, and the decline is likely to have continued. Sun's farm is a precious living collection of endangered food.

'This one we call *hong zui nuomi* [red mouth glutinous rice],' said Sun as he knelt down and stroked a string of seeds. They looked like delicate dewdrops suspended from the tip of the grass. It was September and the rice, which had been planted in the spring, was almost ready to harvest. Hidden inside the husks were grains with a crimson tip, the 'red mouth' of the rice. The rice took its time growing, Sun said, but its flavour was unforgettable, and its texture glutinous and sticky. These features hold secrets from rice's past.

Over thousands of years, early rice farmers in China (like the wheat farmers in the Fertile Crescent) selected plants with non-shattering grains. They also transformed the colour of these grains. In the wild, rice is red, but as a cultivated grain, it lost this colour as the pericarp (or husk) gradually became whiter. The people who noticed these colours weren't the farmers (grain colour isn't obvious on a plant still in a field) but the cooks. Whiter grains became more popular as they required less water and labour, and so were easier to prepare and cook. As a consequence, over millennia, this cereal went from being mostly red to mostly white.

Red-coloured rice is still grown in parts of the world, in Africa for instance, where domestication followed a different path, and also on isolated farms across Asia, such as Sun's, where landrace varieties have been saved and traces of the rice's ancient past have survived. Science has now shown us that red rice contains more nutrients than white, so it's a far healthier food. This is significant because rice is the primary food of three billion people.

But the global rice crop has lost more than essential nutrients. Like wheat, as yields were pushed higher, diversity declined, and the world has lost – and continues to lose – some remarkable plants.

Rare rice varieties have been found that are flood-tolerant, capable of surviving after being submerged in water for weeks (as if the plant is holding its breath); others are able to grow in saline soils (salt is usually lethal to rice plants); some are even able to absorb nanoparticles of silver from soil which accumulates inside the grain. This silver-absorbing rice is used in India to treat stomach complaints (in Western medicine, before antibiotics, silver was also used to treat infections and burns, and is once again the subject of medical research). There are also types of rice that instead of having the usual single grain inside each hull, have two or three (making them super-productive plants). Most of these unusual varieties are grown by just a handful of farmers in the poorest parts of Asia. Some of them survive in the hands of a single farmer. The tragedy is that this rice diversity will be impossible to recover in our lifetimes. These genetic riches took thousands of years to create.

The domestication of rice was as remarkable as that of wheat. Hunter-gatherers in southern China foraged seeds of wild rice plants along the Yangtze River as well as wild species of peas and beans, berries, nuts and acorns. Then, around 13000 BCE, the climate started warming and glaciers melted. As wild rice grew in waterlogged areas, the plants proliferated and spread far and wide across the Yangtze River Valley in the wetter climate. And as the supply of wild grain increased, so did the hunter-gatherer population. Around 7,000 years ago, instead of relying on nature, they engineered wetlands. They dug oval pits (the size of a small dinner table, archaeologists tell us), filled these with water and used them to grow rice plants, which is how the paddy system was born.

These proto farmers also noticed how the most productive plants, the ones with most seed, grew on the margins of wetlands, land that tended to dry out as the seasons changed. By occasionally draining water from the rice pits they copied this pattern. Done at a certain time, depriving plants of water places them under stress and sends them into survival mode; to increase their chance of reproduction they begin to produce as much seed as possible. The rice paddy was born out of these careful observations, and it became the most productive food system ever devised.

All of this was only possible because the rice plant itself is so unusual: through its leaves it absorbs oxygen which it takes down beneath the water to its submerged roots. As most other plants can't survive in these anaerobic underwater conditions, rice paddies also provide a form of weed control. And even in places where soils are too acidic or alkaline to grow other crops, everything falls into balance within the paddy, as a steady pH of 7 is maintained by the standing water. Paddies can be self-fertilising too because decaying plants and animal waste break down in the water, producing nitrogen which nourishes the crop. The paddy system is so productive that, throughout human history, the world's densest populations have been rice-growing cultures. The surplus food generated allowed people to conceive of a future, plan ahead and divide labour, so that some people were free to craft objects, create art, own possessions or gain prestige. As farmers domesticated rice, they shaped civilisation.

The rice we're familiar with today is the result of three separate waves of domestication. Out of the Yangtze River basin came *japonica*, a rice with short, round grains (the type used in sushi). Japonica then spread into northern China, Korea and Japan, where it diversified even more. A second wave of domestication took place further south, around north-eastern India, Laos, Vietnam and Thailand. The rice that evolved here was *indica* which had long, thin grains (this is the most widely grown rice in the world today). Meanwhile, in the Bangladeshi delta, a third wild species called *aus* (pronounced owsh) was domesticated, which had smaller, thinner grains. The genes of these different species started to mix as people travelled and traded and, around 2,000 years ago, somewhere in the foothills of the Himalayas, aus and japonica hybridised, creating some of the most prized varieties we know today: the aromatic varieties, *basmati* and *jasmine*.

In addition to these major rice groups, an extra level of culinary diversity evolved. Long before rice domestication, hunter-gatherers noticed some plants produced grains which, when cooked, were stickier than others (the earliest cooking pots found in China are 18,000 years old). This 'stickiness' was the result of a genetic mutation, and because grains which contained this mutation had been part of diets, and enjoyed, glutinous types of rice were later selected for domestication. Today, a strong cultural preference for sticky rice exists only in certain parts of Asia. In Yunnan in south-western China, for example, it remains the main rice used in all types of dishes. Outside this region, sticky rice is mostly reserved for dim sum and sweet dishes.

The legacy of this long process of domestication and selection by farmers and cooks all over Asia was greater diversity. On the edge of the largest lake in the Philippines, Laguna de Baý, south-east of Manila, in an underground, earthquake-proof vault are 136,000 individual samples of seeds, the largest collection of rice in the world. These grains, with their potential to create a rainbow of colours and intense aromas, each uniquely adapted to a different ecosystem, now mostly exist inside freezers in this seed bank, absent from farmers' fields.

Whereas the global Green Revolution was largely steered by American science and finance, China's push for greater food production was more self-contained. Both efforts happened more or less in parallel. Mao's attempt at rapid industrialisation, the 'Great Leap Forward' in the late 1950s, forced farmers off their land, leading to famine and the death of millions. Soon after, an agricultural researcher, Yuan Longping, was given the task of helping China's recovery by increasing the supply of rice. Based in a lab in Hunan, Yuan, like Borlaug in Mexico, spent years working with landraces and crossing varieties in meticulous experiments. By the early 1970s, he had developed Nan-you No. 2, a hybrid rice so productive it had the potential to increase food supply by nearly a third. Farmers were told to replace the old varieties with the new, and by the start of the 1980s, more than 50 per cent of China's rice came from this single variety. But, as with Borlaug's wheat, Yuan's rice depended on huge amounts of fertilisers, pesticides and lots and lots of water.

In the 1960s, in another part of Asia, a team of scientists were also breeding new rice varieties. What became known as the International Rice Research Institute (IRRI) in the Philippines was funded by the American Rockefeller and Ford Foundations. The IRRI's plant breeders also made a breakthrough drawing on the genetics of a dwarf plant. This new pest-resistant, high-yielding rice, called IR8, was released across India, Pakistan and Bangladesh in 1966. Using the Green Revolution package of irrigation, fertilisers and pesticides, IR8 tripled yields and became known as 'miracle rice'. As it rapidly spread across Asia (with the necessary agrichemicals subsidised by Western foundations and governments), farmers were encouraged to abandon their landrace varieties and help share the new seeds with neighbours and relatives in other villages. Social occasions, including weddings, were treated by Western strategists as opportunities to distribute IR8. A decade later, rice scientist Gurdev Khush, the son of an Indian rice farmer, improved on the 'miracle rice' (IR8 wasn't the tastiest rice to eat and had a chalky texture). A later iteration, IR64, was so productive that it became the most widely cultivated rice variety in the world. But while most of the world was applauding the increase in calories created by the new rice varieties, some people were sounding a note of caution about what was also being lost.

In July 1972, with the Green Revolution in full flow, the botanist Jack Harlan published an article entitled 'The Genetics of Disaster'. As the world's population was increasing faster than at any time in history, Harlan said, crop diversity was being eroded at an equally unprecedented rate. 'These resources stand between us and catastrophic starvation on a scale we cannot imagine,' he argued. 'In a very real sense, the future of the human race rides on these materials.' Bad things can happen at the hands of nature, Harlan reminded his readers, citing the Irish potato famine. 'We can survive if a forest or shade tree is destroyed, but who would survive if wheat, rice, or maize were to be destroyed? We are taking risks we need not and should not take.' The solutions being developed in the Green Revolution would be as good as they could be until they failed – and when they did, the human race would be left facing disaster, he warned. 'Few will criticize Dr Borlaug for doing his job too well. The enormous increase in ... yields is a welcome relief and his achievements are deservedly recognized, but if we fail to salvage at least what is left of the landrace populations of Asia before they are replaced, we can justifiably be condemned by future generations for squandering our heritage and theirs.' We were moving from genetic erosion, he said, to genetic wipe-out. 'The line between abundance and disaster is becoming thinner and thinner, and the public is unaware and unconcerned. Must we wait for disaster to be real before we are heard? Will people listen only after it is too late?' It may be nearly too late, but, fifty years on, people are listening to Harlan.

One of them is Susan McCouch, Professor of Plant Breeding and Genetics at Cornell University and an expert on rice genetics. Her research includes the less familiar aus rice which evolved in the

Bangladeshi delta. 'It has the most stress-tolerant genes of all the rice we know,' says McCouch. 'It grows on poor soils, survives drought and is the fastest species to go from seed to grain.' And yet aus is endangered. Most farmers in Bangladesh have abandoned it and switched to more commercial varieties. Only the poorest people have saved the rice, farmers who couldn't afford to buy fertilisers and build irrigation systems. Its genetics are so rare because, unlike japonica and indica which travelled far and wide, aus stayed put. 'The people who domesticated it never left the river delta,' says McCouch. 'They weren't empire builders, didn't have armies and never enslaved populations.' But by bequeathing the world aus, they have left their mark.

In 2018, McCouch, along with researchers from USDA, released a new rice called Scarlett. It was, the team said, a rice with nutty rich flavours but also 'packed with high levels of antioxidants and flavonoids along with vitamin E'. To create it, McCouch had crossed an American long-grain rice called Jefferson and a rice that was discovered in Malaysia. The reason the new rice was packed with nutrients and called Scarlett was because the Malaysian plant was a red-coloured wild species. One person who would have been unsurprised at the special qualities of these coloured grains was Sun Wenxiang, the farmer I had visited in Sichuan.

Inside a room on his farm, Sun was packing up small parcels of his special red rice to send to customers in Beijing, Shanghai, Chengdu and Hangzhou. They order his red mouth rice on WeChat, the Chinese social media app used by more than a billion people across Asia that is part Twitter and part PayPal (and so much more). Some have told him they buy it for its taste or intriguing colour, but most buy it for its health properties.

For farmers such as Sun working to save China's endangered foods, help is at hand at the Centre for Rural Reconstruction, a modern day iteration of a movement founded a century ago to empower peasants and revitalise villages. In the 1920s a group of intellectuals and smallholders set up the original Rural Reconstruction Movement to develop farms, improve crops, establish co-operatives and sell more produce in China's towns and cities. After the revolution, and during Mao's rule, it disappeared, but in the 1990s was resurrected. A former government economist named Professor Wen Tiejun believed rural communities across China faced serious decline as manufacturing boomed and millions of people migrated from thousands of villages. By 2010, the country had experienced the largest and most rapid rural-to-urban migration ever witnessed in human history. Professor Wen began to ask what this meant for the future of China's small-scale farmers and the food they produced and, as a result, he launched the *New* Rural Reconstruction Movement.

The garden surrounding the two-storey training centre 50 miles north of Beijing is a statement of intent: its raised beds are fertilised with night soil, the nutrients processed from a row of eco-toilets (an ancient technique, as Chinese farmers enriched their fields using human and animal waste for thousands of years). The idea came from a book written a century ago, not by a Chinese agricultural expert, but an American one. *Farmers of Forty Centuries* by Franklin Hiram King has become essential reading matter for some students at China's Centre for Rural Reconstruction.

In the early 1900s, King, an agronomist from Wisconsin, worked at the United States Department of Agriculture, but he was regarded as a maverick, more interested in indigenous farming systems than the agricultural expansion the department had been set up to deliver. Convinced that he could learn more from peasant farmers than the scientists in Washington, King left the United States in 1909 and set out on an eight-month expedition through Asia. 'I had long desired to stand face to face with Chinese and Japanese farmers,' he wrote in the book's introduction, 'to walk through their fields and to learn by seeing some of their methods, appliances and practices which centuries of stress and experience have led these oldest farmers in the world to adopt.' King died in 1911 before he had completed his book and the work was pretty much forgotten until 1927, when a London publisher, Jonathan Cape, discovered the manuscript and published it, ensuring it remained in print for the next twenty years. It went on to influence the founding figures in Britain's organic movement, Albert Howard and Eve Balfour. The farmers who visit the Centre for Rural Reconstruction and come across King's book, will read an account of how food was produced in China's villages a century ago. Crops grown then, now endangered, are also being resurrected.

Inside a storeroom at the centre, now a bank of some of China's rarest foods, I was shown boxes full of seeds and jars and packets of ingredients all produced by farming projects in villages supported by the New Rural Reconstruction Movement. All were distinctive products that were helping to increase farmers' incomes. There was dark green soy from Yunnan in the south; red-coloured ears of wheat from the north; wild tea harvested from ancient forests; and bottles of honey-coloured rice wine. And among other varieties of landrace rice was Sun Wenxiang's red mouth glutinous grains.

'When we lose a traditional food, a variety of rice or a fruit, we store up problems for the future,' Professor Wen told me. 'There's no question China needs large-scale farms, but we also need diversity.'

With 20 per cent of the world's population, China encapsulates the biggest food dilemmas of our times. Should it intensify farming to produce more calories, or diversify to help save the planet? In the long run, there is no option but to change the system. China suffers from wide-scale soil erosion, health-harming levels of pollution and water shortages. As a consequence, land has become contaminated, there are algae blooms around its coastline and high levels of greenhouse gas emissions.

There are signs of change. In September 2016 China ratified the Paris Agreement on Climate Change. Among the specific targets it set was zero growth in fertiliser and pesticide use. To conserve more of its genetic resources and crop diversity, China is one of the few countries investing heavily in new botanic gardens to protect and study endangered species. The Chinese Academy of Agricultural Sciences has also built a collection of half a million samples of landrace crops, varieties now being researched for future use. This is what Jack Harlan might have called the genetics of salvation. It's a long way from King's *Farmers of Forty Centuries*, but there is clear recognition that China's current food system can't go on as before.

'We need to modernise and develop, but that doesn't mean letting go of our past,' said Wen. 'The entire world should not be chasing one way of living, we can't all eat the same kind of food, that is a crazy ideology.' And then he shared the famous quote attributed to Napoleon: 'Let China sleep, for when she wakes, she will shake the world.' 'Well,' said Wen, 'we have woken up and we've started to *eat* more like the rest of the world. We need to find better ways of living and farming. Maybe some answers can be found in our traditions.'

8

Olotón Maize

Oaxaca, Mexico

In the early 1980s, an American plant scientist called Howard-Yana Shapiro climbed thousands of metres to reach remote villages in the eastern highlands of the Mexican state of Oaxaca. The area is home to the Mixe people. No one knew when or how the Mixe had settled in the rugged mountains, and there is little archaeology to explain their history. The soldier and explorer Hernán Cortés, who had conquered the Aztecs, was thwarted by the Mixe. 'Their land is so rocky that it cannot be crossed even on foot,' he wrote in 1525, 'for I have twice sent people to conquer them, who were unable to do so because of the roughness of the terrain, and because the warriors are very fierce and well-armed.' By the 1980s, just a few Mixe villages were still left in isolation, and when Shapiro reached the top of his climb and walked into one, he was confronted with the strangest plant he had ever seen.

The plant was a type of maize known as Olotón, but it grew nearly twenty feet high and had a bizarre, captivating root system. Most plants grow with their roots underground, but this plant also had them sprouting from high up its thick stalks, reaching out into the open air. From these bright orange, aerial roots, shaped like fingers, there dripped a glistening gel. The maize was oozing mucus. Also remarkable was that any maize could grow so high up the mountain and in such poor soil. The Mixe village was so remote that no chemical fertiliser could ever have made it there. The local farmers weren't even growing the maize in a milpa (from the Aztec term for 'maize field'). In this traditional system beans are grown alongside the cereal to fix nitrogen into the soil. Somehow, these alien-looking plants were feeding themselves.

At least, that was the hunch Shapiro left with; that the strange mucus dripping from roots growing above ground was providing the plant with all the nitrogen it needed. The theory seemed unlikely. It broke all the rules. If it was true then this could be a game changer. Fertiliser costs farmers around the world billions of dollars a year and has great environmental costs, from the energy used to make it, to the greenhouse gases it releases, and the rivers and oceans it pollutes. The problem was that forty years ago, Shapiro had no means of testing his hunch.

Other scientists also made the climb up the 'scorched hill', but still no one could figure out the glistening mucus. Meanwhile, at the University of Wisconsin a microbiologist named Eric Triplett, who hadn't seen the maize, or even known of the Mixe village, published a scientific paper in 1996 which set out a radical hypothesis: the 'holy grail' of cereals – maize that can take nitrogen from the air and feed itself – was biologically possible and could evolve. Such a discovery, he added, 'would be of enormous economic value' and would 'improve human health' as it would decrease the amount of nitrate in our water and in our food. For years, Triplett's theory remained just that, a theory. He did, however, have some advice for any plant explorers setting off in search of this holy grail. Echoing Vavilov a century earlier, if something this extraordinary did exist, he said, it would be found close to the origins of maize, in its centre of diversity where its gene pool was greatest: southern Mexico.

If you were to compare a wild wheat or wild barley with a domesticated version, you would be able to see that they were relatives. Maize is different. Teosinte (wild maize) looks nothing like corn on the cob. This wild grass has thin, skinny ears 5cm long and holds just a dozen seeds, each one locked inside a hard case, like a tiny walnut shell. This protective layer is made from silica and lignite, the building blocks of glass and wood. Chew on it and you'd break teeth. But however unpromising teosinte looks to us, about 9,000 years ago hunter-gatherers in south-western Mexico started to interact with this plant and began the long, slow process of domestication.

The hunter-gatherers in the Central Balsas River Valley (in today's state of Guerrero) lived in small groups (most likely of twenty to fifty people) and moved with the seasons, following different wild foods as they came and went. Among these were teosinte seeds, which the foragers ground up into flour. Seeds from the teosinte plants most attractive to these nomadic hunter-gatherers would have been scattered as they harvested, and so by the time they returned to the same location months later, a process of unconscious selection was under way. Eventually, they settled and became farmers. The transformation of teosinte into modern maize, over thousands of years, is one of the most astonishing human feats ever undertaken. Selection by three hundred generations of farmers resulted in kernels coming free of their stony cases, but remaining attached to the plant, making harvests easier. Teosinte's bushy plant, full of dozens of tiny ears, each one the size of a cigarette butt, became a single, straight stalk with just one or two plump ears, 30cm long. At a chemical level the protein content of the grain reduced, but the carbohydrate increased, turning maize into a source of quick energy that was also storable. This transformation didn't just take place over a very long time, it happened over a vast geographical area, beginning in Mexico but eventually involving farmers in the Amazon in the south and all the way up into North America. After 9,000 years of continuous cultivation, the size of maize's seed had increased by 80 per cent, the number of grains by 300 per cent, and the cobs were 60 times larger. These separate pockets of domestication, all working in parallel, resulted in maize becoming incredibly diverse. The process also left the plant entirely reliant on farmers for its reproduction, and farmers, in turn, became entirely dependent on the grain.

Most religious ceremonies and origin stories in early Meso-American culture revolve around maize. According to the Mayan *Popol Vuh*, the first humans were created from white maize hidden inside a mountain under an immovable rock. A rain spirit split the rock open using a bolt of lightning which burned some of the maize, creating three grain colours: yellow, black and red. The creator took this grain, ground it into dough and used it to make humans. For the Hopi in New Mexico, who are experts in growing maize in bone-dry soil, the creation story is a little different: the first humans were offered a choice of blue, red or yellow maize, some with big ears, others small. The biggest and plumpest maize went first, but the Hopi, who were slow to choose, ended up with a small ear of blue maize. With this came three gifts: a bag of seed, a planting stick and a gourd filled with

water. 'You have selected wisely,' the spirit told them, 'your life will
be difficult, but your people will walk the earth forever with this
maize.' The Olmec bound the heads of their newborns to elongate
their shape. This Meso-American civilisation revered the cereal to such
an extent that some archaeologists have interpreted this as an attempt
to evoke an ear of maize.

By 1492, maize's reach had extended south to Chile, and north to
Canada. The genetics of the plant made it extraordinarily versatile,
able to adapt to the desert landscape of Arizona, the mountainous
cold of the Andes and the humidity of cloud forests in Guatemala,
where it spread as a 24-foot creeper with stalks so thick they could be
used as fence posts. No other crop can rearrange its genome around
so many stresses and different environments.

This biological diversity translated into culinary diversity too. Some
kernels were selected for their colour (whites and blues through to
purple and copper), and others for their distinctive textures. One village
might have selected a maize because its grains were plump, making
it good for roasting, while others opted for grains with tough outer
layers so when heated the starch within would explode (popcorn in
other words). In rural communities in southern Brazil, 1,500 different
populations of maize landraces have been identified (including 1,078
landraces just used for making popcorn). Other types of maize were
better for brewing beers, or alcoholic 'pox' made from ground and
fermented maize mixed with sugar cane. But the real culinary
expression of maize diversity lies in the thousands of varieties that
were ground into flour, turned into dough (masa) and cooked as
tamales and tortillas. One type of maize will make thick, spongy
tortillas while another can make dough so elastic it can be stretched
into discs 50cm wide. Inside the world's biggest maize seed bank, held
by the International Maize and Wheat Improvement Center (CIMMYT)
in El Batán, Mexico City, underground bunkers contain 24,000 samples
of maize.

As with all cereals, maize wasn't just adaptable; its grains could also
be stored and transported, which is how it eventually crossed continents. The Columbian Exchange saw wheat and rice travel from the
Old World to the New, while maize went the other way, arriving in
Spain in 1493. By the end of the sixteenth century, maize had been
planted in China and Africa and been adopted by both the Ottoman

Empire and Indian dynasties. What wasn't transported along with the grain were the farming and processing techniques, and for many North Americans and people in the Old World, Europeans in particular, this proved to be disastrous.

The milpa system has been described by the maize scholar Garrison Wilkes as 'one of the most successful human inventions ever created'. To outsiders, a milpa looks like a busy hotchpotch of competing plants, but this mess of diversity is in fact a complex system that creates balance, not just botanically but also nutritionally. In the milpa system, maize is planted with its companions, beans and squashes, its stalks creating a frame for the beans to climb and the broad leaves of the squash giving ground cover, conserving moisture in the soil and suppressing weeds. But the most important feature of the milpa is what happens below ground; the leguminous roots of the bean are host to microbes which fix nitrogen into the soil and help fertilise the other crops. Combined on a plate, these plants also add up to a nutritionally complete meal. Maize provides carbohydrate, the beans essential amino acids such as lysine and tryptophan (without which we're unable to synthesise proteins), and the squash lots of vitamins.

Once harvested, indigenous farmers would then take maize through an ingenious process called nixtamalisation. The word itself comes from two Nahuatl (ancient Aztec) words: *nextli* (meaning ashes) and *tamalli* (a word for maize dough). Nixtamalisation involves breaking down the tough layers around the maize kernels by soaking them in a chemical solution, made from ashes or, more commonly, mineral lime (calcium hydroxide). This not only softens the grains, so that masa can be shaped and tortillas made, but also releases nutrients otherwise locked up inside the kernels. Evidence of nixtamalisation dates back 3,500 years. The first North Americans and Europeans to take maize away with them ignored the food and farming knowledge that had evolved with the crop. Because they didn't grow maize using the milpa system or adopt the practice of nixtamalisation (dismissing both as primitive), they paid a heavy price. Essential nutrients were missing from their new maize-filled diets and many died of the debilitating and excruciating disease pellagra, caused by deficiency in the vitamin niacin.

Nevertheless, with hard lessons learnt, maize was eventually turned into a global staple. So global, you can map the world through maize.

In mountainous northern Spain, a landrace maize called Arto Gorria is grown by Basque farmers and used to make flatbreads baked over the embers of fires. In Italy, in the Comune di Rimella in Piedmont, a buttery polenta called *màgru* is made by toasting the kernels of a landrace called Ders Malp. In the Philippines, a drink that looks like coffee is made by burning maize flour (*sinunog bugas mais*). And in the US, in Charleston, South Carolina, there's Jimmy Red corn, a blood-red, flint-hard grain once favoured by bootleggers because it makes the best whiskey. None of this global maize diversity is any match for what existed in Oaxaca, one of the world's biodiversity hotspots and home to sixteen ethnic groups, including Zapotecs, Chatinos, Amuzgos and of course the Mixes, each with their own languages, religious beliefs and maize.

Trying to make sense of this diversity is complicated. One approach, developed in the 1940s and still in use today, organises Mexico's thousands of maize varieties into 'races', based on the shape of the ears, the colour of the kernels and the structure of the plant. Among the sixty or so 'races' is Bolita, found mostly in Oaxaca. Its name means 'little ball' because its cobs are so small and round. Some Bolita varieties can be ground down and boiled to make a sticky, gelatinous dessert called *nicuatole*. Thought to be even older is Pepitilla, so named because its long, narrow, sweet-tasting grains look like pumpkin seeds. And a type found in Chiapas as well as Oaxaca is Olitillo. The tortillas it makes are fragrant and as soft as pillows. In ancient Zapotec cave burials, urns have been found with depictions of Olitillo's long, slender, cylindrical cobs. Then there is Olotón, a maize suited to growing at higher altitudes, 2000 metres and more. Included in this 'race' are the plants oozing the strange mucilage in the remote villages of the Sierra Mixe now so rare they're mostly found growing in isolated communities. To understand how all of this diversity came to be endangered, we need to cross over the border into the US.

Long before the Green Revolution transformed wheat, a succession of plant breeders had already revolutionised maize. The first step was the result of a fluke; a chance encounter between two different types of maize. In the 1800s, in the north-eastern United States, indigenous people were growing a landrace maize so brittle and hard it became known as 'flint corn'. Meanwhile, a second type of maize had arrived north of the border from Mexico, care of the Spanish. This had been given the name 'dent corn' because of a tiny indentation on the crown of each kernel. Over centuries, these two different types of maize travelled along different paths, passed from farmer to farmer and were planted from one town to the next. Their paths eventually converged in the Mid-Atlantic states, including Virginia, where the two plants – flint and dent – were hybridised to create a new type of maize. It was high-yielding and, as a result, so popular among pioneer farmers that in Indiana, Ohio and Illinois, the hybrid became known as 'Midwest dent'. By the 1890s, varieties such as Reid's Yellow Dent were being planted on such a scale it transformed the landscape of America's Midwest into the 'Corn Belt'. The US quickly became a major exporter of maize to Europe.

The next steps in maize's transformation both happened in 1908. One was Fritz Haber's breakthrough in synthesising nitrogen, the gateway to industrial fertiliser. The other took place at the Carnegie Institute's research station at Cold Spring Harbor, New York. Plant breeder George Harrison Shull discovered that by continually inbreeding two lines of maize and then cross-pollinating these lines, extraordinarily productive plants with abundant kernels could be created (a phenomenon called hybrid vigour). These explosive yields happened only once as the following generation of maize reverted back to less desirable, less productive traits inherited from the plant's 'grandparents'. The appeal was obvious. This first filial generation of seed, known as 'F1 hybrids', was ready to harvest in just three months (some landrace maize took six); they could be planted in larger, more dense monocultures; and yields per acre were increased by 25 to 50 per cent. For farmers, F1 maize meant more grain; the downside was that they could no longer save and replant their own maize. Instead, they became dependent on the products of a new booming industry: the seed companies.

Shull's research on maize changed America. At the beginning of the twentieth century farmers were growing around one thousand different open-pollinated varieties. After the Second World War, hybrids dominated. As the manufacture of explosives declined, a surplus of ammonium nitrate (an ingredient in fertiliser) became available and Fritz Haber's invention began to play a crucial role in the production of food. Applied to vast monocultures of F1 maize the new supply of fertiliser bolstered America's position as the world's pre-eminent exporter of grain. By the end of the century, American-grown F1 hybrids accounted for 50 per cent of globally traded maize. From the tens of thousands of landrace varieties, just a handful now made up the commercial crop. Echoing Jack Harlan's warning, Garrison Wilkes has likened this to 'taking stones from the foundation of a house to repair the roof'.

The maize boom produced more calories but helped to make the global food system more uniform, less diverse and increasingly brittle. Evidence for this came in dramatic fashion in the early 1970s. At the time, 85 per cent of the crop grown in the Corn Belt shared a single genetic trait susceptible to a fungal disease (a form of leaf blight). The disease spread rapidly through corn fields, resulting in the loss of one billion bushels of maize at a cost of $6 billion to farmers. 'Never again should a major cultivated crop be molded into such uniformity that it is so universally vulnerable to attack by a pathogen, an insect, or environmental stress,' the USDA plant scientist Arnold Ullstrup wrote at the time. Diversity, he said, needed to be maintained for all important crop species.

After seed companies developed a new generation of hybrids, yields increased again. All the extra maize needed a home. This is when maize started to turn up in the most unexpected places: as a sweetener in Coke; as a component in the plastic bottles containing that sugary drink; in toothpaste, soap, paint and shoe polish. It also helped fuel the revolution in livestock production: if you consume milk or eggs, chicken or beef, the animal is likely to have been fed maize. Meso-American civilisations had believed they were people of maize, but now we all are. In 2008, researchers in America tested five hundred different hamburgers, fries and chicken sandwiches from a range of fast-food chains: all the chicken and 93 per cent of the beef came from animals on corn-fed diets, and the fries had been cooked in corn oil. Even the cars people drive to buy these foods are partly fuelled by maize (around a third of the crop produced in the US is now converted into ethanol). Eventually, the American maize revolution crossed the border to reach the birthplace of maize itself.

Someone who has tracked the impact of American maize on Mexico is Alyshia Gálvez, anthropologist and professor at the City University of New York. Gálvez has spent years visiting markets in Mexico City, talking to farmers in Puebla and sharing meals in Oaxaca to understand the politics of maize. The focus of her research has been NAFTA, the North American Free Trade Agreement, which came into force under the Clinton administration in 1994. The deal removed trade barriers to ease the flow of goods between the United States, Mexico and Canada. It also resulted in the biggest change to Mexican food and farming for five hundred years. NAFTA was expected to result in the industrialisation of more of the Mexican economy. The forecast was that half a million people would stop farming, leave Mexico's rural areas and go to work in factories. In reality, says Gálvez, it was closer to 10 million who left the countryside. Many were subsistence farmers, who headed not just to Mexican cities, but also north over the border and into the USA.

Land that had been farmed for thousands of years, where seeds had been saved and traditions preserved, was abandoned with landraces falling into decline. NAFTA opened up Mexico to exports of dent corn from the Midwest, a quarter of America's total crop, all propped up by billions of dollars of US government subsidies. The Mexican diet changed as meals based around milpa-grown, highly nutritious maize varieties were replaced by processed foods made with Midwest dents, 'a high-starch commodity, grown mostly for animal feed and for sweetening sodas', says Gálvez. Following the introduction of NAFTA, every indicator of public health in Mexico worsened. By the early 2000s, the country had one of the highest obesity rates in the world and had become the number one consumer of sodas, drinks mostly sweetened by high-fructose corn syrup. NAFTA had overlooked so much: that food is also culture; that *how* maize is farmed matters; that traditional can be healthier. Maize was just maize, a commodity to be traded. Health, heritage and identity weren't even in the footnotes of the deal. 'Is this what agricultural progress looks like?' says Gálvez. 'Sky-high rates of diabetes, a killer of 80,000 Mexicans a year, and tens of thousands more lost to obesity.'

Exactly how much maize diversity in Mexico has been lost in recent years isn't fully known. One rare attempt to measure the decline focused on samples of landraces collected from farmers in the state of Morelos, north of Oaxaca, in the mid-1960s. Ninety-three seed samples had been deposited in the CIMMYT genebank near Mexico

City. In 2017, researchers from CIMMYT tracked down the farmers, or, in most cases, their descendants, to find out how many of the landraces were still in cultivation. It turned out only one-fifth of the farmers had saved the seeds and a quarter of the families were no longer involved in agriculture. The main reason for giving up their landraces, the farmers explained, had been the arrival of new varieties, hybrids that were seen as more productive and more profitable. The downside, the farmers told the researchers, was they now had to buy expensive seed each year.

Despite the long-term decline, an enormous amount of maize diversity still exists in Mexico. Landraces are planted by an estimated two and a half million small-scale farmers, usually on plots no more than three hectares in size, mostly for home consumption in tortillas, tamales and atole. But the future of this maize is precarious, as the simple fact is that saving this diversity brings little financial reward.

Alfonso Rocha Robles, a member of Slow Food Mexico, watched the impact of NAFTA and falling farm incomes unfold on the streets of his home city, Puebla. Here, in the centre of the country, he saw waves of indigenous people arrive each day from the south. Most often he saw them standing at traffic lights offering to clean cars and begging for money. When he stopped to talk with them, they usually told him they had left their villages because it was impossible to survive as a farmer any more. 'They had travelled for fifteen hours by bus, all to live in a room with ten other people and spend their days in a desperate struggle to earn enough money for food. When I talk about diversity and people say to me "it's only maize", I tell them about these farmers.'

The grassroots movement Sin Maíz, No Hay País (Without Maize There Is No Country) was founded in 2007, in part to defend Mexico's maize culture and to combat the decline in traditional agriculture. It argued that in losing local landraces and being exposed to global markets, rural communities had lost income and autonomy and so it has called for a renegotiation of NAFTA and the promotion of domestically produced maize.

Meanwhile, some of Mexico's most influential chefs are trying to boost the value of maize diversity. One is Enrique Olvera, who now works with sixty indigenous farmers, each growing different landrace varieties. 'It's possible to think about landrace maize in the same way as wine,' he says. 'They grow in different soils at different altitudes and they have such different tastes.' Olvera pays the farmers more than ten times the price of dent corn from the Midwest. 'That's maize we don't cook with,' says Olvera, 'it belongs in a bag of corn chips.' By giving maize the status it deserves, and paying farmers the money they need, he is giving Mexico's endangered landrace maize varieties a lifeline. This matters not just to farmers in Mexico, but to all of us.

Nearly four decades after Howard-Yana Shapiro encountered it, a team from the University of California, Davis, solved the mystery of the Mixe maize, after making the trek to one of the remote villages in Oaxaca. 'When we saw those plants, we knew for sure we weren't in Iowa,' says Alan Bennett, Professor of Plant Sciences at Davis, who led the research. 'The plants were towering above us, and three feet above the ground were the weird roots.'

New techniques for sequencing DNA and advances in chemical analysis enabled Bennett to analyse the mucilage dripping from the maize. What he found was a community of thousands of different species of bacteria and hundreds of different complex sugars. It all formed part of an evolutionary trade-off: the bacteria helped to feed the plant and the plant produced sugars to feed the bacteria. Different groups of microbes all played their own specific role. Some specialised in breaking down sugars to give energy to other bacteria, which in turn were busy taking nitrogen from the atmosphere and converting it into plant-friendly ammonia. Meanwhile another group of bacteria made an enzyme called nitrogenase (necessary for all life on earth). As nitrogenase is a sensitive compound (it dies on contact with oxygen), the plant had evolved to ooze out a thick mucilage to act as a barrier, stopping O_2 getting through.

In addition to the maize plant and the bacteria, a third party had been involved in the evolution of this process: humans. The Mixe people had planted and tended the maize over thousands of years, and as the world (and maize) had changed around them, they saved the plant from extinction. Many communities surrounding the village where most of the maize is found had given up their landrace varieties and opted for F1 hybrids. New roads had made seeds and fertilisers available to Oaxaca's farmers. 'We got there just in time,' says Bennett, who is now doing more research on the self-fertilising maize. 'If we'd been too late, that would have been a loss for the entire world.'

The extraordinary potential of the maize with its aerial roots, gooey mucilage and microbes raises a fundamental question about these increasingly rare genetic resources: who will benefit from them? The maize grown by the Mixe might well prove to be the agricultural discovery of the century. The researchers, working with Mars Inc. (the privately owned food business), have signed an agreement with the village to share any financial benefits if the maize is eventually commercialised. 'It's a fifty–fifty arrangement,' says Bennett. If the plant's traits prove to be world changing, we'll have generations of farmers in the Sierra Mixe to thank.

Saving diversity

While the Millennium Seed Bank in Sussex is the backup for the Earth's wild plant diversity, the seeds of the world's landrace crops, the legacy of 12,000 years of agriculture, are preserved on the Arctic island of Svalbard – about as far north as a commercial plane can fly.

In January 2008, the first boxes of seeds flown to Svalbard were carried down the tunnel chiselled beneath a mountain through 135 metres of solid rock. Beyond the huge steel doors, the seeds were taken along a corridor and through an airlock past which the temperature is kept at –18°C. This is the environment created for the white-walled storeroom, 30 metres long, 10 metres wide and 5 metres high. All around are shelves and shelves of boxes containing one million seeds.

The vault was the idea of American botanist Cary Fowler. Forty years ago, he read Jack Harlan's prophecy that a mass extinction was under way in our fields. 'The idea stayed with me,' says Fowler, 'that we were losing precious genetic diversity.' Fowler never forgot Harlan's exact words: 'These resources stand between us and catastrophic starvation on a scale we cannot imagine.' It inspired his fascination with crop diversity and gave him his life mission: to create a safety deposit box for all the seeds of every known food plant.

Fowler convinced governments and organisations to back him. Svalbard was the coldest, most secure, most remote location he could find. 'The only threat was the polar bears roaming outside.'

The seeds here represent a co-evolution between crops, climates, environments and the work of hundreds of generations of farmers over thousands of years. They hold a record of everything our food crops have experienced and adapted to. 'They also represent everything our agricultural system can be in the future,' says Fowler, 'a repository of traits and of diversity. The contents of that vault gives us options.'

Inside the Svalbard vault there are seeds of wheat, barley, rice and maize from nearly every country on Earth, including countries that no longer exist. Fowler watched as the first boxes were carried inside. 'That was pretty close to a religious experience,' Fowler told me. 'My ancestors had a role in saving and passing down those seeds and yours did too.' The enormity of that idea can overwhelm some visitors when they enter the vault, he says, 'which is why they leave with tears in their eyes'.

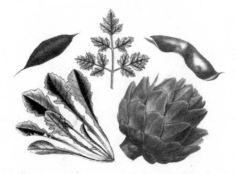

Part Three
Vegetable

Most plants taste better when
they've had to suffer a little.

Diana Kennedy

The first farmers didn't live by cereals alone. The birth of agriculture was a package deal; as wheat, rice, corn and the other cereals were being domesticated, so too were other wild plants. Legumes (beans and peas) played an important role in farming from the start. Perhaps hunter-gatherers observed that grasses and leguminous plants were often found together in nature – take a walk through a wild habitat, a forest in the tropics or a European meadow and you'll find vetches and clover growing as part of the ecosystem. These and other legumes have a special relationship with a bacterium called rhizobium which, attracted by sugars, attaches itself to roots. In the process, it adds or 'fixes' nitrogen from the air into the soil, so helping other plants to grow as well as the legumes. Neolithic farmers might have realised the cereals they were domesticating produced more grain when grown together with leguminous plants. In the Fertile Crescent, chickpeas, lentils and fava beans were domesticated at the same time as wheat and barley. Long before Haber and Bosch invented industrial plant food, microbes and legumes were fertilising the earth.

In traditional farming systems, this same pattern, the pairing of a cereal with a legume was repeated all over the world. The milpa system of Meso-America, as we've seen, put corn with lima and pinto beans; in China, millets grew together with soybeans; in India, millets were planted with mung beans; and in Africa, sorghum went with cowpeas. As well as making soil more productive, this combination of legumes and cereals made a nutritionally richer meal, with more protein and micronutrients than would have been provided by cereal alone.

This agricultural and nutritional harmony has shaped culinary traditions around the world. The great gastronomic cultures all feature combinations of cereals and pulses. Indian *dal bhat* pairs millet with lentils; Japanese miso unites soybeans and barley; *minestra di farro*, a Tuscan stew, marries wheat (emmer) and cannellini beans; Palestinian *maftoul* mixes bulgur wheat and chickpeas; in Mexico there's *frijoles con tortilla*; and West African *waakye* combines rice and peas. There's even a modern British food version: baked beans on toast.

This natural system of growing and eating inspired Sir Albert Howard to found the organic movement. In the 1940s, while serving in India as the British government's chief botanist, he carried out field observations. 'Mixed crops are the rule,' he wrote. 'In this respect the cultivators of the Orient have followed Nature's method as seen in the primeval forest.' Elsewhere, farmers alternated their crops rather than mixing them, growing cereals one year and legumes the next, a 'rotation system' that made harvesting easier but still boosted soil fertility.

Other wild plants that grew around the margins of cereals and legumes also came to be domesticated – including many of the vegetables we eat today. In the Fertile Crescent these included artichokes, asparagus, carrots, onions, lettuce and beetroot; in the Americas, pumpkin, squashes, potatoes, peppers and tomatoes; in India, aubergines and cucumbers; and in Africa, okra. These crops helped to add nutrients to diets as well as texture, flavour and colour.

Like cereals, vegetables (a term which I'm using in the broadest culinary sense, rather than the botanical one, hence my inclusion of tubers and legumes) also diversified as they spread into different regions where they adapted to different environments and were selected by different cultures. In this way they became 'landraces', local populations of a particular crop selected over time for their ability to thrive in a specific location. These landraces were all open-pollinated (which means insects, birds, animals, the wind or human hands did the cross-pollinating) and their offspring were mostly identical to their parents; they *bred true*. The *mostly* part is important: adaptations allow a plant to continue evolving and genetic mutations create yet more diversity.

Imagine if you and I were farmers with access to the same seed. Each time you save your landrace it will further adapt to your local conditions and so you'll end up pushing it along a particular cultivated path until it looks significantly different to mine. To add even more diversity to our fields, we might swap these unique sets of landrace seeds with each other. This would have been common practice for thousands of years. As the farmer and poet Thomas Tusser described the tradition in sixteenth-century Suffolk, 'One seed for another to make an exchange; / With fellowly neighbours seemeth not strange.' However, a century after Tusser's words, the street markets of the Strand in London became home to a thriving trade in vegetable seeds supplied by local nurseries (one was on the site of the Royal Albert Hall). By the 1820s, seed merchants Messrs Sutton and Sons were publishing hundred-page seed catalogues with prices and descriptions of cabbages (145 different varieties), peas (170 varieties) and onions (74 different kinds). In the 1830s, the United States government saw it as a public duty to distribute diverse seeds 'of the choicest varieties' for free through the US Postal Service to farmers and homesteaders. In the space of two decades, the Federal government posted over a million seed packets to American farmers from a selection of 497 varieties of lettuce, 341 varieties of squash, 288 varieties of beets and 408 varieties of tomato. By the end of the twentieth century, only a tenth of that diversity had survived.

Following on from George Harrison Shull's work on corn, by the 1920s F1 hybrids of vegetable crops were being developed. For the promise of higher yields, farmers sacrificed control over seed, along with diversity in their fields. The commercial power this created over food crops transformed the seed industry. In the 1950s, most seed supply in Europe and the United States was in the hands of thousands of small businesses, usually family-owned, all assisted by publicly funded research to help improve crops. Today, more than half of the world's seed supply is in the hands of just four companies.

One of these is Corteva, formed out of a $130 billion merger in 2017 between two American giants, Dow and DuPont; another is ChemChina, a state-owned operation headquartered in Beijing, which bought the Swiss giant Syngenta for $43 billion in 2017; and then there is the German company Bayer, which took over the American business Monsanto in 2018 for $63 billion. The fourth is BASF, also based in Germany. These companies started out as chemical manufacturers that rode the wave launched by the Green Revolution, but since the 1980s have turned their attention to the seed industry, expanding quickly by buying up small seed businesses. They sell a complete 'agricultural package', not only seeds, but also the pesticides and herbicides farmers need to grow them.

Many of these seeds are patented, meaning the companies have legal control over their sale and use around the world. Genetic modification (transgenics and now gene-editing) has also resulted in greater corporate control over seed. Farmers might have cultivated a crop over thousands of years but adding or changing a single genetic trait can result in a version that is private property. More of the world's seeds – the foundation of the food system – are becoming intellectual property and highly profitable commodities.

Movements exist around the world to counter this trend and preserve open-pollinated seeds. In the early 1970s, as Jack Harlan was warning of 'the genetics of disaster', a British writer and gardener Lawrence Hills also noticed that many landrace vegetable varieties grown for centuries were quickly disappearing. The situation was made worse by new laws introduced across Europe requiring all seed varieties to be registered, an expensive process that favoured larger seed companies. This made it illegal to buy and sell many traditional landraces.

Hills wrote a letter in a national newspaper urging people to help prevent what he saw as enormous genetic and cultural loss. Readers responded in their hundreds, offering their support, and many posted him the seeds of their favourite vegetables. The collection became the Heritage Seed Library, a charity with a membership of 20,000 gardeners and allotment owners all helping to preserve and share thousands of vegetables at risk of extinction (it's illegal to buy and sell these seeds, but not to share). Many members do it to save diversity, others do it because of flavour, the reason these seeds were saved in the first place, and because of the stories the seeds encapsulate. The endangered vegetables we're about to meet are all grown from seeds that have been lost and then found.

9

Geechee Red Pea

Sapelo Island, Georgia, USA

In the American South, along a 200-mile stretch of the coast of South Carolina and Georgia, there is a scar on the Earth's surface so big it can be seen from outer space. Starting in the seventeenth century, more than 40,000 acres of land were cleared here and 780 miles of canals dug, all to produce food. This is just one mind-jolting legacy of centuries of punishing labour by enslaved people. Most motorists who travel along this part of the Lowcountry are probably unaware that what they're passing is as close as anything America has to a Great Wall of China or the Great Pyramids of Giza.

This land was cleared for rice, which grew in abundance in the eighteenth and nineteenth centuries, traded mostly through the nearby city of Charleston, then home to many of America's wealthiest farmers. Carolina Gold rice was shipped around the world. English importers described it as being the weightiest, largest and whitest rice in the habitable world, with a taste of hazelnut and a luxurious melting wholesomeness. It commanded extraordinary prices in the markets of Paris. After ripening in the Southern sun, ready for harvest, it was said to take on the lustre of an antique wedding ring. This glorious rice had a companion, a far humbler food, a tiny pea. This legume not only helped to nourish the soil on which the rice grew, but it also fed the enslaved people who laboured in the rice fields. All three – the people, the rice and the pea – came from Africa.

Between 1619 and 1860, 12.5 million enslaved Africans were transported along the Mid-Atlantic Passage to the Caribbean and the Americas. Ten and a half million survived the 4,000-mile journey and were put to work on prairies and plantations to grow tobacco, corn, sugar, cotton and rice. Most were taken from West Africa, from Senegal down to the Ivory Coast. Seeds travelled with them. Some stories suggest that the seeds – tiny enough to be hidden but important enough to risk being smuggled – were brought by the Africans themselves, concealed in their hair. A seed could be a life-saving resource on a journey into the unknown, the theory goes. Others argue that if seeds made it on board a slave ship, they would have been placed inside a hold, bounty collected by botanists and seen as potential crops for the New World and a food source for the enslaved.

'Slave traders understood that good labour depended on good health,' says the food historian Jessica Harris, and so they stocked up on supplies of cowpeas and rice at West African ports, knowing the enslaved people were more likely to accept them than other foods. 'Refusing to eat was the only control the Africans had left,' says Harris. 'It is generally believed that the slaves do best with the food of their own country,' said a close observer of the trade, a botanist called Anthony Pantaleo who travelled to Ghana in the 1780s for the British government to identify useful crops, 'every slave ship takes out a large quantity of beans as food for the slaves.' Alexander Falconbridge, a surgeon who travelled on four slave voyages, told a committee of MPs in 1785, 'The negroes were fed with beans and rice,' adding that the quantities of food provided were 'barely sufficient to support nature'.

Slave ships carried Africans to the Americas not only to put them to work on the land but also for their agricultural skills. The farming knowledge of the enslaved, and the food it produced in the New World, including rice and sugar, helped make the industrialisation of the world possible. Culinary historian Michael Twitty has made the case that white owners paid a premium for men and women from regions in West Africa where rice and peas grew. Before the invention of chemical fertiliser, knowing which pea or bean to plant where and when meant the difference between farming success and failure. The people brought from West Africa knew this.

The 4,000-year-old charred remains of a pea, *Vigna unguiculata*, have been found in rock shelters in Ghana, surrounded by fragments of pearl millet and oil palm. The pea was a food of the savannah, a plant adapted to life in the marginal dry and hot places where most other crops failed. Its value wasn't only in its high-protein seeds, but also in its bushy edible leaves, rich in vitamins and beta-carotene. Still today, in the region radiating out from that cave, millions of West Africans depend on this tiny pea species for nutrients for themselves as well as to feed the soil. Traditionally farmers intercropped them with cereals, including indigenous varieties of rice, so to European and American farmers these legumes became known as 'field peas'. Because they were fed to livestock too, the name 'cowpea' stuck.

In the parts of the New World where enslaved Africans were sent, you can find cowpeas served with rice: in Brazil, *baião de dois*; in Puerto Rico, *arroz con gandules*; in the Caribbean, *moro de guandules*; and in the American South, Hoppin' John. Every community that grew peas would have had their own prized landrace varieties (30,000 different samples of cowpea are held in seed banks around the world, most about half a centimetre long, and they come in a kaleidoscope of colours, from earthy browns to vibrant purples).

After cowpeas arrived in the American South and were taken up by plant breeders, the legumes became essential ingredients in farming and food. Their various names hint at their different uses. The no-nonsense-sounding iron pea and clay pea were soil improvers while the more refined lady pea was, according to a nineteenth-century plant breeder, J.V. Jones, 'a delicious table pea'. Black-eyed peas, Jones claimed, were so chalky they were 'more valuable for stock making'. Lists of these Lowcountry peas go on and on. People grew to know their late locust from a flint crowder, and a relief from a shinney (the prince of peas, according to Jones).

By the 1830s, rice, corn and cotton had been cultivated so intensely that Southern soils had become exhausted. An agricultural crisis loomed, and experts called for a concerted effort to rebuild the soil before it became so depleted that economic collapse would be inevitable. The solution was to plant more cowpeas and practise crop rotation; with their nitrogen-fixing powers, peas put back the fertility lost from intensive farming. And so, African peas combined with rice grown in the Carolinas became the cornerstone of Southern cooking and continues to be so to the present day. Rice and peas cut across all barriers, social, economic and racial. 'If you were poor you would have had a breakfast of rice and peas,' explains heritage grain expert Glenn Roberts, recalling a saying from his childhood in the South, 'and then when you came home after working in the fields, you had a brand-new meal: peas and rice.'

While rice farming was booming in the nineteenth century, some rarer landrace peas were cultivated by enslaved Africans in secret gardens which contained forbidden food, such as varieties of African red rice, beloved by the enslaved but deemed a threat by slave owners who saw them as a potential contaminant of their fields of lucrative white rice. In these gardens, Africans also grew varieties of sweet potato, benne (sesame), kale, okra, collards, watermelon and sorghum, which had all somehow found their way from Africa into the American Lowcountry. Always in these secret gardens, without exception, were cowpeas. But there were parts of the South where the enslaved didn't need to hide their crops away. On an isolated Sea Island off the coast of Georgia called Sapelo, Africans had more freedom and were allowed to grow their own crops. There, unique landrace plants evolved, including sugar cane and citrus, but perhaps the most remarkable of all a tiny, red-brick-coloured pea.

Seen from a map, the south-eastern coast of the USA looks as if it's crumbling away into small pieces. Here, splinters of land, around a hundred in total, form a chain of islands. Over thousands of years they have been home to different cultures: indigenous Native Americans; French colonists; American plantation owners; and enslaved Africans, followed by their freed descendants. Three hundred years ago, some of these Sea Islands were points of arrival and of quarantine for slave ships from Africa. Some of the enslaved men and women stayed on these islands which, surrounded by swamp and marshland, were rich breeding grounds for insects and disease. The harsh conditions and relative isolation of the Sea Islands perhaps explain why the Africans here had more autonomy over their food than enslaved people in other parts of the South. The tiny red cowpea they grew became an essential ingredient for people forced to work from sunrise to sunset. The pea was cooked long and slow in cast-iron pots and turned into a gravy which was served up with local rice. Constant cooking of this gravy, day after day, year after year, stained red rings onto the insides of metal pots (markings that can still be seen on now antique plantation cookware).

The descendants of the enslaved Africans of Sapelo (as well as other Sea Islands and parts of the Lowcountry), describe themselves as Geechee. It's likely the name is derived from the Kissi (pronounced Geezee) tribe in West Africa. Sapelo is still remote; unlike neighbouring

islands with bridges to the mainland, you can only get there by boat
or aircraft. This is why the community has retained uniquely strong
links to its West African roots. The way some people on Sapelo speak,
how they cook and the way they dance have closer cultural connections to Sierra Leone, Ghana and Senegal than to African American
culture on the US mainland.

The Geechee of Sapelo were among the first freed slaves to purchase
land and set up autonomous communities. This led to the preservation
of African foodways and farming practices, including the planting of
the Geechee red pea which has continued to this day. The survival of
that pea in recent years is thanks in part to one woman, Cornelia
Walker Bailey.

Her family had always grown the red peas, and for much of her
life Bailey thought nothing of it. She and her husband Frank sowed
the seeds early in spring (to a growing moon, she said) and harvested
them during the summer. Her life seemed to run to the rhythm
of the pea, from the saving of its seed in the autumn, to the big get-
togethers when the islanders would cook up pots of red pea gravy
and rice, a must on New Year's Day. The pea carried a lot of history,
and pain, but it also spoke of being Geechee.

In the last few decades, things around Sapelo have changed quickly.
In the 1950s, developers began to buy up land on the other Sea Islands,
attracted by their pristine white beaches and dense forests. Then
interest turned to Sapelo. As plot after plot on the island was bought
up by outsiders, the last of the Geechee retreated to Hog Hammock,
a part of Sapelo that became something of a refuge. But even here
house sales to the wealthy sent property taxes higher, pushing the
African descendants out. In 1910, five hundred Geechee people lived
in Hog Hammock, by 2020 there were no more than forty. As their
numbers kept dropping, Bailey feared for the survival of her people.
Cultural genocide she called it.

Bailey began to see the red pea as a means of saving Geechee
culture. People who left the island always asked to be sent supplies,
and it grew so easily on Sapelo, maybe it could generate an income
and so help Hog Hammock remain a place for Geechee people. In
2012 Bailey began planting the crop, helped by her sons, Maurice and
Stanley. It was touch and go; supplies of the seed were so low that

one summer when a drought hit the island, they had to go door to door asking people if they had some red peas stored away for safe-keeping. But the crop started to grow, and word spread to African American farmers interested in finding out more about their food history.

One of these was Matthew Raiford, a farmer on the mainland. His great-great-great-grandfather Jupiter Gilliard was born into slavery in 1812 in South Carolina and became a landowner in 1874, buying 476 acres of farmland for $9 and taxes in Brunswick, Georgia, just north of Sapelo. As a young man, Raiford wanted nothing to do with the South and most definitely not its soil. In the years after the civil rights era, the message had been loud and clear: 'Don't be a farmer, become a doctor or a lawyer instead,' he says. Farming was tough and, for some, working on the land was too bound up with the history of slavery. In 1910, African Americans made up about 14 per cent of America's farmers; today that figure is less than 2 per cent.

Raiford joined the military and then worked as a chef, but in the 1990s his grandmother persuaded him to return to the family farm. One day, he came across the story of Cornelia Bailey. He remembered his grandparents had grown a red pea and so he made the journey to Sapelo Island to meet 'Miss Bailey'. Walking onto the island was like going back in time, he says. People spoke in Geechee dialect and used expressions his grandmother used, like the midday sun feeling 'hotter than fish grease'. Bailey was working a hoe on an acre of peas when he found her. 'And I'm looking at her thinking, is it really that easy?' he says. 'Baby, this pea don't need no fuss,' she told him, 'the pea knows what it wants to do, all you've got to do is break the soil, drop in a pea, cover it and give it some water, it'll grow.' She was right. The plant is tough, and it now grows on Raiford's family farm near Brunswick.

Someone else who came from the mainland to help bring back Sapelo's red pea was Nik Heynen, a professor of geography at the University of Georgia who was converted to farming by Cornelia Bailey, 'one of the most important people in my life'. When Bailey died in 2017, still hoping the pea was going to save Geechee culture, Heynen worked with her children to keep the crop growing. 'If we lose the pea, we lose a variety of something that helps us understand the world,' he says. The pea tastes different to anything else, not a thousand times better than anything else, just different, and because he helps to grow it on Sapelo, for him the pea comes from an emotional landscape as much as a physical one. 'The tiny red pea is infused with so much history and culture,' Heynen says. Which is why he can't imagine letting it go extinct.

10

Alb Lentil

Swabia, Germany

The mountains, valleys and caves of the Swabian Jura in south-western Germany have a special place in human history. Here, on the eve of war in 1939, two archaeologists found hundreds of broken pieces of mammoth ivory in the inner chamber of a cave. When these were finally pieced together in 1969, they formed a 30cm tall figure of a powerfully built man with the head of a lion. The carving was at least 40,000 years old, which makes the Löwenmensch figure of the Stadel cave the oldest known depiction of an imagined being. In caves nearby, ancient musical instruments were discovered – carved hollow wing bones of swans and vultures punctured with holes along one side. The hunter-gatherers who made these objects were among the first modern humans to reach Europe, to coexist with Neanderthals and then to replace them. Thirty thousand years later, when seeds of plants domesticated in the Fertile Crescent were carried across the Balkans and along the Danube, farming got underway in the Swabian Jura (also known as the Swabian Alb or Alps). Among the crops they grew were einkorn, emmer and barley (the ancient cereals we met earlier) and lentils.

Over thousands of years, lentils growing here evolved into a landrace known as the *Alb-linse* (or Alp lentil). Swabian farmers planted this legume in fields mixed among the cereals. The small, bushy plants, just 40cm tall, were supported by taller stalks of wheat and barley and in return the lentils fertilised the soil for the cereal. This tiny legume adapted to everything the Alps could throw at it. In thin and rocky soils it grew where nothing else could, and in bad years where there was little else to harvest, it could always be depended on. Settlements within the Alps were often cut off by snow and ice, so the lentil proved to be a lifeline. But life was so tough in the eighteenth and nineteenth centuries, thousands of people left the Swabian Alps in search of better (and possibly easier) lives in the New World.

The Swabian Jura remains one of the most isolated parts of Central Europe. Among Germans, the Swabians are known for their fierce work ethic and for being innovators (Daimler and Mercedes-Benz originated in Swabia). The people also have a strong sense of identity, and their own language. As one Swabian saying goes: '*Wir können alles. Außer Hochdeutsch.*' ('We can do everything. Except speak proper German.') For centuries, that identity also included food. The crops Swabian farmers harvested provided the ingredients for the 'national dish' of *Linsen mit Spätzle*, the dark green landrace lentils served with wheat noodles. During more affluent times, and in prosperous homes, sausage was added. The unique Swabian lentil was much loved for its thick, creamy texture and its deeply satisfying mineral flavour. But in the 1960s, it went extinct.

One reason for this was economic. The manufacturing boom in 1960s West Germany pulled people off the land and into factories. The second reason was global changes to farming. India had been the world's biggest grower of lentils, but when Borlaug's Green Revolution wheat arrived it replaced other crops and sent lentil cultivation into decline. At the same time, farmers in the Canadian province of Saskatchewan started to experiment with growing lentils.

To begin with, lentils were seen as a cheap way of fertilising their soil, but by developing their own high-yielding variety, the crop became a serious commercial opportunity. Within a few years, millions of hectares of prairie had been cleared and planted with monocultures of green and red lentils. Today, Canada produces more lentils than India and America (the world's other main producers) combined. When these lentils were exported around the world, farmers growing local landrace varieties couldn't compete. Why bother, when you could cook up a dish of *Linsen mit Spätzle* with cheaper lentils imported from across the Atlantic? The *Alb-linse* which had evolved in the mountains over thousands of years was suddenly gone.

The extinction of the Swabian lentil played on the mind of one Swabian farmer, Woldemar (Wolde) Mammel. The *Alb-linse*, he believed, was more than just a lentil. He saw it as part of a much bigger system, which offered self-sufficiency and had helped create a distinctive way of life. In the early 1990s, Mammel decided he would bring the landrace lentil back. But it had been decades since any farmer had planted it, and no one had saved any seeds. Neighbours told him the rescue mission was the craziest idea they'd ever heard.

Mammel started looking at lentils most similar to the *Alb-linse,* including in the Puy region of south-central France, home of the famous green-marbled, peppery lentils. They were good, but they didn't have the taste people remembered, and they didn't grow so well in the mountains. For ten years, he searched in the attics of old farmhouses and in barns, hoping he might come across a seed or two in the cracks and gaps of rafters and floorboards. He contacted seed banks in Germany, USDA's seed library in Colorado, the Vavilov Institute in St Petersburg, and the keepers of the world's biggest collection of lentil seeds in Syria. But no one had even heard of, let alone seen a sample of, the *Alb-linse.*

In 2007, Mammel and a small group of Swabian farmers travelled to Russia to look through the records of the Vavilov Institute, thinking that at least they might have other landrace varieties they could grow in the Alps. As Mammel thumbed through the records with one of the curators, one index card stood out. For a decade three letters and a filing error had stood in his way: the lentils had been listed as *Alpen-linse* instead of *Alb-linse.* The Russians couldn't understand why the famers were so excited about this one lentil, there were thousands of different varieties stored away. It was the only one they cared about, Mammel explained, because it was the variety that had been part of their history. Back home, he used the seeds from the Vavilov collection to grow a crop of lentils, the seeds of which he shared with other like-minded farmers. Mammel had succeeded in bringing back one of the thousands of unique lentils once grown across Europe, now mostly lost.

Hunter-gatherers would have collected wild lentils from stringy bushes that twisted and climbed their way around other plants. In the wild, legumes have pods that open explosively, flinging their seeds far away (in some leguminous trees with large pods, these explosions sound like firecrackers). A gene mutation left the seeds stuck in the pods of some lentils (the equivalent of the mutation in wheat that led to non-shattering grains), making harvesting easier. This transition can be

seen in the contents of a cave in southern Greece excavated in the
1960s. The Franchti cave plots changes to food and farming over 30,000
years as different groups came and went. The earliest people to shelter
beneath the rock were hunter-gatherers. They left the bones of wild
pig and ibex in the archaeological record. By around 13,000 years ago,
wild lentils start to appear, along with wild almonds and wild pistachios. Then, 7,000 years ago, there is evidence of farming in terraces
built near the opening of the cave to grow oats and wheat, mixed
together with (by now) domesticated lentils. Lentils spread around
Europe, both as a source of food and a means of fertilising soil.
Thousands of landrace varieties evolved, among them the *Alb-linse* of
Swabia.

We know about these landrace varieties, even the extinct ones,
because of work done in the 1930s by the Russian botanist Elena
Barulina. After growing up in the port city of Saratov on the River
Volga, she moved to St Petersburg where she spent decades sifting
through thousands of lentil seeds collected from different parts of the
world. She was racing against time to catalogue diversity because the
arrival of chemical fertilisers was seeing the crop fall into decline
across the industrialised world. As fast as Barulina could record
Europe's landrace varieties, they were disappearing. Nearly a century
on, her research, set out in a 319-page monograph, has remained the
standard work on the legume that helped shape the modern world.
Her name should be better known, as should the man who helped
collect many of the seeds she studied: Barulina's husband was Nikolai
Vavilov.

When Vavilov was imprisoned by Stalin in 1940, Barulina fought
for his release and sent him food parcels. These packages never arrived.
Vavilov, as we know, died of starvation in a Soviet jail in 1943, and his
wife and son spent years living in poverty. In 1955, after her husband's
reputation had been restored, Barulina began sorting through the huge
collection of unpublished papers Vavilov had left behind about his
seed-collecting expeditions. But she died in 1957 before she was able
to complete her work.

Barulina's catalogue of landrace lentils, together with the example
set by Woldemar Mammel in the Swabian Alps, have inspired other
communities across Europe to bring back their own lost legumes,
and a lentil movement now exists. A Swedish farmer called Tomas

Erlandsson has revived beans, peas and lentils that were extinct on the island of Gotland, among them the *Gotlandslinsen*. This 'blonde' lentil had adapted to Gotland's alkaline soil and cool temperatures. Books handwritten by monks on the island in the Middle Ages make reference to the *Gotlandslinsen*. For centuries it was used to make stews and turned into flour for flatbreads. By the 1960s, it was gone. It was seen as '"poor man's" food,' says Erlandsson. After some detective work, he found two elderly farmers on the island who still had seeds. 'What I found was remarkable. The lentils taste amazing.'

The story of Swabia's *Alb-linse* also reached a team of researchers based on the east coast of England. In 2008, Josiah Meldrum, Nick Saltmarsh and William Hudson were trying to design a new food system for cities, one that would be more climate-resilient and less destructive to the environment. They quickly realised that pulses (the seeds of leguminous plants) would be crucial to making any new system work, needing few, if any, resources to grow and being great for soil as well as highly nutritious. After hearing about the work in Swabia, they looked at what had been grown in Britain, and found that all the way back to the Iron Age, pulses were an indispensable crop, even featuring in the first English recipe book, *The Forme of Cury*, written in Old English in 1390. 'Take benes and seeþ hem almost til þey bersten' were part of the instructions for benes yfryed. Among the poems by Thomas Tusser they found, from 1570, 'A Hundreth Good Pointes of Husbandrie', a set of planting instruction for farmers: 'In Feueryer [February], rest not for taking thine ease: / get into the grounde with thy beanes, and thy pease.' Fava beans and lentils were important staples in Britain for at least 3,000 years, but as people began eating more meat and dairy, pulses were considered inferior foods. Rhymes even captured the monotony of poverty and pulses – 'Pease porridge hot, pease porridge cold, / Pease porridge in the pot, nine days old.' Where ancient crops such as fava beans continued to be grown in the UK, they were fed to animals or exported overseas. In 2012, Meldrum and his friends set up a business called Hodmedod (an old East Anglian word for something round or curled up, such as the climbing vine of a legume). Award-winning and successful, it has brought pulse-growing back to Britain, including lentils.

*

Woldemar Mammel's way of getting his fellow Swabians to join his mission was to ask them to eat the lentil, telling them, 'It tastes and feels like nothing else.' He also taught farmers to intercrop the lentils among wheat and barley which feeds the soil. The final touch was a machine, designed and built by Mammel, that separates the lentils from the other grains, making harvesting much easier. One hundred and forty Swabian farmers now grow the lentil, and demand for the *Alb-linse* outstrips supply. Proof that it is possible to bring a food back from extinction.

II

Oca

Andes, Bolivia

'Can you see the foetus?' my companion Loritano shouted, pointing to a small gap at the top of a boulder. We were 3,000 metres up a mountain in search of a sacred stone. Among cactus, bushes of Andean mint and tall, spiky bromeliads, a skeleton about the size of a pet cat was perched inside a crevice of rock, its head and spine just visible. It looked as if an animal had slowly shrivelled away in the heat. The llama foetus was an offering, explained Loritano, and the ten-metre-high rock was part of a network of giant stones that led towards a temple higher up the mountain. The baby llama was going to help make this year's harvest a good one.

We were in the Cordillera Apolobamba mountain range where Bolivia borders Peru. The villages here are mostly inhabited by indigenous Aymara and Quechua people. It had been snowing and the only movement around us were the alpacas grazing on the edges of mud tracks. Beyond the stones were ice-capped mountains, their peaks 6,000 metres high. At this altitude, even on the sunniest days, it can be bitterly cold.

Loritano is a Kallawaya, one of a dwindling group of shamans who have practised traditional medicine in the Andes for 2,000 years. Originally a distinct ethnic group that occupied the northern shore of Lake Titicaca with their own language (now extinct), today they're dispersed in villages across the Andes. Their role as healers has continued and, over the centuries, plants used by the Kallawaya have been absorbed into Western medicine, including coca. Whereas the Kallawaya used the leaves of this plant to treat dysentery and headaches, European doctors in the nineteenth century extracted the alkaloid – cocaine – to make anaesthetic. Another medicine that was widely adopted was the dried bark of the cinchona tree utilised by the

Kallawaya for more than a thousand years as a treatment for malaria, and then put to the same purpose across the British Empire (quinine is a compound found in the bark). In the 1890s, when workers on the Panama Canal began dying from malaria and yellow fever, Kallawaya healers travelled thousands of miles to provide treatment. But by the 1930s, with the arrival of physicians from the West, the Kallawaya were being branded as 'witch doctors'.

Loritano, in his early thirties, is one of the last of the Kallawaya. He inherited his knowledge and powers from his father, also a Kallawaya. 'The birthmark on my face was a sign,' he says. 'Among my brothers, I was the chosen one.' His role as a shaman goes far beyond providing plant knowledge and being a living pharmacopoeia; the Kallawaya are also the chief communicators with the most important entity of all, Pachamama, or Mother Earth. In the Andean cosmology, an illness or a poor harvest might be caused by a disturbance in the relationship between humans and nature. Farmers call upon the Kallawaya to avoid this happening.

Loritano was dressed in a poncho woven from alpaca wool, in bright red, green and yellow stripes. As we talked, his right hand frequently disappeared into a *chuspa* hanging from his neck to pluck out dried coca leaves which he chewed in the side of his mouth. At the sacred stone, he took six of the leaves and placed them at the base of the rock, followed by a sprinkle of liquid from a bottle. This was powerful Andean moonshine, a spirit made from potato. With the gifts for Pachamama now in place, Loritano was ready to pray. 'This way, food will come.'

As I watched him in this world of snow and rock, 3,000 metres up the mountain, I realised why farmers still looked to the Kallawaya for blessings. This is one of the highest, coldest, toughest places on Earth to live, and somehow humans have managed to survive here for thousands of years. Throughout this history, the Kallawaya, with hundreds of wild medicinal plants at their disposal and botanical knowledge passed down through generations, helped make that existence possible.

From the rock, Loritano and I crossed stepping stones over a fast-flowing river and entered a plateau. Ancient stone terraces stretched up the mountainside like a staircase made for giants. Growing beneath our feet was another essential element of life in the Andes – one of the plant kingdom's ultimate survival foods: tubers. Ornate stone walls held each section of soil in place, an ingenious design which made farming viable in an otherwise impossible landscape. With a stick, Loritano dug into the earth beneath a small-leaved green plant and eased out a potato.

Early humans wouldn't have been able to just dig up potatoes and cook them for food; first they had to deal with the toxic compounds that made these wild plants inedible. The plant is a member of the deadly nightshade family and its toxins act as a defence against attacks from harmful organisms, including fungi, bacteria and hungry animals. Even cooking fails to break down these chemical defences. An ancient fix for this was to make a 'gravy' of clay and water, the tiny mineral particles of which extracted the poison (some varieties of Andean potato are still sold with small packets of soil). Over thousands of years of domestication, farmers not only dealt with the problem of toxins, they also selected tubers that were bigger, tastier and more nutritious.

Loritano then dug out a different-looking tuber, coloured bright yellow, bumpy and bullet-shaped. This was an oca. The terraces around us, and all the different tubers that filled them, had supported pre-Columbian civilisations for millennia, from the Chiripa and the Tiwanaku through to the Inca Empire in the thirteenth century. Nowhere else in the world at this altitude, not even in Tibet or Nepal, has farming been so successful or sustained populations as dense as those in the Andes.

Whereas roots anchor plants in soil and supply them with nutrients and water, tubers are more like underground energy banks. These storage organs can be called upon during times of stress, when temperatures fall and rains don't come. What evolved as a means of survival for plants, a package of carbohydrate, calcium and vitamin C, in turn became a means of survival for humans. Protected beneath the soil, tubers can provide food when other crops fail. They can also be treated as a living food depository, happy to be left underground for more than a year and dug up in times of need. During conflicts, when grain stores might be at risk of being seized by enemies, tubers are safely hidden. The Hadza wouldn't be able to survive without *ekwa* and *do'aiko*, the tubers they dig up from the African savannah; and the same could be said of the Aboriginal people and murnong in pre-colonial Australia.

With the Columbian Exchange, potatoes made it to the Old World, a crop that, per acre, provided four times as many calories as wheat or barley and which went on to feed millions of Europeans. Without the potato, it's questionable whether industrialisation on the Continent or imperial expansion from there would have been possible.

This world-changing tuber was domesticated in the Andes 7,000 years ago. This is the centre of diversity for the potato, its birthplace if you like, and that of many other tubers too (including *mashwa*, *papalisa* and oca). No population anywhere in the world has as many diverse tubers as the people of the Andes. There are 4,000 Andean varieties of potato alone, which are grown in rotation with beans and corn. This diversity was created in many tiny settlements across the Andes, where each tuber adapted to a particular altitude, microclimate and soil. All share that same package of nutrients: carbohydrate, calcium and vitamin C. Most of us alive today have a reason to thank the hunter-gatherers who started that domestication process because, after wheat, rice and corn, the potato became the fourth most consumed crop in the world.

As a double insurance policy, people in the Andes developed a special technique for turning potatoes into a food that could be stored for years: *chuño* and *tunta*. Resembling smooth, small pebbles, these are potatoes preserved in the cold of the altiplano. On the high plateau there are three hundred nights of frost per year, and when the temperature falls below −5°C, farmers arrive here with thousands of small round potatoes they've grown. These are spread across the landscape, making it look as if a beach has been created in the middle of the mountains. This is the first stage in making *chuño* and *tunta*. After the sun sets, the potatoes begin to freeze which draws water out of them. As the sun rises, the tubers thaw and more moisture evaporates. Families watch over this vast potato carpet as the daily cycle of freezing and thawing gradually dries the potatoes. During the day, they brave the cold to walk across the tubers, pressing out every last drop of moisture with their bare feet. When fully dehydrated, the now dark-coloured *chuño* can be stored away for years. When they're needed, they can be turned into flour or rehydrated in stews, where they take on the look and texture of gnocchi, the Italian potato dumplings. The white-coloured version, *tunta*, involves an even more arduous stage in which the potatoes are stored in water-filled pits dug into the earth. Weighed down with stones and packed with hay (made from a tough grass called *pajabrava*), they're left for a month before they join the *chuño* potatoes in the freeze-drying process.

This technique is at least 3,000 years old and was used by the Tiwanaku, one of the early farming civilisations that flourished across present-day Bolivia, Chile and Peru, all with the help of preserved tubers (meat jerky, or *ch'arki* in the Quechua language, was preserved in a similar way). Warehouses filled with *chuño* made it possible for the Incas in the fifteenth century to feed large populations even in the highest outposts of the Andes (as well as the one million people who lived around Lake Titicaca). But white-coloured *tunta* remained a prestigious food: like white rice and white flour in other cultures, this more refined version was reserved for the elite.

Even after the Inca Empire fell, *chuño* endured. 'Many Spaniards have enriched themselves ... merely by taking these chunus to sell at the mines,' wrote a conquistador, Pedro Cieza de León, in 1590, adding, 'They have another food called oca which is also profitable.' Around the same time, a Jesuit missionary, José de Acosta, described how mine owners protested over the price being demanded for the *chuño* they needed to feed their workers. These dehydrated tubers not only made Andean survival possible, they also sustained empires and created fortunes.

But my main interest was in the second tuber Loritano had found, the oca, which was domesticated further north. In the Guitarrero Cave in Peru's central highlands, pieces of charcoal, wood and tiny fragments of textiles 10,000 years old had been preserved, along with plant and animal remains. In the 1960s, when archaeologists dug deep through the strata, they excavated one ancient diet after another. Cobs of corn, bean pods, chilli and seeds of the tomato's wild relative all showed up, but among the few foods that appeared in all the layers, from the oldest to the most recent, was oca.

Oca (called *khaya* in Quechua) hasn't travelled the world like the potato, but in parts of the Andes it's just as cherished. It is hardy, it can tolerate sub-zero temperatures, it is highly disease-resistant, it can grow in poor soils and it is perfectly in tune with the extreme diurnal conditions in the Andes (summer by day, winter by night). It's so perfectly adapted in fact that it struggles when it's too far away from here. The plant produces edible tubers when temperatures are cool but not too cold, and the days are short and nights long (tuber production is triggered by darkness). Few other places – New Zealand being one exception – match these exact conditions for large scale cultivation. This is why varieties of the more adaptable potato became the world's favourite tuber. But just like the potato, there are hundreds, possibly thousands, of varieties of oca across the Andes (oca's lower global status means it hasn't been as deeply researched).

When you travel through the Andes, you see the spectacular diversity of oca in vibrant colours (chalky white, yellow, red, purple and black) with flavours that range from aggressively tangy to addictively sweet. Oca contains a complex compound, oxalic acid, part of the plant's defence mechanism against pests and diseases. High levels of this acid make some oca varieties so astringent they're impossible to eat until they have been left in sunlight for a week, allowing sugars to build up which counter the acidity. Only then are they ready to be boiled, baked or fried, giving out an intensely nutty sweet-potato flavour.

As with *chuño* and *tunta*, it was preserved oca that became an essential food of the Andes. To see it being preserved, I said goodbye to Loritano and headed higher up the Andes to one of the historic Incan outposts, a small village 4,000 metres up the Apolobamba mountain range. Ayllu Agua Blanca is home to one hundred families who, for several months of the year, live surrounded by frost and fog. Dried *khaya*, the oca equivalent of *chuño* and *tunta*, is their daily bread here.

I followed a group of Quechua women from the village up a mountain path towards their fields. The altitude made it a struggle for me to keep up as they marched ahead. They were dressed in the traditional *cholita* outfit: heavy, multi-layered petticoats, blue skirts, dark brown bowler hats (the *borsalino*) and beautiful woven red and yellow shawls. It didn't look like an outfit designed for climbing mountains or for farming tubers, but they made it look effortless. The villagers plant tubers in fields and terraces spread around the valley. This might seem impractical, what with all the climbing and walking involved in getting from one plot to another. But this way they can spread risk; if frost or disease hits one field, they can fall back on another at a different altitude and soil. They also plant different crops each year, including oca, *papalisa* tubers, beans and quinoa. Across the community this adds up to a collection of hundreds of different varieties. 'Rotation is important,' one of the women said. 'The soil needs to rest.'

At one of the fields, they harvested sacks of oca which they then carried on their backs to the Pelechuco River, a forty-minute hike. The riverbank looked as if it had been bombed; several metre-wide holes pitted the earth, each one dug so close to the other you needed to tiptoe along their narrow ridges to avoid falling in. Each of the pits was filled with water, hay and handfuls of *muna* (Andean mint). The sack of oca was lowered in and weighed down by stones where it would be left for at least a month. Over the loud rush of the Pelechuco, one of the women, Vasillia, lifted out some of the rocks, reached her arm into the cold water of the pit and pulled up one of the older sacks. Pinching a tuber that was losing its skin, she shook her head. 'Not yet,' she said, 'another week.' It needed to be soft and feel like a sponge. By then, the sourness of the acid would have leached away.

From here, the oca that are ready are taken further up the mountain and spread out across the ground like *chuño* on the altiplano. For around a week, the oca goes through the cycle of freezing and thawing. 'When they start to look as if they are rotten, we press them,' Vasillia explained. And so, on the freezing mountainside, they walk barefoot to force out the last of the moisture. When they are dry, flat and dark in colour, the tubers are taken to the village.

Inside a small kitchen, the women took pieces of dried oca – like charred pieces of blackened wood – and ground them down to make a dough. A strong, sweet smell of farmyard (a legacy of the fermented hay placed inside the pits) hung in the air as salt, herbs and sugar were added to the dough which was then moulded into mini-burger-sized pieces. Fried in corn oil, they became hard chewy discs that tasted part treacle, part liquorice and part barnyard.

On the day I left the Apolobamba, the village held an *atapi*, a communal meal that brought all of the surrounding villages together. Some had walked for miles so they could swap news and share food. Spread over blankets were the various tubers the communities had brought with them; fifty or sixty types of oca, *chuño*, *tunta* and native potatoes of different shapes, sizes and colours. Each tuber was adapted to its village, some higher up the mountain, some lower, making the feast a celebration of diversity.

There are people who have dedicated their working lives to understanding this diversity. Among them is Eve Emshwiller, an American botanist, who has spent nearly thirty years travelling through the Andes, much of that time trying to find forgotten and endangered varieties of oca, helping the Peruvian and Bolivian governments conserve oca's diversity. As a student in the 1970s, she took an interest in the music and language of the Quechua people, but by the 1990s had turned her attention to their food, focusing in the end on the little-studied oca. Today, she's considered the world expert on this tuber. In most of the villages she has visited over the years, both in Bolivia and Peru, farmers have been growing a range of different oca, including varieties found nowhere else. But with each new research trip, she notices the same thing: fewer and fewer people are growing oca. Some farmers have said this is because their oca crop had been attacked by pests. 'They told me the climate was changing and their crops had been destroyed.' In other places she was told that all of the young people had gone to find work in the cities and that no one was left to grow food. In the first decade of this century alone, one-third of Bolivia's entire population migrated from rural areas and into cities. El Alto, adjacent to La Paz, has tripled in size to 900,000 inhabitants in just over two decades. As a result, the villages are being emptied.

On one expedition to a village in Northern Peru famous for its oca, she barely saw any oca being grown or eaten. She and the conservationists she was with asked around, trying to find an explanation, but the scarcity of oca remained a mystery. On their journey home, they pulled in at a fuel stop and started a conversation with a truck driver who was transporting potatoes to the city nearby. These were called *yungay*, he said, a big, yellow variety of frying potato that had become really popular in the city. As the city became more populated, wholesalers needed to increase supply of the potato and so the driver found a job going from village to village handing out seed potatoes. The unintended consequence was that the Andean farmers were abandoning traditional varieties of tubers and, on large plots, growing the yellow potato instead. Whatever they grew, the truck driver promised to buy. And so, the farmers became *yungay* growers.

Across the Andes, Emshwiller has seen other farmers abandon rotation systems for monocultures in which they attempt to grow the same crop on the same land year after year. This usually results in them using more pesticides and, as the soil becomes exhausted, they have to bring in fertilisers. In this way, they had lost not only ancient varieties of oca, but also the complex system that had given them self-sufficiency. Many just give up and leave for the shanty towns on the outskirts of cities. Working alongside government agronomists, Emshwiller is collecting every variety of oca she can find, helping to safeguard oca diversity in the Andes for future generations.

Andean communities need food and farming resilience more than ever. Weather patterns are becoming more erratic, communities are being affected by intense droughts, floods and frosts, temperatures are warming, and ice is melting causing glaciers to retreat and disappear (and with them, ancient supplies of water used for irrigation and to supply cities such as La Paz). Even making *chuño* and preserving oca has become more erratic as the frosts don't appear as regularly as before. Warmer temperatures are also taking crop diseases to ever greater altitudes, forcing farmers to climb higher in search of safe, fungus-free soil. Many plants won't be able to adapt to such rapidly changing conditions and the increasing range of pests and diseases, but some can. This is why saving diversity across the Andes, and supporting farmers there, is so important.

'The Andes are like a living laboratory for understanding climate change,' says Stef de Haan, senior scientist at the International Potato Center (CIP), a research station over the border in Lima where 4,600 different Andean tubers are being preserved. Some of these might possess traits needed in future, but more are likely to exist in the thousands of remote communities where landrace varieties are still being grown and are continuing to adapt. This idea led to the founding of the Parque de la Papa, or Potato Park, in Cusco's Sacred Valley, close to the Peruvian–Bolivian border. Six thousand indigenous people live in this sprawling reserve, conceived as a way of saving cultural identity, medicinal plants and farming knowledge, as well as many varieties of tuber. In 2017, 650 of these varieties were sent from the Potato Park to Svalbard as backup.

The science behind saving this kind of diversity is becoming clearer. In 2011, scientists mapped the genome of potato and oca, which helped explain why some tubers are more prone to disease than others – and why the blight that caused the Irish potato famine was so devastating.

This genome is helping to identify resistance to that blight, which is still wreaking havoc around the world, ruining crops and threatening global food security. Research is pointing to rare landrace varieties of tubers, including oca, as a source of resistant genes, as well as wild relatives of oca (found growing in Bolivia's cloud forests, the birthplace of the tuber). The more diversity we can preserve the better, not only for communities in the Andes, but also for farmers across the globe. 'We overlook this at our peril,' says de Haan. 'Andean farmers are the guardians of a genetic resource for the world.'

12

O-Higu Soybean

Okinawa, Japan

One thousand miles to the south of the Japanese mainland, right in the centre of the Pacific island of Okinawa, Kenichi Kariki, a slight man in his early seventies, tends what might be the world's smallest plot of soybeans. On this one-metre by five-metre clearing surrounded by a tropical wilderness, Kariki is attempting to bring back one of Japan's rarest varieties of soy. Rare soy? How can that be? Newspaper headlines remind us of the problems caused by too much soy growing. Deforestation in Brazil's Cerrado, the Yungas 'cloud forest' of Argentina and Bolivia's Gran Chaco is most often blamed on the rise and rise of *Glycine max*, the small, yellow, oval bean we call soy, a legume so packed with protein it's the number one ingredient for most of the chicken and pig feed on the planet. In 2020, demand for the global crop grew at its fastest rate in years.

But Kenichi Kariki's bean is rare. So rare that even though he's been growing it for three years, he hasn't dared to eat a single bean. One day he hopes to have enough seed to share with farmers and bring the bean back for good. And so he saves each one, as if each tiny bean were a precious artefact, which in Kariki's eyes it is.

Before Okinawa was turned into a Japanese prefecture in the 1870s, it had been an independent state, the Ryuku kingdom, for centuries, with its own emperors, dynasties, language, culture, religion and soybean. This landrace soy was called the O-Higu, and it's the one Kenichi Kariki is trying to grow. What Kavilca wheat had meant to people in eastern Turkey, or the *Alb-linse* to the inhabitants of the Swabian Alps, the O-Higu was to people on the island of Okinawa: survival, identity and self-sufficiency. Since the fourteenth century, farmers would plant the bean in the spring, at the first sight of the cherry blossom. O-Higu grew faster than other varieties of soy, which meant that by the time the rainy season arrived, the beans could withstand their biggest threat, the insects brought by the hotter, humid weather. So farmers saved and passed on its seeds.

The origins of soy lie in northern China where, 6,000 years ago, farmers began domesticating the plant. Three and a half thousand years ago, during the Shang dynasty, the bean first appears in written records as fodder for animals and as an ingredient in porridges for humans. Even after hours of cooking, the legume has a tough outer layer and an intense bitter taste. Early converts to soy overcame this problem through fermentation, allowing bacteria to break the bean down. First came a basic condiment called *jiang* which, with the addition of salt, rice or barley, evolved into miso. But the real masterstroke that turned soybeans into the equivalent of 'daily bread' for many Asian cultures was the invention of tofu, an almost miraculous seeming transformation of bitter beans into white blocks of tasty food. A mural inside a 2,000-year-old tomb in Henan Province, central China, depicts the steps in tofu making: first, making a 'milk' by cooking the beans, then coagulating the liquid by adding sea salt and, when it's sufficiently thick and silky, pressing it into blocks. The expansion of Buddhism and its vegetarian principles out of China into other parts of Asia also spread soybeans and tofu. In the twelfth century, Japanese Shinto priests were placing tofu offerings at holy shrines. By this time, soybeans had arrived on Okinawa.

The Ryuku kings governed from the magnificent red-tiled Shuri Castle built in the capital city of Naha, in the south of the island, and this was the destination for the *sakuho-shi*, China's imperial ambassadors. China, the giant empire across the sea to the west, was the greatest influence on the kingdom at that time; it granted the Ryuku kings their power, provided much of the island's trade and shared its seeds and culinary techniques. This is how the O-Higu bean arrived on Okinawa, as well as *shima-dofu* (island tofu), a softer, silkier form of tofu than is found on the Japanese mainland, closer to the Chinese tofu tradition. A 'Survey of Japanese People's Diets' recorded in the late nineteenth century – by which time Okinawa was under the control of Japan's Meiji dynasty – found that a typical Okinawan meal consisted of tofu and 'sweet potato and miso soup with plenty of vegetables' for breakfast, lunch and dinner. Their mostly plant-based, soy-rich diet led to Okinawa later being listed as one of five blue zones – regions of the world in which people live exceptionally long and healthy lives. But, in the mid-twentieth century, a strange and unexpected shift took place in their diet. By the 1960s, the people on Okinawa were still eating tofu, but the O-Higu bean had gone extinct and the soy they ate instead was grown in the American Midwest.

Of all the seeds humans have domesticated and cultivated for food, what makes the soybean so exceptional is not so much the compounds it contains, but the quantities involved. Roughly 20 per cent of a soybean is oil and 35 per cent is protein, high proportions as far as legumes go. Soy had been of interest to American scientists since the eighteenth century and by the 1850s it was one of the legumes used as a rotation crop in the American South. But it was only in the early twentieth century that the real potential of its protein and oil started to be exploited, in most part thanks to an incongruous combination of plant collectors, entrepreneurs and religious leaders.

Soy's great ascendancy in the West started to build in the early 1900s, when the United States Department of Agriculture began to send botanists, including the legendary seed collector Frank Meyer, to Japan, Korea and China, to build up a collection of soy varieties. The 4,500 soybean samples sent back were put to the test in experimental field trials. Around forty were approved for commercial use by the USDA and posted to farmers for cultivation. As the supply of the bean increased, so did demand for soy products. The Seventh-Day Adventist Church endorsed soy as an ingredient suited to the strict vegetarian regime its members were expected to follow. One of these, the food entrepreneur John Harvey Kellogg (of cornflake fame), believed the bean had great potential for improving human health. Kellogg had already developed soy products that had similar textures to meat – precursors of the lucrative meat 'alternatives' made today – and launched 'Corn-Soya Shreds'. 'There's no other cereal like it!' ran the ads.

Meanwhile, industrialists were also busy using soybeans to make paint, soap, textiles and plastics. While physicists were splitting the atom, chemists in the USA were deconstructing the soybean, extracting constituent parts and finding uses for its abundant oils and proteins. Henry Ford was an early evangelist of the legume, building the body of a car completely out of chemically processed soy, spraying it with paint made from the bean and stuffing the seats with soy-fibre. The food industry fell in love with soy as well, processing it into ever greater quantities of margarine and cooking oil. Another component of soy, lecithin, became the most widely used emulsifier, and a crucial ingredient in ready meals, salad dressing and chocolate. By the 1950s, the United States was growing so much soy (including American-bred varieties, such as the fattier, higher-yielding Lincoln bean) that it had enough of a surplus to export. One of its biggest customers would be Japan.

In the spring of 1945, US marines and the Japanese Imperial Army clashed in the Battle of Okinawa. The 82-day battle is known on the island as *tetsu no ame* ('the rain of steel') because of the ferocity of the bombardment. Ninety thousand combatants died and Okinawa's population was halved. Hundreds of farms on the island were left devastated and others were cleared to make way for what would become one of America's largest overseas military bases, with more than 50,000 US troops. Under US occupation, more sugar cane was planted as a cash crop, replacing the diverse foods farmers had grown for islanders. Instead, Californian rice, wheat from Kansas, tinned American pork (Spam) and soybeans grown in Iowa were imported. There was little incentive to save the O-Higu as huge amounts of soy were imported to Asia, not only from the USA but, increasingly, from other parts of the Americas.

But in the 1970s the soy boom really intensified. This boom has a lot to do with a diminutive fish. For decades, vast shoals of anchovy were caught just off the Peruvian coast and used as the major protein source in the poultry and cattle industries. But in 1972, a combination of overfishing and El Niño led to Peru's anchovy harvest dropping by nearly 90 per cent. A protein panic rippled out across the agricultural world. To protect its own industries (and prevent meat prices going up), the Nixon administration restricted exports of American soy. This, in turn, had an impact on Japan, by now heavily dependent on American supplies. Realising just *how* dependent and vulnerable it had become, Japan began to put a long-term plan in place. There was no other big supplier to turn to, and so it had to create one. Brazil had been a marginal player in the soy business, but with Japanese investment and the clearance of virgin forest, including parts of the

Cerrado, it became a giant. In 1960, Brazilian soy production was less than 300,000 metric tons. In the 1980s, helped by newly developed soy cultivars suited to the Cerrado's acidic soil, this increased to around 20 million tons. The 2020 harvest, of 130 million tons, broke all records and exceeded the size of the American crop putting Brazil on course to become the undisputed world leader of soy cultivation.

As this soy boom was taking place, behind the scenes, transformation of the global seed industry was also under way. The $4 billion soybean seed market became the major battleground. Already, soy grown across the Americas was based on a small number of genetically uniform varieties, all grown in monocultures, making them vulnerable to pests and diseases. The solution was genetically modified soy. In 1996, Monsanto launched Roundup Ready soy, a plant resistant to the glyphosate-based herbicide (or weed-killer) of the same name. The product had been developed after a chance discovery; a bacterium spotted growing inside one of Monsanto's waste ponds was found to have resistance to Roundup, and genes from this bacterium were transferred to create a new variety of soy. Syngenta followed with its own version, VMAX, then, not to be outdone, Bayer with a variety called Liberty Link. By 2014, more than 90 per cent of all soy grown across North and South America was GM.

Consolidation wasn't only a feature of the soy seed business; the global trade in the bean also became heavily concentrated among a small number of companies. For many years this was the so-called ABCD group: Archer-Daniels-Midland, Bunge, Cargill and (supplying the D from its middle name) Louis-Dreyfus Company. These companies and the soy they trade have helped to turn food production into the 'complex, globalized and financialized' business it is today. Food prices, deforestation, land and water use are all influenced by their activities. In 2016, the picture changed (slightly); Asian companies, including one owned by the Chinese government called COFCO, started to exert more control over much of Brazil's soy exports and China became the main driver of soy expansion in South America, to feed a rapidly growing population of pigs and chickens. The future of the Cerrado depends to a great extent on Chinese diets.

In 2012, I paid a visit to the C of the ABCD group, Cargill. It owns the biggest soy-processing plant in the UK, the Seaforth refinery, a large, anonymous-looking building on the waterside of Liverpool's docks. There, I met the operations manager who showed me through a network of large open spaces, with a snake of steel pipe winding its way through the entire building, joining up vast, unfathomable blocks of machinery. One of these was sending out a hum as it turned the round beans into flakes.

Apart from the manager, there were only a handful of other people here, as most of the work was automated. Nearly a million tonnes of soy a year were being processed at the site, the equivalent of three square miles of soy plantation every day. Once a month, a ship arrived from Brazil containing 60,000 tonnes of beans which needed five days just to unload. Turning it into oil, protein and lecithin took a lot less time, about four hours. This was mostly done through 'solvent extraction' in which hexane (a chemical side product of the petroleum industry) dismantles the bean's compounds, putting every possible molecule of protein and oil to use. This happens inside a tower, forty feet wide and twenty feet tall, and involves a massive piece of equipment that emits an ear-punishing drone. As we followed the pipe network, we reached the 'de-solventiser', which removed the hexane and made the soy edible. From his pocket, the manager pulled a small vial filled with a sample of thick yellow oil to show me what was being made. In the hands of food processors, this product is used to make cooking oil, salad dressing, mayonnaise and margarine. At the end of the production line were big, yellow dumper trucks parked up next to what looked like a sand dune made of yellow powder. Forty-eight per cent protein, I was told, and destined to be turned into animal feed.

Soy protein has made a greater impact on our planet and transformed diets more fundamentally than any other plant material in recent history. Around 70 per cent of the world's soybean protein is used to feed poultry and pigs, and most of what remains goes to cattle, sheep and farmed fish. Since the soy boom, the global pig population has more than doubled to a billion, while poultry numbers have increased more than sixfold to more than 22 billion. In the case of fish, feed from soy has helped a new species to flourish: farmed Atlantic salmon. But what soy has given the world in food abundance, it has taken away in biodiversity, including the loss of virgin forest. A soy moratorium introduced in 2006 reduced deforestation in the

Amazon, but since President Jair Bolsonaro took office in 2019, levels have increased again and thousands of square miles of forest cover have been lost. The moratorium was never extended to the Cerrado. Just 20 per cent of Brazil's tropical savannah remains undisturbed. Soy also exerts a huge influence on geopolitics. In the summer of 2019, when a trade war broke out between China and the USA, one of the first industries targeted by tariffs was the soybean trade.

On Okinawa, most memories of the O-Higu and its tofu had faded into obscurity and the last known seeds belonged to a farmer who died in the 1970s. At the beginning of the twenty-first century, Kenichi Kariki started looking for Okinawa's O-Higu seeds. Some had been sent to the Vavilov Institute, but there were too few in the collection to send any out to an experimental farmer on Okinawa. The paper trail from the Vavilov Institute took Kariki to a seed collection at Okinawa's Ryuku University where, fifty years before, one of the university's botanists had stored seeds away for safekeeping. It is those seeds that are now growing in Kariki's small soy patch.

I visited Kariki on Okinawa in 2018, when there were just enough seeds to be shared out with farmers around the island. 'When we eat island tofu again made with O-Higu soy it will be a big day,' he told me. 'It's a food no one has tasted for more than half a century.' During the Second World War, Shuri Castle, the physical symbol of the Ryukyu kingdom, had been burnt down, but that had been relatively easy to restore. Reviving a lost food culture isn't so simple; it's less tangible, more complicated, but no less important. 'Okinawa deserves to have its own crops back,' Kariki said. To outsiders, O-Higu might appear an insignificant bean. 'But to many Okinawans, after colonialism and occupation, its return feels like an act of resistance and a celebration of who we are.'

Seed power

Vegetables generate a different kind of emotional response in us than other crops. Cereals are often seen as fuel: a rich source of carbohydrate. Vegetables, however, in their many shapes, colours and textures, offer more obvious displays of beauty and diversity. As flavour-filled packages of essential vitamins and minerals, vegetables, more than meat, are what have sustained most humans. And they can be grown on small patches, unlike the large open spaces needed for wheat and other grains. So vegetables are the usual starting point for those in search of greater self-sufficiency. This was one of the reasons Esiah Levy began to grow vegetables. But his interest in these edible plants developed much further.

From his home in south London, he sent seeds around the world. Envelopes that had once held letters, bills and circulars were recycled and filled with a spoonful of landrace seeds: varieties of squash he'd discovered through his Jamaican relatives; jumbles of different corns, sweet, popping, red and 'painted'; seeds for beetroot, rhubarb and peppers. He produced these seeds by growing plants wherever space allowed – in allotment plots; on the balconies of friends' homes; along and up the garden fences of neighbours; inside an old shoe he had found; in the flower beds around his mother's house. 'It was like walking into *The Secret Garden*,' says Levy's sister Syreeta. When he ran out of pots, he filled supermarket carrier bags with soil and grew seeds in those. He believed it wasn't lack of space that prevented people growing food from seed, but lack of knowledge and desire.

It all began when a friend at work gave him a handful of seeds from a Blue Ballet squash. He planted them and watched them grow. 'The flesh was amazing,' he remembered, 'best roasted, so that the sweetness filled your mouth.' Inside his first home-grown squash he found hundreds of seeds and it didn't feel right to throw them away. So, he began to give the seeds to other people. Before long, he was sharing his wonder at this miraculous journey from seed to plate with his two young children, and then with like-minded people online. By day, he worked for London Underground, where he looked after the signals, but at night he took to Instagram where he posted pictures of his open-pollinated seeds and the landrace vegetables from his miscellany of garden treasures. 'I want to use what nature provides,' he posted to followers around the world. 'Seeds are plentiful, and importantly, they're free.' All his followers had to do was ask and he would post them seeds – to Georgia, Germany, Jamaica, Morocco, Ghana, 'to the world and beyond', he once said, and maybe it wasn't a slip of the tongue. When he watched stories of disasters on television news, he sent packets of seed to the communities affected. 'When we care, we are at our most creative, and our imaginations are unlimited.'

Many sent him seeds in return: Aztec broccoli came from a gardener in Poland, red sweetcorn from a follower in Canada, bean seeds from Holland, and more from Japan and America. People took inspiration from the pictures he posted and the promise of hope they contained. 'Magic, pure magic,' said one of his followers in thanks. Levy thought so too. Where he lived fresh produce wasn't always easy to find. Instead there were fried chicken shops and plenty of poverty. Seeds offered a means to a better life and a source of empowerment, one that you could see, touch and taste.

Esiah Levy died aged just thirty-two in January 2019 of sudden adult death syndrome. But through the thousands of seeds he posted around the world, Levy lives on. 'I want everyone to share seeds and to grow them,' he once said. 'Everyone has a part to play in the security of our seeds.'

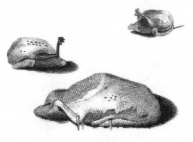

Part Four
Meat

The time will come when humanity will extend its
mantle over everything which breathes.

Jeremy Bentham, *Principles of Morals and Legislation* (1789)

Inside the Smithsonian's National Museum of Natural History in Washington DC is a tiny piece of fossilised bone less than 2cm long. FWJJ14A-1208 (as it's labelled) has two sets of indentations on its surface; one made by a large scavenging animal, the other by a stone knife wielded by a human. The bone (which most likely belonged to a type of antelope) was found near Lake Turkana in East Africa, north of the hunting grounds of modern-day Hadza. It is 1.5 million years old, making FWJJ14A-1208 among the earliest pieces of evidence so far discovered of hunting by our ancestors. It heralds the ascent of meat in human diets.

Hunting for meat led to all kinds of changes. It led our ancestors to travel more widely and become explorers. Because tracking animals depended on cooperation between members of a group, their communication skills became more sophisticated. And locating dead animals by watching vultures circling overhead pushed them to create more complex mental maps of their world. Meat eating changed human physiology; brains grew bigger and guts smaller (as digesting large quantities of plants was no longer necessary). Then, around 12,000 years ago, instead of hunting and killing animals, some humans brought these creatures closer into their world and began to change them.

Out of the 150 or so potential candidates, our ancestors domesticated fourteen mammals. From within that group, a 'big five' emerged: sheep, goats, cattle, pigs and chickens. Each fulfilled six important criteria: they weren't too aggressive (unlike the zebra); their diets weren't too complicated (unlike the anteater); they grew quickly (unlike elephants); they bred easily in captivity (unlike pandas); they followed leaders (unlike antelopes); and they didn't become too stressed in confined spaces or when brought face-to-face with predators like us (unlike gazelles). As agriculture spread out of the Fertile Crescent and China, so too did domesticated animals, and in the same way that crops adapted in different environments to become landrace varieties, so animals adapted and evolved as breeds.

This continued haphazardly for millennia until in the eighteenth century an English Presbyterian farmer began running experiments in animal genetics on his farm in the Midlands. Seeking to satisfy the growing demand for meat in industrialising England, Robert Bakewell's groundbreaking work led to him breeding bigger, faster-growing animals.

Before Bakewell's radical advances, animals had been too valuable to be raised just for their meat. Sheep and goats were kept for wool and skins; cattle for milk, as beasts of burden and for manure; chickens for their eggs; and pigs were living stores of surplus food, fed during times of plenty, saved until winter and slaughtered when other food ran low. In many parts of the world, certain breeds of animals were kept because they had a sacred or important cultural status. With Bakewell's new breeds, meat production could become the primary goal. He visited farms in different parts of England to better understand how varied farm animals could be and to draw from the widest gene pool possible. In each area, he noted the slightest differences in the cows, pigs and sheep he saw so he could select specific qualities. He dissected dead farm animals to study their anatomy, analyse their skeletal structure and see how their muscles worked. Until this point, breeding farm animals had been a random business. Bakewell turned it into a science.

In his system, males and females were separated to prevent less systematic breeding and instead he adopted a principle of 'in-and-in breeding' (inbreeding the animals that had the traits he wanted and culling those with undesirable characteristics). Through this approach he transformed ancient breeds of cattle into animals which built up fat and muscle more quickly; he thinned their hides, reduced their bone structure, even changed the colour and texture of their meat. He developed sheep with 'the greatest weight of mutton for the least expenditure of food in the least possible time'. His breeds became the most expensive and sought-after and his techniques spread around the world. Darwin would later cite Bakewell's work to illustrate his ideas on selection. There was no turning back. Our relationship with animals, and with meat, was changed forever.

In the last sixty years, Bakewell's principles have been sent into overdrive. In that time, global meat production has quadrupled and the number of animals slaughtered each year has reached 80 billion. To achieve this we have changed the physiology of animals more fundamentally, and at a faster pace, than at any other time in history. The Green Revolution created such a surplus of cereals it could be used not only to feed humans but also livestock. A third of all the grain we grow now is eaten by animals and this has helped to accelerate their growth and productivity. Since the middle of the twentieth century, the body mass of the average chicken has increased fivefold, its lifespan shortened to as little as five weeks. While a dairy cow in 1900 might have been expected to deliver between 1,500 and 3,000 litres of milk per year, by the end of the century the expectation was more like 8,000 litres. To achieve these increases, animals were taken on the same path as food crops: we narrowed diversity on a global scale to suit our needs. More than 95 per cent of America's dairy herd is based around one breed of 'super cow', the Holstein (and most of these animals can be linked back to a handful of males). In much of Europe, including the UK and Germany, the Holstein makes up around seventy per cent of the dairy herd. Just three breeding lines dominate global poultry production, and most pork is based around the genetics of a single breed, the Large White.

Advances in technology helped speed up what Bakewell had set in motion. In the 1950s, artificial insemination and the invention of frozen straws of sperm allowed a narrow gene pool to spread around the world. A single bull in Wisconsin can now father half a million off-spring in fifty different countries. The global meat industry has been built on this uniformity; fast-food chains are able to guarantee every burger tastes exactly the same and supermarkets can fill counters with cuts of meat identical in shape and size. Where nature creates diversity, the food system crushes it.

With cereals and vegetables we have seen how monocultures increase vulnerability and create risk. The animal equivalent, large-scale intensive farms where thousands of genetically identical animals are kept in close proximity, can also bring vulnerability (animal diseases), harm to the planet (lakes of effluent pollute rivers and soils) and misery to the lives of millions of creatures. This book is focusing on diversity, not animal welfare, but the two are closely connected.

The diversity we are losing in our race to produce more and more meat is frightening. Many livestock breeds becoming extinct are indigenous and adapted to local conditions over thousands of years, each a part of an intricate and interconnected food system. They hold genetic traits we can't afford to lose. Yakutian cattle in northern Siberia were selected over millennia to survive in the coldest inhabited place on Earth, where temperatures fall to –50°C. Less than a thousand are left, dispersed among three villages. Then there are the Swiniarka sheep of Poland, so light-bodied that the animals can graze on fragile grasslands that would easily be destroyed by heavier animals. Pantaneiro cattle live in tropical wetlands of Brazil, Bolivia and Paraguay, and can tolerate food shortages, see off diseases and pests that would knock out high-yielding breeds developed for intensive farms, and cope with summer temperatures of 40°C. After the Spanish introduced European cows to South America, it took five hundred years of selection by farmers here to create this breed. Now endangered, it could be lost in the space of a decade. According to the United Nations Food and Agriculture Organisation, of the 7,745 recorded livestock breeds, around a quarter are at high risk of extinction. But as a global census doesn't exist, far more could be at risk or already gone without us realising.

For the majority of the 12,000 or so years of animal domestication, the relationship between humans and animals has been far more complex and co-dependent than it is now. In early wall paintings and religious iconography, we see the awe and respect our ancestors had for the creatures which fed them. Although this reverence has now mostly disappeared, it can still be found in remote communities and on small-scale farms. But for the mainstream, animals have been made into commodities, anonymous units of production hidden away in sheds and slaughterhouses. Biodiversity and precious genetics have become endangered, as has our sense of the true origins, meaning and value of meat. In this part of the book, I want to take you to four very different places, to meet people and animals who can show us it's not too late to regain a more respectful, more caring relationship with the animals that provide most of the world with meat.

13

Skerpikjøt

Faroe Islands

'When we go inside, don't panic. You'll see mould all over the place and something that'll make you want to run away rather than eat.' The wind was blowing in this barren landscape, but luckily (I thought) I had been promised lunch. Stepping through the creaking doorway of the wooden shed, I glimpsed my meal in the half-light, hanging by a hook from a rafter. As my companion, Gunnar Nattestad, put it, 'It looks like part of a dead animal I found in the road.' The hunk of meat was coated in a thick layer of mould, with patches of creamy yellow, chalky white and an ominous dark brown. 'Don't worry, I'll wash it a little before we eat.'

Nattestad is a farmer, shopkeeper, carpenter and butcher, his string of professions reflecting the inescapable self-reliance needed for life on the Faroes, an archipelago of eighteen islands in the north Atlantic. To the north is Iceland, further east is Denmark (of which the Faroe Islands are an autonomous outpost) and two hundred miles to the south are the Scottish isles. The 50,000 people who live on the Faroes are easily outnumbered by some 80,000 sheep. I was looking at a piece of one of these animals. From the shape of it, I recognised it as a leg, but its colour and texture made it look more like a mass of old parchment or decayed leather. There was a strange beauty to it, like a fallen rotting tree that had grown patches of moss on its bark. Two forces had exerted their influence on the carcass; one was time, the other was fermentation. The sheep had been slaughtered the year before, in September. It was now May and in those nine months, bathed in air salted by the sea, the meat had become dense and solid to the touch. This strange object meant survival to generations in a land where few crops could grow.

The full history of the island is sketchy but we know that Celtic explorers arrived in the sixth century followed by Irish monks and

Vikings in the ninth and tenth centuries. They discovered a treeless place of bleak beauty, a green-and-grey landscape dotted with fjords where steep volcanic peaks descended to bubbling, rocky streams and on to the cold, crashing ocean. The settlement of the Faroe Islands is an epic story of endurance. Of the men and women who didn't survive the harsh conditions, legend has it that 'They were laid in their graves with seaweed in their mouths', a reference to the desperation of slow deaths from starvation. Few historic buildings exist on the wind-battered Faroes. The most important piece of cultural heritage here might well be the knowledge and skills required to survive.

Crucial to the process of preserving the meat I was looking at was the wooden shed itself, called a *hjallur* (pronounced chatler). This ingeniously designed rectangular building has long horizontal beams from which food can be hung, protected by the building's sides which are made of vertical wooden laths with a thumb-sized gap between each one. Unlike every other building on the Faroes, the *hjallur* is designed to let in the brutal Atlantic winds. 'The winds are exceedingly uncertain and violent,' wrote one visitor to the Faroes in the 1840s, 'storms ... overturn houses and ... move blocks of stone, making it necessary for the traveller to throw himself on the ground in order not to be carried away.' And there was something particular about the Faroese winds, the visitor added, 'sea mists of the Faroe Islands contain salt particles in considerable quantities ... salt crusts cover the face after a trip in a boat'. The *hjallur* is designed to turn this assault from the sea into a means of preservation.

Trees, and most other vegetation, stand no chance of prospering on the exposed landscape of the Faroes. With no trees, and therefore no firewood, it wasn't possible to preserve sheep with smoke, or by boiling seawater to create salt. Instead, the islanders built their drying huts and fermented their sheep meat with the help of salt blown in from the sea. '*Skerpikjøt* wasn't invented,' Gunnar Nattestad told me. 'It was given to us by the islands. They make this meat.'

Keep a sheep's carcass in a wooden shed somewhere else in the world and things will not go well. 'Most likely it will become rotten and full of maggots,' Nattestad said. 'But here, over time, the wind from the sea turns the flesh into *skerpikjøt*.' This Faroese word refers to meat that has reached a specific stage of fermented funkiness, a sweet spot on its journey into decomposition. Over time, the salt air draws moisture out of the hanging meat, while a community of microbes break down the proteins, month by month, sometimes over years. Everything about the *skerpikjøt*, the way it looks, the way it smells, speaks of endurance. 'For centuries, the population here remained small,' said Nattestad. 'If someone on the island could find a way to leave, they usually did; if they stayed and survived, most likely they had *skerpikjøt* to thank.'

The humans who lived here were tough, but the animals they farmed were tougher. The early Faroese sheep were an ancient animal, agile, hardy and short – what the Victorians would have referred to as a 'primitive breed'. A tiny number of similar ancient breeds have survived in remote parts of Europe, such as on the uninhabited Scottish island of Soay, which gives its name to one of these breeds. The wool of these 'primitive' animals could be plucked rather than shorn, a genetic trait more commonly found in pre-domesticated animals, one that allowed them to shed their coats naturally. Humans selected sheep that kept their fleece, which made 'harvesting' wool easier (here I see parallels with the way Neolithic farmers selected non-shattering wheat). The primitive sheep also behaved differently; instead of flocking like modern breeds, they scattered and would have been more difficult to herd (on islands where there were no predators, they were happy to graze on their own or in small groups). And on the Faroe Islands, beneath their chestnut-brown wool, they had generous layers of intramuscular fat that helped them endure extreme weather conditions.

The sheep the early settlers brought with them could take all the energy locked up in thousands of acres of grass (the one thing that did grow in abundance on the islands) and convert it into life's necessities: wool for clothing; milk and butter for food; tallow to make candles for heat and light; and dried dung for fuel. The importance of the animal gave the archipelago its name, the Faroe Islands, 'Sheep Islands'. The earliest known document on the Faroes is the thirteenth-century 'Sheep Letters', which set out the island's laws, from land ownership to grazing rights, and helps to show the value of sheep to the people here. For the island's inhabitants, wool was currency. The oldest Faroese proverb, *Ull er Føroya gull*, means 'wool is Faroese gold'.

Meat was a by-product, an important one, but still a by-product. The last thing you would want to do as a settler on the islands was kill the animal that gave you everything you needed to survive; not until it had given you all it could. And so, by the time the sheep were ready to be slaughtered and their meat turned into *skerpikjøt*, they would have been four or five years old, possibly more. This mature meat, marbled with fat and strongly flavoured, is known in most countries as mutton. Sheep are still allowed to live long lives on the Faroe Islands, a practice that was common across most of Europe from Neolithic times until just over a century ago. Eating an animal as young as a lamb is a modern phenomenon.

Until the start of the early twentieth century, mutton was as popular as beef. It was served in royal palaces with capers and cream or inside hot pies sold to workers by street vendors. 'Sticky, rich, gelatinous and unctuous,' is how the chef Fergus Henderson, the master of 'nose to tail' cooking, describes it. Mutton is a far more beguiling, noble and complex meat than lamb. It was served as the last lunch on the *Titanic* in 1912 and cooked as a birthday meal on Captain Scott's last expedition the same year. Arthur Conan Doyle flavoured sixteen of Sherlock Holmes's adventures with mutton, while Charles Dickens (a serious cook) not only had his characters feasting on mutton, he even invented a recipe of baked leg of mutton stuffed with veal and oysters.

Mutton was the meat that fuelled the Industrial Revolution, but its popularity began to fade. By 1900, nearly 50 per cent of all sheep meat eaten in Britain was being imported in refrigerated ships from the New World, particularly New Zealand and Australia. Because of this new and extraordinary abundance of livestock across the empire, it became possible to raise sheep primarily for their meat and to kill them at a younger age – lambs to the slaughter quite literally. By the middle of the twentieth century, mutton was considered too fatty, too strong-tasting and too time-consuming for cooks. Palates now favoured younger animals, and more tender, less flavourful meat.

In Britain, butchery skills and processing techniques centuries old went extinct. On Shetland, a type of preserved mutton called *vivda* (Norse for 'leg meat') was lost. As Shetland is close to the Faroes, it's no surprise that descriptions of *vivda* resemble *skerpikjøt*. Shetlanders even had their own version of the *hjallur*, square stone buildings called *helyar* or *skeos* which had open vents to allow air to breeze through and cure the mutton hanging inside. Across the rest of Britain it was as if mutton was wiped from the nation's culinary and cultural memory. In the 1960s, following the rise of synthetic fabrics such as nylon, wool prices collapsed, and the British Ministry of Agriculture stopped bothering to record the market price of mutton. For farmers, it made little financial sense to keep a sheep alive beyond a year; their real value was now lamb not wool. This led to changes in animal breeding; by the 1970s, most of the multi-purpose breeds that once existed across Northern Europe were either extinct or endangered, replaced by a larger, more muscly and meatier breed from the Netherlands, the Texel. The hardier, 'primitive' breeds now account for just 0.3 per cent of the gene pool and continue to decline. On the remote Faroe Islands, however, the more ancient attitude towards sheep and meat has survived – just.

While legs or shanks of *skerpikjøt* slowly mature in the *hjallurs*, the Faroese eat their way through every other piece of meat they can extract from that sheep's carcass. For example, *seyðahøvd* is a sheep's head (its brain removed). This is cut in half, dried and then boiled. The animal's blood is turned into black puddings. Everything is used except the gall bladder, which is bitter-tasting and toxic.

When you eat a piece of *skerpikjøt*, you can taste decay, just a hint. The fermentation process makes the fat a little rancid which can catch the back of your throat when you swallow. 'To us, that is a nice sensation,' says Nattestad. 'It's a twisted taste but a good taste.' For the Faroese who know *skerpikjøt* well, appreciation comes with experience. 'It is like wine. If the sheep has spent its life up in the hills, it has a particular taste; if it lived sheltered within a valley, it will have another.' The taste of the meat also depends on the location of the drying shed and the direction of the winds.

A strange kind of poetry describes the various stages in the fermentation of *skerpikjøt*. First comes *visnaður*, or wilting, which is when the meat starts to break down and become tender. After three months inside the hut, cured by the sea air, it becomes *raest* (half rotten), 'like the cells inside the meat have been filled up with juice and the bacteria are getting the fermentation process under way'. Nattestad describes this stage with a knowing smile. 'For outsiders, this is scary food.' *Raest* has a pungency described as somewhere between Parmesan cheese and death. Through the winter, however, as fermentation slows down and fiercer winds bathe the meat in salty mist, things begin to calm down. This is when the meat finally becomes *skerpikjøt* – the moisture recedes, it becomes drier, firmer and the flavour mellows out.

Another important source of animal protein on the Faroes comes from the seasonal *grindadráp*, the annual whale cull. Every summer, the island explodes into action when pods of migrating pilot whales swim so close to the shoreline it's possible for fishermen to surround them in boats and herd them towards the beach. Nearly a thousand whales can be slaughtered in one day, turning the swirling waters of the Atlantic blood red. Church records from the seventeenth century show that in the years when the migrating whales didn't arrive, the island's population fell sharply as people left or starved. In such years as these, having *skerpikjøt* hanging in a *hjallur* would have been a lifesaver.

Getting other traditional sources of meat involved death-defying feats of bravery. On a coastal path close to the *hjallur*, Nattestad pointed over the edge of high cliffs to places where generations of hunters had risked their lives in search of birds' nests. Using ropes, people would climb down to find baby gannets or puffin eggs. Every family seemed to have a story to tell of a relative who had slipped to their death in search of this food. Further along the coastal path, we reached a group of houses, their roofs sprouting thick grass for insulation. Dried fish were hanging from their eaves like wind chimes. *Ræstur fiskur* is the aquatic version of *skerpikjøt*, made by tying pairs of cod together and leaving them to dry and ferment in the salt air. Breaking the solid fish into pieces and picking out the bones requires a hammer. The flesh is so dry, you have to chew and chew, which slowly brings out the flavour of fresh fish.

When the Faroes came under Danish rule in the fourteenth century these food traditions were viewed with suspicion, *skerpikjøt* in particular. For generations, like a shameful secret, *skerpikjøt* was hidden away, not to be shared with outsiders. After the Second World War, with the arrival of bigger boats and new technology, the Faroese fishing industry developed quickly and gave the islanders one of the highest per capita GDPs in Europe. This meant they could afford to eat food from all over the world. Now, each week, a ship arrives from

Denmark delivering cuts of chicken, pork and beef, and *skerpikjøt* has become an endangered food.

In 2004, a group of twelve chefs across the Nordic region signed a document called the 'New Nordic Manifesto'. It was a pledge to break free from the classical Western European restaurant world where many of these chefs had been trained and to investigate traditions and ingredients closer to home. Among the ten pledges were 'To base our cooking on ingredients and produce . . . in our climates, landscapes and waters' and 'To develop . . . new applications of traditional Nordic food products'. Among the signatories was René Redzepi, whose restaurant Noma, with its use of wild foraged ingredients, went on to be voted the best restaurant in the world in 2010. Another was a chef from the Faroe Islands, Leif Sørensen.

Sørensen had left the islands in his late teens to study in Denmark where, desperate for a taste of home, he used to hang pieces of *skerpikjøt* out of his window. His fellow students complained about the smell and the meat vanished. 'I never found out what they did with it,' he says. After university, Sørensen worked as a chef in Copenhagen, cooking French food in Michelin-starred restaurants. When he returned home a decade later, he found little trace of the food he had grown up with. Nobody touched the mahogany clams that grow so slowly in the cold water some are three hundred years old. Even the juicy mussels waiting to be prised off the coastal rocks were overlooked, as were sea urchins and langoustines. Monkfish was thrown back in the sea, while the taste for seabirds, puffin and razorbill was fading with the older generations. Wild, wind-cured *skerpikjøt* was now viewed as revolting, poor man's fare on a cash-rich island. Sørensen set about changing all that.

He opened a restaurant dedicated entirely to the food traditions of the Faroes. He called it Koks, meaning to become obsessive in search of perfection. On the menu were fulmar and razorbill, birds that live along the craggy coastline so that their flesh tastes of the sea; the bright green, perfumed, subarctic herb angelica; and, of course, *skerpikjøt*. Reviving these foods hasn't been easy, even in his own home. 'My wife doesn't understand *skerpikjøt*,' says Sorensen, 'but then again, she is a Dane.' His father-in-law refuses even to be in the same house as the meat.

Koks has since been handed on to a new Faroese chef, Poul Andrias Ziska, and Sørensen has moved on to work on another of the manifesto pledges, to use old food traditions to create new foods. Ziska has kept *skerpikjøt* on the menu at Koks.

Raest – the strongest and 'most twisted' phase in the *skerpikjøt* process – is the name of another restaurant, tucked along a narrow lane in the capital Tórshavn ('Thor's Haven'). Here I met the young, golden-bearded chef Kari Kristiansen working on that night's menu, one dedicated entirely to traditional Faroese fermented foods, including *skerpikjøt*. 'We are no longer embarrassed by our food,' he said. 'It's time to say, "This is who we are, and this is the food that comes from our part of the world."'

Back at the *hjallur*, Nattestad served me lunch. We started with black, chewy pieces of cooked whale blood, which tasted of caramel and iron. Next, was a cube of its blubber, preserved like a block of Turkish delight, tinged pink. It coated my fingers in a fine grease. Then came the *skerpikjøt*. Nattestad's pride was clear as he passed me a thin slice of the meat he had raised, slaughtered and preserved. It was as refined as a piece of prosciutto and tasted sweet, salty and musty with a kick of acid (the 'twisted' taste Nattestad had promised).

'Outsiders criticise us for killing whales and wild birds, and they laugh at us for eating what they describe as rotten sheep,' Nattestad said at the end of the meal. 'But I believe we are the ones who know the truth of what it means to kill an animal and eat its meat.' Across the world images seen of the *grindadráp* and the bloody ocean had led to Faroe Islanders being accused of brutality. 'But the whales are free until the point of death, and our sheep are allowed to grow old. In your world, animals are trapped inside buildings and hidden away from view. Why is our meat any crueller than the slaughter of millions of animals inside industrial abattoirs no one ever gets to see?'

Above our heads hung the ugly-beautiful leg of *skerpikjøt*, the product of a thousand years of history. The drying shed was filled with the sights and smells of death, and yet it was full of reverence and care too.

14

Black Ogye Chicken

Yeonsan, South Korea

There was little sign of such reverence for the dead when I visited one of the UK's largest slaughterhouses, a block of buildings hidden by a ring of security fences. I was following the journey of a single lorry-load of birds, 6,000 of them, along the production line. A forklift truck carried blue plastic crates stacked eight high from the vehicle and onto a conveyer belt, each crate packed with birds, their white feathers just visible through the mesh. The crates were shunted along and into a chamber in which the chickens were first gassed and then had their necks sliced open by a robotic machine. Everything was automated and in constant motion – 180 birds a minute across the site, 2.5 million a week. Each dead chicken was hooked onto a pulley system that travelled above our heads and through the plant, a space so vast it took fifteen minutes to walk from one end to the other. Along the route was a tunnel filled with steam where hot jets of water from either side scalded feathers off the birds' now limp bodies. The staff lining the chickens' route stood on platforms that put them at eye level with the birds. Wearing plastic aprons, wellington boots and rubber gloves and against a relentless wall of industrial noise, they occasionally nudged a carcass as it went by, making sure each chicken stayed in its correct position.

This lorry-load, one of the many arriving at the slaughterhouse that day, represents a tiny fraction of the nearly one billion chickens slaughtered in the UK each year (double the number slaughtered two decades ago). Set against the 69 billion dispatched globally, that barely registers. Whatever the future success of lab-grown proteins and meat-free meat and however good it looks and tastes, the rise and rise of this bird looks set to continue long into the future. The mass of the 23 billion chickens alive at any given moment is greater than that of all the other birds on Earth combined. We are living in the age of the chicken. One of the geological markers of the Anthropocene is expected to be the copious amounts of chicken bones left behind in the fossil record. 'The signal of our civilisation is already being recorded,' says Carys Bennett, a geographer at Leicester University, 'and that signal is the modern chicken.'

Although it hasn't been given such a memorable title, a change as seismic as the Green Revolution also took place for the chicken, and it happened roughly in parallel. By the time the transition was complete, it was safe to say no other animal in history had undergone a biological change as fundamental or as rapid. Its lifespan was shortened to as little as thirty-five days (a few days longer than that of a housefly) and its body mass made to grow so quickly that if a human grew at the same rate, they would weigh twenty-four stone by the age of two. As a story of food production, this was an astonishing success. But this transformation should also fill us with foreboding. In just a few decades, the world has become dependent on increasingly homogeneous birds, produced in an increasingly uniform way on a vast scale. It's a strategy full of risk.

How humans first came to interact with chickens is a mystery, but a detailed analysis of the bird's genome, published in 2020, at least provides a time and a place for the start of the domestication process. Over a twenty-year period evolutionary biologists collected the DNA of almost a thousand different types of chicken indigenous to Asia and Africa, and that of their common ancestor, the red jungle fowl. They concluded that the origins of the modern chicken can be found in a region that includes southwestern China, northern Thailand and eastern Myanmar. Here, sometime after 7500 BCE, people started to tame the jungle fowl. One theory gaining ground is that humans didn't go in search of this bird but the bird came and found us: that long after cows, pigs, sheep and goats had been domesticated, farmers in this part of Asia attracted the attention of this timid, treetop bird. Rice cultivation was spreading, and for these wild birds, paddies presented an opportunity: weeds, seeds and insects. Drawn to rice farming, this ancestor of the chicken came into regular contact with humans, and as their dependency grew, they became tamer. For farmers there were benefits too: the birds helped control pests; they provided a source of fertiliser; and, of course, they laid eggs that could be eaten. Perhaps the humans also had aesthetic reasons for tolerating this bird. The red jungle fowl is smaller than today's domesticated chicken, but its plumage is far more spectacular, a mix of greens and reds with metallic-looking tints. In some ancient cultures, wearing feather hats, capes or costumes was regarded as a means of communing with gods. In Hawaii, these ceremonial objects were believed to confer supernatural powers on chiefs in need of a successful harvest or greater prowess ahead of a battle.

The source of the feathers, the birds themselves, were seen as spiritual messengers, divine manifestations that moved between Heaven and Earth. Chickens were both worshipped and sacrificed. The Khasi people in the wild citrus region of Meghalaya believed the bird to be a living vessel that carried all human sin, so they sacrificed them as an act of purification. Elsewhere, traditional healers and shamans looked to different parts of the chicken for remedies: meat, bones, organs, feathers, combs and eggs. The chicken served as a walking pharmacy, with potential cures for ailments that ranged from migraines and epilepsy to asthma and insomnia. Meat and eggs were just two of the many attractions of chickens. In some cultures they provided entertainment in the form of cockfighting, while in others observing the bird's behaviour was a means of telling fortunes. Cocks of certain breeds were prized for their crowing abilities, some so loud and long they were taken on voyages across the Indian Ocean to warn other boats to keep away. By 1000 BCE, domesticated chickens had been introduced into the Near East and by 800 BCE further west into Europe. The Romans took the chicken into every part of their empire, including Britain. The bird's biological future was now firmly in the hands of humans, and through selection and breeding, this genetically elastic animal became many different things.

In Quebec, the Chantecler chicken was developed by a Trappist monk called Wilfred Chatelain, who managed to breed a bird so hardy it produced eggs even in the depths of the harshest winters. In Brazil, the *galinha caipira* is a black chicken with golden neck feathers. Its dark meat and bones are used to make a broth flavoured with coconut called *pirão de parida*. In Egypt, the Bigawi chicken lays small, cream-coloured eggs considered to be an aphrodisiac and which are eaten during the springtime festival of Sham El Nessim. The poule de Barbezieux of France is a giant of a chicken. In *The Physiology of Taste* the famous gastronome Brillat-Savarin described eating one of these birds stuffed so full of truffles and foie gras it was fit to burst.

In Asia, birthplace of the chicken, more ancient, smaller and slower-growing breeds still exist, including the Yeonsan Ogye in South Korea, one of the rarest chickens on Earth. The bird is completely black, including its plumage, skin, beak, crest, eyes, claws and bones. The earliest reference to this unique chicken is found in a fourteenth-century poem by Lee Dal-Chung, a *seonbi*, or public scholar. In the seventeenth century, the bird was included in the *Donguibogam*, a 25-volume medical encyclopedia compiled by a Korean court physician called Heo Jun. According to this text, every part of the Ogye (which translates as 'black chicken'), from head to toe, can be used as medicine, even the bird's faeces.

The shape of the Yeonsan Ogye's body is similar to that of the red jungle fowl and, like its wild ancestor, it's an accomplished flyer, so it can reach the branches of trees to peck away at leaves and find insects. Its behaviour also mirrors that of the wild bird, as it will dig away at the ground, enjoy dirt baths and show a preference to feed on grasses rather than grain. Unlike its faster-growing, more productive modern cousins, it might only lay one egg every three to four days. This strikingly beautiful, mysterious-looking creature is an anachronism to the modern poultry industry. In Korea, in the 1930s and 1940s, during the Japanese occupation, faster growing, larger birds were introduced, which is when the Ogye, along with other traditional breeds, fell into decline.

The person protecting most of the last surviving Yeonsan Ogye pure breeds is Lee Seung Sook, whose family have raised the breed for five generations. Their farm is in the town of Yeonsan, 100 miles south-west of Seoul at the foot of the Gyeryong Mountains, known locally as *Chicken Dragon Mountain*. From here, Lee's great-great-grandfather sent Ogye birds to a member of the Korean royal family who had fallen ill. Fortunately, after being fed the chicken broth, Gojong, the 25th Joseon king, recovered and decreed it a special, life-saving animal.

Its status as a medicinal, health-giving bird has survived into the twenty-first century. 'Their bones are hard and their bodies are muscular,' says Lee, 'which is why after the intestines are removed the entire chicken is slowly boiled to make a thick and nutritious broth.' There are other reasons she is committed to saving the Yeonsan Ogye from extinction. 'It is part of the living and breathing history of Korea,' she says. 'This chicken has lived with our ancestors on this land for at least 700 years. If Yeonsan Ogye were to disappear, we would lose a piece of our souls. If it were to become like the dodo, more like a legend and an animal from the past, seen only through photographs or as a stuffed specimen, that would be a tragedy.'

Across the Pacific, American farmers had their own favourite birds. There, as in Europe, well into the twentieth century, although the chicken was prized as a source of eggs, it was marginal in people's diets and to the nation's economy. Pigs and cattle were the central characters in the rise of the mechanised and increasingly centralised meat industry. Chickens barely had a walk-on part, and for a long while their production remained a far more casual, backyard affair populated by a huge diversity of breeds. In issues of the *American Poultry Journal* published in the 1920s, the classified ads listing the different breeds a farmer could choose from ran on for pages: Single-Comb White Leghorns, Anconas, Buff Orpingtons, Black Minorcas, Rhode Island Reds, Speckled Sussex, Silver Wyandottes, Brown Leghorns, Black Langshans, and on it goes.

These birds were reared by thousands of breeders spread around the United States and sold to millions of family farming businesses which raised and sold chickens. Most of these were small-scale, mixed-farm operations, with a range of crops and animals. Just as a farmer would grow a variety of landrace wheat because it suited the environment around them, so it was for the choice of chicken. And just as sheep were kept primarily for their wool and only slaughtered towards the end of their lives, chickens were dual-purpose animals, kept for their eggs and sold for meat only when the hens could lay no more. This is how the poultry industry of America (and the rest of the world) stayed until the 1940s.

Then, around the same time as Norman Borlaug was toiling in Mexican fields in his effort to improve wheat, an equally ambitious initiative got under way with the chicken. The USDA, in partnership with poultry organisations and a retailer, the Great Atlantic & Pacific Tea Company (the Walmart of its day), organised a competition to find the most productive chicken ever seen. Newspaper advertisements called for birds so chunky they could feed a family, with breast meat so thick it could be carved into steaks and large drumsticks of dark, juicy meat – all at low price. A challenge was being laid down to the poultry industry: focus less on eggs, produce more meat and find a way of making it profitable.

The 'Chicken of Tomorrow' competition was a big deal, a nationwide effort that involved scientists, universities, civil servants and farmers from every state in the country competing for a substantial cash prize. In various guises, the competition ran for several years, between 1946 and 1951, time enough for the entrants to fast-track the evolution of the bird and create a breed with all the desirable characteristics set out by the Chicken of Tomorrow wish list: sturdier, meatier and quicker-growing.

In the end, the competition was won by an entry from California, the Vantress Poultry Breeding Farm. Unlike other farmers who had entered pure breeds of chickens (and selected the best from these lines), Vantress had crossed two different birds, the California-Cornish with a New Hampshire. Coming in second was a line of New Hampshire bred by Connecticut's Arbor Acres Farm. The birds created out of the competition were so productive that by the early 1950s nearly 70 per cent of America's commercial meat chickens (broilers) carried their genetics.

As these Chickens of Tomorrow spread rapidly around America, many of the locally adapted birds that had been developed by generations of farmers and breeders became endangered and then, in most cases, extinct, at least in the commercial world. Not only was the chicken transformed but so was the entire structure of the industry. Behind these new hybrids were complex cross-breeding techniques and intricate family trees that would have boggled the mind of Robert Bakewell. In the same way as the arrival of F1 hybrid maize meant that a farmer couldn't save and plant seeds and expect them to breed true, farmers had few options but to keep going back to commercial breeders year after year to restock their sheds with these finely tuned, big, meaty birds. And just as Borlaug's wheat travelled the world, so did the genetics of these new-breed chickens and the more intensive systems used to grow them.

The result is that seven decades after the Chicken of Tomorrow competition, the descendants of those winning chickens make up most of the nearly 70 billion birds slaughtered each year. And whereas the older breeds of chicken had 'open-source' genetic material spanning thousands of years, the birds that came to dominate poultry production are, like a high-yielding variety of maize developed by a seed company, intellectual property.

Tens of millions of pounds are invested each year in maintaining these pedigree lines. By the early 2000s, three companies dominated the world's poultry genetics, Cobb, Aviagen and Hubbard. In 2018, this number was effectively reduced to just two after Aviagen took over Hubbard. Cobb and Aviagen own the genetics behind the world's most dominant broiler breeds including the Cobb 500, the Ross 308 and the Hubbard Flex. All are capable of growing to around 2 kilos in around 35 days. This means the greatest amount of meat is produced using the least amount of feed in the shortest amount of time. However, faster growth rates can contribute to increased risk of lameness and higher levels of mortality and birds less likely to display natural chicken behaviour (including foraging and dust-bathing). This is why, particularly in Europe, slower growing breeds of commercial chickens are gaining ground.

The lifespan of the bird isn't the only feature of the poultry industry that has been fast-tracked. In the US, slaughterhouses can run at speeds as high as 175 birds per minute (faster than EU law allows). This delivers cheaper and cheaper chicken, but it has created a system in which some poultry plant employees in the United States have claimed the pressures of the production line led to them wearing diapers instead of taking bathroom breaks.

When something goes wrong in large and intensive systems, in which sheds house thousands of genetically uniform birds, it can go wrong on a frightening scale. In developed economies, years of research and investment have resulted in highly advanced biosecurity measures, with close veterinary supervision, but this industrial model of poultry production is now being rolled out in places where these resources and skills are in shorter supply. This, some animal disease experts argue, is how more zoonotic illnesses could be incubated. Things can go wrong even in more advanced economies. In South Korea, home of the Yeonsan Ogye, in October 2020 an outbreak of avian flu began to spread with a ferocious speed through the country's commercial flock. Within the space of a few months, farmers had to cull more than 20 million birds. Chickens in all systems are vulnerable to avian flu. However, when a virus finds its way into large-scale intensive systems, as this example shows, its spread between birds can be rapid.

The homogenisation of chicken is happening just as we're recognising how much poultry diversity matters. Around 1,500 locally adapted indigenous breeds are thought to exist globally. These birds are genetically diverse, highly adapted to their surroundings and have evolved to scavenge in a wide range of different environments. In less developed economies, these indigenous birds still provide around half of all the poultry meat and eggs people eat, but as commercial farming operations spread further around the world these local breeds are being lost. In an increasingly unpredictable world, facing the impact of climate change, we would be wise to preserve the diversity of these animals. We might need to call on their wider gene pool one day.

There is no Millennium Seed Bank or Svalbard for chickens. Instead, there are people such as Lee Seung Sook, the saviour of the Black Ogye in South Korea, on her farm in Yeonsan. Without the efforts of small-scale farmers and amateur enthusiasts in different parts of the world, hundreds of breeds of chicken would have been lost long ago. Fortunately, diversity is out there, but it's mostly being stored in back gardens. Bigger efforts include the British National Poultry Collection, located in an out-of-the-way field under a flight path in north Somerset. This modest set-up is where some of Britain's most endangered breeds have been preserved. I was shown around the collection by the great poultry expert Andrew Sheppy, who pointed out birds admired in their day, including Nankim Bantons, near-extinct Brussbars and the once famous Ixworth. 'None suited to the intensive system,' said Sheppy, who passed away in 2017. Asked which one he would choose for pure taste, he said, without hesitation, the Marsh Daisy. Its feathers were light brown, its legs willow green and it had a rose-coloured comb over its head. 'The flavour's beautiful,' Sheppy told me. Then again, all of the birds were, each in their own different way, beautiful.

If we cannot bring diversity back, what else can we do? The temptation will be to keep intensifying the system, build even bigger sheds and continue to 'improve' the genetics of the bird. Greger Larson, Professor of Evolutionary Genomics at Oxford, an expert on the domestication of the chicken, was once told the story of a poultry shed in Brazil. Inside the enormous building, the numbers and density of the birds had become so great that they had started to turn on each other in acts of aggression, a serious and not uncommon problem in the poultry industry. As a result, chickens were dying, and profits were down. But in one corner of the shed, a group of birds were behaving differently. They were calmer, quieter and there was no aggressive pecking. 'It turned out they were all blind,' says Larson. 'Oblivious to much of what was going on around them.' Could a blind bird be the Chicken of Tomorrow?

The idea was explored in the 1980s, using a line of birds which were born blind due to a genetic mutation. Like the ones in the Brazilian story, the chickens displayed no signs of feather-pecking or acts of cannibalism. 'They did not appear to have any other obvious welfare problems, and they were more productive,' said a review of the experiment years later, adding that the scientists involved 'were of the opinion that blind hens could play a role in future ... This seemed, so to speak, to be a win-win situation: Farmers would make more money and hens would live better lives.' Bigger, faster and, for our benefit, even blind? Among animal ethicists, this is called the 'Blind Hens' Challenge'. We might not have all the information we need when we select some chicken to eat, or perhaps the income to explore every option, but we are all players in the Blind Hens' Challenge and we need to ask ourselves how far are we willing to go? This is why we need to know the history of chickens. We need to be reminded how different our relationship with these animals used to be, when they were highly revered.

15

Middle White Pig

Wye Valley, England

The pig was another unlikely candidate for domestication. Sheep, cows and goats made sense; humans couldn't digest grass, but these animals could and became a source of milk, meat and so much more. In contrast, pigs looked like competition. Their teeth, jaws and digestive systems are closer to ours than those of ruminants and, given the chance, pigs are capable of ruining crops in fields and devouring stores of grain. But around 8,000 years ago, pigs became indispensable to farmers. Agriculture and settlements created food surpluses and waste, from grain husks to 'organic matter', including human faeces. Pigs happily ate it all, converting it into fat and muscle, in turn becoming a living food store for humans. As with sheep and chickens, killing a pig for meat would have been delayed as long as possible. Kept alive, they were a source of something far more valuable: manure that fed crops. Long-distance migration was helped by pig domestication. With these portable living larders, people could travel into the unknown and, with animals they could breed on arrival, avoid starvation. The first humans to settle remote islands in the Pacific, for instance, only managed to do so because they were accompanied by pigs.

Before pigs were brought into human settlements, hunter-gatherers had always tracked and killed wild boar for meat. The first tentative steps towards taming pigs must have happened in the same way as with dogs. Wild boar that came close to humans in search of food but were too aggressive were killed; those that were too timid and fearful didn't make it close enough to access food. But passive boars comfortable in the company of humans were the ones people started to interact with. The pig domestication process took place at different times and in different places. How and where this happened is important, because it explains how the pig became one of the most industrialised and globally traded animals in the world.

Inside the Taosi cemetery in northern China, a sprawling Neolithic site discovered in 1999, archaeologists found evidence of pig domestication buried among the thousands of graves. Along with jade jewellery, exquisite pottery and musical instruments were complete skeletons of pigs. In this society 4,500 years ago, pigs were symbols of prosperity, worthy companions in the afterlife. In a later Han dynasty burial site, 2,000 years old, the symbolism is more sophisticated. Instead of skeletons, clay models of pigs had been placed inside tombs. Both of these sites provide clues to how, for thousands of years of Chinese history, the pig was not only an animal to be kept close in death, but also in life.

Pigs were so important in Chinese societies because rice farming using the paddy system resulted in a great increase in China's population. By the time of the first recorded census during the Han dynasty in 2 CE, more than 60 million people were living and farming in dense settlements around fertile river valleys and the North China Plain. In these highly populated settings, pigs couldn't be left free to roam and forage, putting crops at risk, so they were raised in sties and fed at troughs. Terracotta models made at the time depict pigsties set below homes so that waste generated by humans dropped down to be eaten by pigs. Completing the cycle, the pig's manure enriched soils, helping farmers produce more food and feed more people. The central (and intimate) role pigs played in Chinese domestic life was captured in language; the character 家 (jiā), which means 'family', 'home' or 'house', was designed thousands of years ago by adding one symbol (for a roof) above another (the pig). The word for 'meat' in Chinese (肉, rou) refers solely to pork; all other animal flesh needs to be identified by species, for example 'cow meat' (牛肉) and 'sheep meat' (羊肉).

With pigs an essential part of the ecosystem, farmers created breeds suited to specific environments, mostly round, pale, short-legged and pot-bellied pigs, among them the Meishan, one of the oldest, if not the oldest, domesticated pig in the world. This docile animal was adapted to live at close quarters with humans in confined spaces and it thrived on a diverse diet. Across China, more than a hundred other breeds of pig could be found; their chief role, right through the Communist era under Mao, was to act as fertiliser factories on four legs. Pigs were slaughtered only at times of crisis or celebration, their meat a rare luxury. As with sheep on the Faroes, when animals were finally killed, every part was used. Pig faces continue to be served whole as a delicacy in China and pig brains are cooked to be 'soft as custard, and dangerously rich', as Chinese-food expert Fuchsia Dunlop puts it. The pig's stomach, intestines, tails, ears and jellied blood are also widely enjoyed. Because of their genetics, and the diet they were fed on, the meat from these ancient breeds was fatty, which in turn shaped Chinese cuisine, from *mei cai kou rou* (steamed pork belly with mustard greens) to the rich flavours of vegetables fried in pig fat.

In Europe, humans took pigs on a completely different path. From early efforts in the Fertile Crescent, pig domestication spread west and happened in fits and starts. From the Neolithic to the Bronze Age, human populations in Europe were less dense than in China, so agriculture was less intensified, and deforestation happened at a slower pace. As a result, different European populations independently evolved systems in which pigs were left semi-domesticated (or, put another way, semi-wild). The animals were mostly free to forage in forests, feeding on 'mast' (from Old English *mæst*), meaning beechnuts and acorns. The extent of human involvement was to help fatten the pigs up by knocking more food off branches using long sticks. This 'pannage' system, in the hinterland between tame and untamed, was widespread in Europe. It began to decline during the High Middle Ages around a thousand years ago, as Europe's population more than doubled and the Continent was deforested, but pannage systems survived in isolated pockets well into the sixteenth century. The red woolly Mangalica pig in Romania is a legacy of this ancient and highly seasonal system, as is the pure-bred Iberian in Spain and the Cinta Senese in Italy. In the New Forest in England, pigs still roam free during the 'pannage season', between September and November. By rooting around, they help new plant life to grow and enhance the forest's ecosystem.

Because of this different route to domestication, European pigs looked and behaved differently to Chinese breeds. For one, they still had close contact with boar populations, and so acquired traits of these wild animals; they were more aggressive, more agile, longer-legged and far leaner (they could roam up to four miles a day in search of food). Their litters also contained fewer piglets than their Asian cousins. And people were wary of these pigs. In medieval Europe, hundreds of pigs were executed in animal trials, held following acts of 'murder' by feral boars or sows. Because of these factors, ruminants (cows, sheep and goats) were much more important to settlements, and the pig was a marginal creature. But what happened next helped turn the pig into one of the most intensively reared animals not only in Europe but also the world.

In eighteenth-century England, an agricultural revolution as well as an industrial one was under way. Robert Bakewell's ideas had started to improve livestock, and many pig breeds were developed as farm animals, even becoming a feature of city life (converters of waste in breweries and dairies). But then English breeders hit something of a brick wall. The European pig was neither productive nor suited to larger-scale production. This is when Asian pigs were introduced. Citrus, spices, tea, silk and porcelain had been arriving into Europe from Asia since the early seventeenth century, and in the early eighteenth, animal breeds too. Chinese pigs were mentioned in the 1760 *Farmer's Compleat Guide*: 'The small low bellied hog is hardier and feeds on anything; it produces a great many young and is in many cases preferable to the other [the European pig].' As another farming source explained, the Chinese pigs were also admired 'for the Sweetness of their Flesh' and 'for the delicacy ... of roasting'. English farmers began using the Asian pigs for breeding and in doing this found they could double the number of piglets in their litters, increase the number of teats on sows, lengthen a pig's body (in some cases by two vertebrae), and change the temperament of their existing pigs, making them more suited to being confined. The stage was set to create pigs for the industrial age.

All of the existing British breeds were transformed with the arrival of Chinese pig genetics, including the Wessex Saddleback, a hardy pig that had evolved out of the pannage system of the New Forest. Its numbers grew as dairy industries in the south-west expanded, creating waste for the animals to eat. The Gloucester Old Spot, meanwhile, was an 'orchard pig'; it proliferated as cider and apple businesses developed. In England's grain belt in the east, the Berkshire, a pig with a long pedigree (Cromwell mentioned it in dispatches during the English Civil War), was also cross-bred with Chinese pigs. By the 1850s, with the help of Asian genetics, Britain was the epicentre of livestock breeding. One of the breeds produced during this intense national effort was the Large White (so named because of its white skin), and also known as the Yorkshire after the county in which it was first developed. But a different breed, a variation on the Large White, the smaller-sized Middle White, was then the most popular pig in Britain. Compact and suited to the urban masses, it was also named the London Porker. It fed on household scraps and food waste which is why up until the 1930s, from the backyards of London to the mining villages in the north-east, it was Britain's pig of choice. But by the middle of the twentieth century, like most of the other British breeds, this pig was as good as extinct and the Large White was on course to take over the porcine world.

Soon after the Large White was officially registered as a breed in 1868, British farmers started to export it, first to Europe, then around the world to Australia, Argentina, Canada, Russia and America. In its favour was impressive productivity; it had a long body and put weight on quickly. It was also versatile, happy indoors and out, and produced excellent bacon and pork. Cooperatives set up by Danish farmers were among the first to buy Large Whites as breeding stock, and they used it to produce an even more productive pig, ironically called the 'Landrace'. This pig helped Denmark become the most efficient pork-producing country in Europe, so much so that by the 1930s, British farmers were struggling to compete with Danish imports. Following the war, in a desperate bid to prop up Britain's ailing pig industry, the government set up a committee to tackle the problem. Its conclusion, published in 1955, was that British pig farming was being held back by diversity; there were too many different breeds of pigs. It recommended the nation focus on a single type of pig for commercial production.

And this is exactly what happened. Farmers began to focus on the Large White, or variations of it (including Denmark's Landrace). In the 1970s, following more recommendations from the government, these breeds were modified again as new dietary advice to reduce saturated fat in diets meant the animals had to be made leaner. Older breeds were replaced, leaving a narrow selection of more productive ones. In 1973 (the time of Harlan's 'genetics of disaster' warning), a group of concerned British farmers took action, and set up an organisation to prevent animals going extinct. Among the first of the breeds recognised by the new Rare Breeds Survival Trust was the Middle White. By then, the number of these pigs across Britain had dwindled to double figures.

In search of a Middle White pig, I travelled to the idyllic Wye Valley in the west of England, where Richard Vaughan runs Huntsham Court Farm. The estate dates back to the 1650s, and the family's local roots go back further to the twelfth century. Now in his seventies, Vaughan seems like a country gent from another era, but in his twenties he turned the family farm into one of the most modern and intensive beef operations in the UK. In America he had studied how farmers reared livestock, and with their methods he sped up meat production back on his farm and used new types of high-energy feed. 'I reduced the time from birth to slaughter to less than a year,' he says. 'The poor animals had no chance of a good life but the retailers wanted cheaper and cheaper meat.' A chance conversation changed his outlook on meat production. He happened to phone up the abattoir where he sent his animals for slaughter and from where the beef usually went straight to supermarkets. Vaughan asked the abattoir if they could send him a sample of his beef so he could taste it for himself. 'Roars of laughter came down the phone,' he remembers. 'They told me my meat was worth selling but not eating. It wasn't worth the effort.' The animals had been raised so quickly and slaughtered so young they hadn't only missed out on a life, but also their meat lacked any flavour.

Disillusioned, Vaughan turned his back on the meat business and converted the estate into a farm park. If people weren't prepared to spend good money eating animals, he thought, perhaps they'd be prepared to pay more to pat them. He included some rare breeds, among them Middle White pigs, recommended by the Rare Breeds Survival Trust. When their numbers grew, he had to slaughter some, which resulted in a revelation. 'I had never tasted meat like it,' he says. Unlike the modern breeds, Middle White pork came with good layers of fat, which made it succulent and gave it heaps of flavour. Convinced by nothing more than that memorable flavour, Vaughan decided to become a pig farmer to conserve the Middle White through consumption.

At Huntsham Court Farm, Vaughan took me to see the cosy lamplit stalls where the pregnant sows are kept. There, we watched a new litter of piglets, crowded around their mother's teats on a carpet of hay. She looked like the kind of pig you would see in a children's book, large, sticking-up ears and a shoved-in snout. 'The friendliest pigs you'll find,' said Vaughan. These pigs like to enjoy life in the slow lane, both in terms of how they grow and how they reproduce. 'They get to live a life, which is how all meat should be produced.' The pigs at Huntsham (around sixty sows) account for most of the world's population of Middle Whites, a conservation made possible not only because of Vaughan's stewardship of the breed but also because of growing demand for the meat. Many of Britain's top chefs, captivated by the flavour and the provenance of these pigs, have added the meat to their menus. Set against the modern breeds, rearing Middle Whites is like being in a Formula One race with a Model T Ford, says Vaughan. 'I just can't compete, and I don't want to, pigs are too precious for that.' In a world where high-yielding breeds take precedence, the Middle White is now rarer than the Himalayan snow leopard.

The fate of the Large White couldn't have been more different. It now populates the largest industrial pig units in the world, including America's. These are places capable of housing 30,000 sows and producing 800,000 piglets a year. In units like these, pigs can be immobile for most of their lives, receiving feed and water, vaccinations and antibiotics in stalls where they stand on slatted floors. These floors are designed to allow pigs' manure and urine to drain out into giant lagoons. The state of North Carolina has thousands of these lagoons, and they contain so much waste, no one has yet come up with a solution of what to do with it all. Pregnant sows live in gestation crates that are 2m by 60cm, something the animal behaviour expert Temple Grandin equates to a human living in the economy seat of an aeroplane (sow stalls, used in 75 per cent of American farms, have been banned in Britain since 1999 and Europe since 2013). Researchers say antibiotics used as growth promoters by the industry since the

1950s have contributed to the rise of drug-resistant bugs that are now considered a serious public health risk. The industry says the threat has been exaggerated.

This model of pork production is becoming a global one, all made possible by the genetics of the Large White crossing the world, replacing traditional breeds. The Large White (or the American Yorkshire as it became known) arrived in the United States in the nineteenth century, but farmers only started to develop the breed after the 1940s (around the same time as the Chicken of Tomorrow). The breed helped in the expansion of the pork industry in Illinois, Indiana, Iowa, Nebraska and Ohio before eventually ending up in every state in the US. By the end of the twentieth century, the genetics of the American Yorkshire had become the most studied of any pig as breeders dedicated their efforts to making it even faster growing as well as larger and leaner. Today, from Brazil and India to Vietnam and, increasingly, China, the Large White is being used to create an unprecedented level of scale and homogeneity in the global pig population. For a food system that needs to become more resilient, this is a problem.

In January 2019, a few seconds of footage taken from a mobile phone, reportedly in China, found its way on to social media. The video shows thousands of pigs, still alive, being dropped from a lorry into a deep, wide pit. Some could be seen climbing over others in a futile effort to escape. These pigs are believed to have been destroyed and then buried. This was said to be a snapshot of the desperate measures China was taking to deal with one of the worst outbreaks of an animal virus in living memory. The disease, African swine fever (ASF), decimated China's pig population. By summer 2020, the disease had killed 180 million animals, nearly half of the country's pig population (a quarter of all the world's pigs). According to the World Organisation for Animal Health, the intergovernmental organisation which coordinates responses to disease outbreaks, it had become 'the biggest threat to commercial livestock seen by our generation'.

ASF is a shocking condition. It begins as a high fever, then turns a pig's skin purple before causing bloody diarrhoea and a discharge from the animal's eyes and nose. It is incurable; death follows within days. The virus has brought painful deaths to hundreds of millions of pigs, and for Chinese people it has meant rocketing food prices. The Chinese government has been forced to access its gigantic emergency reserves of frozen meat, and the disease has had a domino effect on global meat prices as China has turned to the rest of the world for pork.

In February 2019, ASF crossed into Vietnam, the world's fifth largest pork producer. There, by the autumn, the virus had resulted in the death of 5 million pigs. It then spread into Laos, Cambodia, North Korea and Mongolia, and by the summer of 2020, the infection had entered Europe. ASF has also reached India. So far, the United States hasn't seen a single outbreak of the disease, though some experts in animal diseases believe it's only a matter of time before it does.

China was forced to quickly rebuild its pig population before meat shortages and higher prices became serious political issues. The only way it could do this was to look to breeding companies in the West and pig genetics based around the Large White/American Yorkshire. These pigs do fly, and in the spring of 2020 more than 4,000 breeding sows were transported by plane from breeders in France and the Netherlands to China. This is just the start of a bigger transfer of pigs from Europe and the US into Asia; the exact reverse of the situation in the 1700s when Asian animals arrived and transformed pig breeds in Europe. The scale of this twenty-first-century exercise is, however, very different. Some reports have put the number of gilts (young females) needed to restock the country at 10 million. Although the Chinese government has created a gene bank (basically a giant freezer of pig semen) in an attempt to preserve the country's traditional breeds, in the coming years many more of China's pig breeds will disappear, and this pig from Yorkshire which was transformed in America will be used to create yet more global homogeneity.

16

Bison

Great Plains, USA

The mass slaughter of bison that took place on the American Great Plains in the nineteenth century was the greatest destruction of any wild animal witnessed in modern history. It began in the 1820s and, after six bloody decades, the creature was as good as gone, a silence falling across the plains. It remains the most chilling example of one animal species directing its destructive powers against another. These bison roamed a vast ecosystem that took up most of the interior of America; 1,500 miles from Montana in the north, all the way down to Texas in the south, stretching from the Rocky Mountains in the west to the lower Missouri River in the east. The Great Plains were the closest America had to the African savannah, a place teeming with wildlife, but with the bison's annihilation, these grasslands were changed forever.

Estimates vary widely. Thirty million bison are believed to have inhabited the Great Plains itself but if you add the animals scattered across the rest of North America, from the prairies of north-western Canada and down into northern Mexico, the total population could have been 60 million. No one really knows. Individual herds were so huge (in some cases twenty-five miles long) it took days for people on horseback to pass them. Their numbers seemed limitless but this was far from the case. In 1883, a group of hunters described watching a herd of 50,000 buffalo moving northwards towards Canada. They expected the animals to be back on the plains within months, and that, to resume hunting, all they had to do was wait. But the bison never did reappear. What those hunters had seen is likely to have been the last of the great herds, and all of them were slaughtered before they even reached Montana.

Conscious of the bison's impending extinction, in 1886 the National Museum in Washington sent the taxidermist William T. Hornaday out west to hunt and kill one of the remaining bison. This way, they figured, future Americans would get to see the animal, even if it was a dead one, stuffed and standing in an exhibition. Hornaday reported back to the museum that he had found and slaughtered three bison: 'The Old Bull, the young cow and the yearling calf were killed by yours truly. When I am dust and ashes, I beg you to protect these specimens from deterioration and destruction.' They went on display in March 1888. Within a few years, fears of the bison's extinction had come to pass; the carnage on the Great Plains had continued and the wild buffalo population, Hornaday calculated, was down to around one thousand animals.

People who would never get to see or feel a herd of 50,000 animals racing through the landscape (literally a ground-shaking experience) could instead stand in front of the artist Albert Bierstadt's ten-foot-wide painting called *The Last of the Buffalo*, completed in 1889. The foreground is filled with dead and injured buffalo. Skulls from older kills litter the landscape. But the central image, surrounded by the vastness of a dry golden meadow and distant mountains, is a man on horseback, a Native American, about to drive a spear down into the neck of a charging bison. The foreground might be an example of skilful realism, but the background is pure fiction; there are bison grazing as far as the eye can see. A book published the same year had a title that told the real story: *The Extermination of the American Bison*.

This was a human tragedy as well as an animal one. Since the last Ice Age, indigenous people and bison had shared the Great Plains, and Native Americans both worshipped and hunted the animal; it was central to their existence. Bison fat and muscle provided food, its skin gave shelter and clothing, its bones were fashioned into tools and its sinews turned into strings for hunting bows. With the disappearance of the bison, Native Americans lost not only a crucial source of food, but also a way of being in the world.

How and why the slaughter happened is still contested. Some argue the extermination was politically motivated, part of a strategy by the US government and army to clear indigenous people off the Great Plains so the West could be taken. Others point to greed, plain and simple; the bison became a commodity to be killed, butchered and sold off by meat packers, hide traders and bone dealers.

A more recent and compelling account adds the cattle industry into the equation. The making of America's modern meat industry, this argument goes, depended on a remaking of the Great Plains, where cows replaced bison.

Today, there are close to 100 million cattle in the United States, most of which can be found in a massive strip that runs down the centre of the country, including all the plains of the Dakotas, Nebraska, Kansas, Oklahoma and Texas. Seen this way, one grazing animal has been replaced by another. This was also the case with humans on the Great Plains as Native Americans were evicted so ranchers could move in. The argument that cattle and beef pushed out the bison has been put forward by historian Joshua Specht who reasons that 'ranchers weren't just the beneficiaries of this process they were also agents of conquest'. It's likely all three of these factors – a state-backed land-grab, capitalism and a growing beef industry – were playing out together. The outcome, however, remains the same: Native American nations were forced onto reservations, the bison were pushed towards extinction and the entire ecosystem of the Great Plains was transformed.

The Great Plains was one of the wonders of the world. 'An American Serengeti, a place of poetry and spectacle, where there were wild horses, gray wolves and coyote,' says another historian of the West, Dan Flores. 'Cattle drives, "Indian wars" and the buffalo hunt, all of this took place here, the history of the West unfolded on the Great Plains.' The bison were there long before any of those human dramas played out. One hundred and thirty thousand years earlier they had crossed a land bridge that ran from the Siberian Steppes to graze alongside mammoths who had been on the Great Plains for millions of years. The bison was a 'keystone species', an animal that helped the entire ecosystem to function. They foraged, aerated the soil with their hooves, fertilised it with their manure and helped spread seeds across the plains. This created habitats for other species; birds such as long-billed curlews and Cassin's sparrows all co-evolved with grasses and vegetation grazed by the bison over millennia. In turn, this bio-diversity sustained millions of wolves, prairie dogs and the deer-like pronghorn. According to Beth Shapiro, an evolutionary biologist who has studied the rise and fall of the bison, the only other invasion of North America that has had such an ecological and environmental impact is that of our own species. Humans migrated along the same land bridge as the bison, perhaps as far back as 20,000 years ago and, until the last two centuries, bison and people managed to coexist.

Spanish conquistadors were the first Europeans to see the Great Plains bison after they arrived in Colorado's San Luis Valley in search of gold. While Native Americans hunted on foot and with bows (it took fifteen arrows to fell a bison), the Spanish changed the balance of power with horses and rifles. Then, in the early nineteenth century, American ranchers set their cattle and sheep loose to roam the prairie, creating a new source of competition for the bison. With more fire-power at their disposal, the ranchers also made a serious dent in bison numbers, but it was during the 1860s that the slaughter intensified. By then, the trade in buffalo robes and bison meat was growing, and an army of bison hunters were working their way across the Great Plains. By the end of the Civil War in 1865 there were 2 million rifles in circulation in the United States, and more than a million veterans trained to use them. Some had nothing to go home to; their farms or homesteads had been burnt out in the conflict, but with a gun and a mule they could become bison hunters. It was the perfect storm. One million individual hides were shipped out of Kansas in 1872 alone. As the West became increasingly weaponised and competition over land escalated, Native Americans were also drawn into the trade, selling hides and meat in order to survive.

Bison hides, supplied by American and indigenous hunters alike, were sent east on the newly built Union Pacific Railroad and then around the world. At their destination they could be turned into anything from insulation for wagons and coaches to drive belts for factories, from material for shoemaking to luxury furniture. Tougher than cattle hide, buffalo skins were sought after by Americans and Europeans alike. Newly invented refrigeration meant bison meat could also be transported further afield, including pemmican, a traditional Native American food made from dried and ground-up bison fat and meat. This product became industrialised, the meat processed in fac-tories, canned and sent across the new frontier. Workers extending the railway out west also created more demand for bison meat, as did the new army camps based along the route. When the trains started to run they brought a new influx of hunters to the Great Plains and shooting bison out of carriage windows became a sport. A railway engineer working on the Santa Fe line that travelled through Colorado and Kansas said it was possible to walk for miles alongside the track stepping from one bison carcass to another. Bison bones were put to use by the fertiliser industry, sugar processors and in pottery making. But most of the slaughter was just a tragic waste; many meat buyers were only interested in specific cuts, such as the tongue and parts of the hump, so countless bison were killed only to have most of their carcass left rotting on the ground.

Towards the end of the 1860s, as the bison population plummeted on the Great Plains, cattle ranching quickly replaced it. By rail, beef could reach Chicago, the epicentre of the meat trade, with ease, and so America's love affair with beef began. The extra supply of meat made possible by clearing the plains was so vast that towards the end of the century, 140,000 tonnes of US beef were being shipped across the Atlantic to England each year. Meanwhile, immigrants newly arrived in America from the Old World (people who would have been used to only eating meat on rare occasions) must have found the displays of beef in markets and butchers' shops overwhelming.

In 1906, the journalist Upton Sinclair published *The Jungle*, one of the most famous protest novels of the twentieth century. In it he captured the experience of exploited meat workers and gave stomach-churning accounts of slaughterhouse filth. The book sent shock waves around America and bolstered the Federal Meat Inspection Act, which was passed the same year. Sinclair had intended his account of the meat industry to serve as a critique of industrial capitalism but this, it seems, was lost on readers, who were more worried about the unhygienic conditions their food was being produced in. Sinclair said later of his book, 'I aimed at the public's heart, and by accident I hit it in the stomach.' As Joshua Specht curtly puts it, 'He hoped for socialist revolution but had to settle instead for better food labelling.'

Millions of Native Americans were by now living on reservations, where cruelty, corruption and incompetence too often led to starvation. Those who survived were sold beef from the cattle now reared on the plains. In a further insult, the meat was of such poor quality, rejected as it was from the slaughterhouses of Chicago, it was barely edible.

There were efforts to save the bison. States including Idaho, New Mexico, Wyoming and Arizona introduced restrictions on hunting and the trade in meat and robes. But the laws came too late, and some were even passed after the animals had disappeared. It wasn't until 1900, with a federal law called the Lacey Act, that trade in wild animals was banned. What really saved the bison from total extinction was a small and incongruous set of people who were spread out across the Great Plains, a group consisting of a Texas cattle rancher, a bison hunter from Kansas, an adventurer based in Canada, a Native American living on a reservation in Montana and a trader working out of South Dakota. Independent of each other, in the 1870s and 80s these individuals realised what was happening to the bison and so, on their ranches, they took in a handful of bison calves to help save the species (the adults proved too difficult to handle). These orphan calves were each paired with a milk cow.

Some of the bison saviours had only conservation in mind (the Texas rancher Charles Goodnight had been encouraged by his wife to try to preserve the bison). Others saw the bison as an increasingly rare and potentially valuable species with a commercial use. This was the view of hunter Charles Jesse Jones (better known as Buffalo Jones). In 1886 a severe blizzard ripped across the Great Plains and wiped out three-quarters of the cattle; the hardier bison came through it unscathed. Jones began to cross the bison he had saved with his cattle to make a new animal that would be as hardy as the bison but with the meat quality of a cow (the hybrid became known as a Cattalo). These preservers of the bison may have had different motivations, but their actions brought the same outcome; most of the bison alive on the Great Plains today are descendants from these five foundation herds, which in 1888 numbered less than two hundred animals combined.

In 1903, William Hornaday, now a determined conservationist, moved some of the surviving bison to the newly built Bronx Zoo (of which he was a director). At first the zoo was a safe haven for the animals, but with the help of President (and fellow conservationist) Theodore Roosevelt, it played an important role in helping to restock the Great Plains. Hornaday and the owners of the five foundation herds were pioneers; considered today as instigators of the first serious effort to save a large mammal from extinction, and so providing a model for much of the conservation work now taking place around the world.

The biggest bison population in America today, the 5,000 within Yellowstone National Park, was made possible because of animals sent from the Bronx Zoo and the other foundation herds. In 2016, more than a century after the Great Plains bison had been all but eliminated, reflecting the place of the bison in the national psyche, President Obama named the animal America's 'first national mammal'.

Although there are thought to be half a million bison in the USA today, only a small proportion of these are pure bison. This is partly a consequence of the early conservationists crossing the wild animal with cattle, a practice that continued into the early twentieth century in an effort to rebuild bison herds more quickly. Now, with gene sequencing and selective culling, cattle genes are slowly being removed. Many projects in which bison are being reintroduced to the Great Plains are on Native American reservations. One is a partnership between Jennifer Barfield, Professor of Animal Reproduction at Colorado State University, and the Kiowa and Navajo tribes. Barfield has spent years increasing the numbers of genetically pure bison. Before the animals are transferred to the Great Plains, members of the tribes give them a blessing. Barfield had been focused on the job of making 'bison babies' (her words) but watching some of the ceremonies forced her to re-evaluate her work. During one, she was standing beside a pen where the bison were being held before their release onto the plains. 'The animals knew something was happening,' she says. 'They were restless and moving their feet.' When the ceremony began and the tribal leaders started to sing their buffalo song to the beat of a drum, all movement stopped and the animals fell silent. She'd spent a year with those animals and knew them really well. Usually when the bison heard unfamiliar sounds, their senses were heightened and they became agitated, but all Barfield could see here were bison eyes peering intently through the spaces of the fence. They were completely still, transfixed by the drums. At that moment she knew she was involved in something that went beyond science, genetics and conservation. 'A different kind of connection was going on between these animals and the tribe,' she says. Perhaps that was palpable. Outside hundreds of people had gathered to watch the bison be released out into the open, some hiking for miles to get there, 'and when the animals burst out into the open and started to run across the ground, people started crying'.

In my own search for bison, I found myself on a sand dune in the San Luis Valley of south-west Colorado, the wind howling around me and grains of sand prickling my face. With thirty square miles of sand dunes, some that tower 750 feet high, the valley is part *Lawrence of Arabia* and part spaghetti western, where trails in the distance disappear through mountain passes. The earliest recorded description of this scene comes from a 27-year-old American soldier, Zebulon Pike, in 1807. Along with twelve frostbitten and hungry companions, he had made it through a pass on foot. With his telescope, he looked down on the dunes that 'extended up and down the foot of the White Mountains ... Their appearance was exactly that of the sea in a storm, except as to colour, not the least sign of vegetation existing thereon.' In the far distance, though, there was plenty of wildlife: short-horned lizards, sandhill cranes and immense herds of bison.

Huge piles of bison bones have been discovered on the edge of these dunes. Eleven thousand years ago hunter-gatherers herded the animals over a precipice and to their deaths, the most effective way of getting their meat. Right up until the 1870s, before Ute Indian tribes were moved onto reservations, Native Americans lived among the bison in this area, shifting their settlements around south-western Colorado as herds migrated through the grasslands. Today, this place is home to one of the most ambitious projects aimed at bringing bison back to the Great Plains. This is Zapata Ranch, a 100,000-acre reserve which was bought in the 1980s by a Japanese-American architect Hisa Ota. His original plan had been to turn the ranch into a high-end resort, but when he started reading about the history of bison in the area, he became fixed on the idea of helping bison return. Ota started buying up bison from private collections and bringing them to the ranch. By the late 1990s, Zapata's bison herd was in the hundreds. This is when he handed it all over to the Nature Conservancy Trust, which now runs the ranch and takes care of the bison.

The landscape around the ranch consists of high plains desert, dry creek sand beds, running springs, vast meadow and, as Theodore Roosevelt had once described, the 'shimmering, tremulous' cottonwood trees with their green leaves set against the dust. My first glimpse of bison was three females drinking from one of the creeks that did have water. Each was as big as a horse, with horns that curled forwards in a C-shape. Winter was coming and their chocolate-brown winter coats were becoming shaggy. They looked powerful but there was something nonchalant about the way they lazily lapped up the water, lifting their heads up every now and then to give me a short stare. 'They're checking us out,' said Kate Matheson, who is Zapata's ranch manager, adding in reassurance, 'Don't worry, they're not aggressive.' Their nostrils were wide and their long triangular heads were covered in fluffy hair finished with the tuft of a goatee. Although they look heavy and cumbersome, bison can, for a short distance at least, hit speeds of more than thirty miles per hour and outpace most horses. Driven by powerful haunches which rise to a hump and then slope down along their back, they look like prehistoric cave paintings made flesh.

As we drove further into the expanse of Zapata Ranch, we passed four male bison calves, each the size of a fully-grown Great Dane, teenagers with awkward-looking twisted horns. Born in the spring, their orange coats were now becoming thick and dark, ready for the winter when temperatures here can drop to as low as −40°C. Nearby was a group of adult males. They would soon be moving off to spend their time in bachelor herds but for now they were still mixing with females, sniffing the air to check if any were 'cycling' and ready to breed. These bulky, tank-like animals weigh around 2,000 pounds. Further on, we stopped the jeep, and a thousand bison surrounded us. I watched spellbound as they looked up and stared, and then, ever so slowly, got back to the business of eating grass.

The plan at Zapata is the same as Richard Vaughan's rescue mission for the Middle White pig: conservation through consumption. Each autumn an audacious exercise in herding takes place as a network of fences is erected around the ranch. Wranglers (modern-day cowboys and cowgirls) then use motorbikes and a small plane to round up bison. Seven of the animals keep Zapata's log cabin restaurant stocked with bison meat for an entire year. The rest of the cull is sold to chefs across the state, raising money for the conservation project and helping to spread awareness of the bison. The meat is tender and a little coarser and gamier than beef, chewier (in a good way).

The extermination of the Great Plains bison took place 150 years ago, but the extinction process of other animals goes on. Instead of targeting an individual species in the way hunters on the Great Plains did, we're destroying entire ecosystems. Since 1970, it's estimated that deforestation and the conversion of wild habitats for human food contributed to populations of vertebrates dropping by 60 per cent on average. The research, published by WWF, provides evidence that biodiversity is being lost at an unprecedented rate. Can we become stewards, rather than the destroyers, of the planet? The story of the bison shows us our immense power to annihilate but also, as demonstrated by the work at Zapata, our ability to restore species and rebuild ecosystems. We humans can get things wrong, but we can make things right too.

Spillover

Covid-19 started as a meat story. The first reports pointed to wild animals as the origin of the virus (specifically bats) which then jumped to an intermediate species (possibly pangolins) before making its way into the human population. Early on in the outbreak, a 'wet market' in Wuhan, central China, thought to be the origin of the virus, was closed down. At markets like these, supply chains dealing in animals from all around the world can converge: live and dead animals, wild and domesticated, legal and illegal, from civet cats and porcupines to wolf pups and snakes (as well as farmed meat and seafood). Many animals are kept alive in confined spaces and under great stress until their slaughter, creating the kind of conditions in which viruses can thrive.

As the pandemic extended around the world, media reports described wet markets as a traditional feature of Chinese food culture. They aren't. The big live animal markets didn't exist before or during the Cultural Revolution. They're a modern phenomenon which took off in the 1980s but only really boomed at the turn of the century. China's new wealth, and with it an appetite for new exotic foods, drew in animal species hunted across Asia, Africa and the Americas, all brought together by a trade network that's as impressive for its logistical dexterity as it may be horrifying in its consequences.

Among experts in zoonosis, the wild animal trade had long been a cause of concern, a new and risky setting for an old problem. Many of our most pervasive and long-running diseases made the leap from animals to humans, including smallpox, whooping cough, mumps, HIV and Ebola. Measles is thought to have emerged after domestication brought humans into close and prolonged contact with cattle. The earliest descriptions of the disease in humans come from the Silk

Road in the ninth and tenth centuries. At that time, urban populations were expanding and people were living close together, creating the perfect environment for a virus. Zoonotic diseases became one of the defining forces of human history. When Europeans carried smallpox and measles with them to the New World, millions of indigenous people died. Disease turned out to be the greatest weapon of the colonialists.

Covid-19 has already reshaped our world in the twenty-first century, and other more deadly diseases could be on the horizon. By extending agriculture's footprint and destroying forests and other habitats, we are breaking down barriers that evolved over millions of years. It's like shaking a snow globe; the wild and the farmed are being disrupted and mixing like never before, and contact between different species is taking place at a speed and intensity once thought impossible. Emerging diseases are now being linked to land-use change. One example of this was seen in Malaysia in the 1990s, when the country's pig industry was becoming more intensive, with new farms built to house more animals. These buildings encroached on wild habitats, where land was also being cleared to plant orchards. Wild bats started to come into closer contact with the pig farms, attracted by the fruit nearby and because their other food sources had been depleted by deforestation. In early 1998, droppings from these bats contaminated the swill being fed to the pigs with a disease called Nipah virus which then infected the pigs. It led to the near collapse of the billion-dollar pig industry in Malaysia and the deaths of 105 people. As the science writer David Quammen puts it, when we disrupt ecosystems, we shake viruses loose from their natural hosts. 'When that happens, they need a new host. Often, we are it.' And so they spill over from wild animal populations and into human ones. Perhaps Covid-19 will prove to be a wake-up call. We now have the most selfish of reasons to save biodiversity: our own welfare.

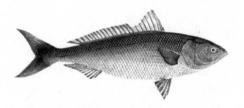

Part Five
From the Sea

'Some shoals were the width and breadth and depth of
towns, which meant weeks of enormous catches ...
They were eternal, a natural plunder that would never
fail. But they did fail.'

Jane Grigson

In her 1951 book, *The Sea Around Us,* the marine biologist Rachel Carson wrote that, 'even with all our modern instruments for probing and sampling the deep ocean, no one now can say that we shall ever resolve the last, the ultimate mysteries of the sea'. Seventy years on, many of these 'ultimate mysteries' still haven't been solved. The chapters in this section of the book also explore mysteries of the sea, including the severe decline and near extinction of several creatures. Some disappearances we can explain, but there are many we can't. And although we're not even sure exactly how many life forms are at risk of extinction, we do know one common factor in their decline is us.

To help get a sense of the problem, in the summer of 2007, three hundred scientists from more than ninety countries set out on an impossible-sounding task: to catalogue the total number of known species living in the oceans. Impossible-sounding because the surface of Mars has been more thoroughly mapped than the deepest parts of the Earth's oceans. Estimates of the number of species range between 700,000 and 2 million.

Over a decade into the big count (part of a project called WoRMS, the World Register of Marine Species), the number so far stands at almost 240,000. This changes on a daily basis as new species are added to the list, from molluscs to mammals and from fish to crustaceans. 'We don't think we'll ever have the full picture,' says Tammy Horton, one of the scientists working on WoRMS (she's in charge of some of the crustaceans, 10,000 species and counting), 'too many species are going extinct before we can count them.'

It took billions of years for life to evolve in the oceans, followed by millions of years for a mind-boggling amount of diversity to be created. But it's taken us little more than a century to dismantle it. Since the advent of industrial fishing the decline of some fish species has been truly shocking; Pacific bluefin tuna down 97 per cent from historic levels; and Mediterranean swordfish, 88 per cent. In more recent times, keystone species such as the Pacific sardine have seen populations crash by as much as 95 per cent.

The global fishing effort that's driving much of this decline is worth around $100 billion a year, and illegal boats net a further $10 billion to $23 billion worth of fish. Our activities out at sea are so wide reaching that two-thirds of all ocean areas have been 'significantly altered' by human action; in other words, marine wilderness itself is disappearing.

We believed the oceans contained a limitless supply of food, and we became far too good at extracting it. Steam-powered trawlers joined sail-powered fishing boats in the 1880s, followed in the early 1900s by diesel-powered vessels capable of going further out to sea to fish in deeper waters. The invention of nylon in the 1920s didn't just revolutionise how we dressed, it transformed how we fished, being used to create fishing lines and nets that could stretch for miles. At the same time, it became possible to fast-freeze fish on board boats, meaning fishers could stay out on the oceans for longer. When sonar technology designed to track submarines in the Second World War was deployed against shoals of fish, it was as if a new underwater war was being waged against wildlife. In 1954, one of the world's first factory trawlers was launched, the *Fairtry*, capable of processing 600 tonnes of fish a day. It became a floating gold mine and others soon followed. There are 4.6 million fishing vessels in the world today – China alone has up to 800,000 boats including a 17,000 strong deep water fleet – many of which would make the *Fairtry* look like small fry. There are fewer and fewer places for fish to hide. Deep below the ocean, some trawlers can emit momentary pulses of electric current that cause fish to cramp their muscles and become motionless, making them an easy catch for the nets that follow.

From a purely selfish point of view (thinking of the sea as a source of human food) this is a problem; 3.3 billion of us depend on the oceans for protein. Global consumption of fish per person has doubled on average since 1990 and the rate looks set to continue increasing. But from a planetary point of view, extracting life from the sea in such quantities is proving disastrous. By targeting so many large adult fish, we have depleted the ocean of eggs, fry and food for other species. The same applies to the smaller fish we catch to feed farmed salmon, seabass and bream. Entire ecosystems are being disassembled and complete food chains demolished. And with this decline in marine life, something fundamental to our very being also goes.

Before our ancestors became meat eaters 2 million years ago, early humans were finding food from the sea, catching fish and foraging for molluscs. Fishing is most likely the oldest, most widely practised and continuous form of food gathering in our history. For *Homo sapiens* it led to the creation of coastal communities and riverside settlements, and food from the sea shaped cultures and forged identities. Each of the four endangered foods in this section reflect some of that cultural history, and they also illustrate how many traditional societies, like the fish they depend on, are now endangered.

This isn't the first time we've had to rethink our relationship with the sea. One thousand years ago, people in Northern Europe were living through a fishing crisis. Excavations of fish bones from that time show how, in the space of just fifty years, the population was forced to make a major shift from eating freshwater fish caught in lakes and rivers (pike, bream, trout and salmon) to marine fish such as cod, plaice and herring. Freshwater stocks had been overexploited and as a result people began building bigger boats and bigger nets and headed out to sea in search of new species. The team of scientists at York who identified this shift called it the 'fish event horizon' and 'the ultimate origin of today's fishing crisis'.

History teaches us that we can preserve and not just decimate fish stocks. In the thirteenth century, King Philip IV of France raged over the decline in fish stocks, declaring, 'Each and every river and water-side of our realm, large and small, yields nothing due to the evil of fishers ... the fish are prevented by them from growing to their proper condition.' He ordered nets to have larger meshes so that young fish could escape, and protected miles of rivers and streams. Today we need to adopt more ambitious, global measures, but as Philip understood eight hundred years ago, we need to catch less and conserve more. We also know the problem today is far more complex than the 'evil of fishers'. Climate change is diminishing marine populations, in some areas by one-third, as increased carbon dioxide levels in the atmosphere are acidifying oceans, threatening the complex web of sea life.

The chapters which follow show us the forces at work that are reducing the rich diversity of ocean life, some of them little known. There are diseases and disappearances that can't be easily explained; we can see evidence of their impact, although we don't fully understand what is happening. Carson might be right: we may never resolve 'the ultimate mysteries of the sea'.

17

Wild Atlantic Salmon

Ireland and Scotland

Atlantic salmon are paradoxical fish. On the one hand they now count among the rarest of the ocean's animals: few of us will ever get to see one (or eat one). Yet, thanks to fish farming, the Atlantic salmon is also one of the most ubiquitous animals in the world. Within a few decades, aquaculture has taken the salmon from being an exclusive delicacy to a global commodity and the single most traded fish on the planet. It could be that 10,000 years after we began to tame cattle, pigs and sheep, we are taking a fish species along the same path, a domestication process in which the animals disappear from the wild but flourish in captivity, in this case occupying the ocean inside underwater cages. But we must worry about the fate of the wild Atlantic salmon. As a natural barometer of the state of the Earth, this fish has no rival. Its ability to transform itself from a freshwater creature to a saltwater one and then back again means its life cycle takes it from inland rivers, out to the ocean and then home again. Through the salmon we can see the cumulative effect on the natural world of a host of human activities, from deforestation, dam building, pollution, overfishing and the drivers of climate change. Its decline is an alarm being sounded for what's happening on both land and sea. If we want to save the salmon, we have to stop destroying the planet. It's that simple.

The life cycle of this enigmatic fish seems miraculous. In the gravel of its home stream, a female will lay a cloud of around 8,000 eggs which males then compete to fertilise with their milt (sperm). Eight weeks later, tiny alevin hatch out of large, golden-yellow eggs and for the next thirty days live off the contents of their yolk sac. From small fry, they grow into larger parr, by which time they're big enough to leave the shallows of their gravelly home and swim out to deeper and more dangerous parts of the river. Here, a salmon has to survive for up to three years and find enough food to grow to 15cm in length and become a 'smolt' with enough muscle to enable it to make an epic ocean journey. This involves thousands of miles of endurance swimming in the Atlantic to reach the rich feeding grounds in the north. Then, if it's lucky enough to have survived predators and storms, two or three years later it will swim against the current, overcoming any obstacles in its way, to return to the exact spot of gravel from which it hatched. Here, in the place that marks the start and the destination of its journey, it will spawn. Of the original 8,000 eggs laid, just two can be expected to live long enough to complete the salmon life cycle, one of the most astonishing in nature.

To leave their freshwater river home and swim into the salt of the ocean, the salmon undergo a physical transformation called anadromy, a trait that evolved millions of years ago as the oceans cooled and became a richer source of food. This enables the salmon to 'smoltify'; its body becomes more streamlined and its skin more reflective and silver, better camouflaged for the sea. Highly territorial and aggressive as a river fish, its temperament mellows as it moves into deeper water and congregates with other salmon to form a shoal. Further down-stream towards the sea, it will get its last chemical 'fix' of the water it's about to leave. It is believed this 'imprint' helps it to find its way back home after thousands of miles at sea. In estuaries, where fresh and salt water meet, the salmon transforms its gills and its breathing changes to suit a new environment so it can swim out close to the surface of the ocean. Here, it will feed on crustaceans, squid, small fish and large zooplankton such as krill. But these hunters also become the hunted. Among their predators are cormorants, sharks, sea lions, seals and, of course, humans.

This incredible undertaking happens right across the North Atlantic, involving salmon populations in the 2,000 or so rivers and tributaries that thread through Europe and North America. Atlantic salmon can be found from Norway in the north to Spain and Portugal in the south, Russia in the east and Canada in the west. But wherever their origins, Atlantic salmon converge around the same feeding grounds, on the west coast of Greenland and off the Faroe Islands. Here, each fish doubles in size and builds up reserves that will insulate it from the cold of the North Atlantic and fuel its return home.

Much of this life cycle should be included among Rachel Carson's 'ultimate mysteries'. We don't really understand how the salmon finds its way back to its river (it could be a combination of memory, smell, solar navigation and use of the Earth's magnetic fields), or how it knows it is time to return. We do know that the salmon will do anything to get back home. Along the forty-mile run of the River Finn, near the town of Cloghan in County Donegal in Ireland, the salmon come up against what appears to be an impossible barrier. Water gushes down a waterfall ten feet high, a violent deluge over hard rock. From the pool at the bottom, the fish move forward and then attempt leap after leap. Some seem to bounce their way up in stages, tail flipping off the water or the surfaces of rocks, while others manage heroic leaps that appear to get them clear in a single effort. At this stage in its journey home, the fish is living off its reserves. Once back in the river, for the days, weeks or months it takes to get back to its birthplace, it stops eating. But years spent feeding out at sea means the fish is at the peak of its powers, and for predators waiting on the riverbank (humans and other animals) the condition of the salmon on its return can't be bettered.

The poet Seamus Heaney, an angler from childhood, fished for salmon to the east of the Cloghan falls in County Donegal. He would watch their still-silver bodies, with blue-green scales and torpedo-like heads, breaking the surface of the water, driven on, he says, by the pull of their home water. When Heaney's poem 'The Salmon Fisher to the Salmon' was published in 1969, the total population of wild Atlantic salmon was around 10 million. Today, it's less than 2 million. To put that into perspective, a different species, the Pacific sockeye salmon (from the same evolutionary pool 20 million years ago), returns to its rivers in the tens of millions. This is why the decline of its Atlantic cousin is so scary. Fifty years ago, for each of the one million salmon that left rivers around the Atlantic, half returned to lay eggs and complete their life cycle. Today, only 30,000 will do so. Despite a global effort to understand what is happening, we're still not entirely sure why the fall has been so colossal. For any species, there comes a point at which the number of individuals becomes so small its future is problematic, which is why the extinction of wild salmon from much of the Atlantic and its river systems is a real possibility.

*

Plotting the earliest encounters between humans and any species of fish is complicated; soft bones and skin don't leave many clues in the archaeological record. Some of the oldest evidence of human inter-action with salmon comes from a cave in Georgia in the Caucasus, where Neanderthals left behind a cluster of large salmon bones dating back to around 45,000 years ago. By around 25,000 years ago, *Homo sapiens* were not only catching and eating salmon, they were cele-brating them in cave art. In the Dordogne region of France near the town of Les Eyzies on the Dordogne River, a hunter-gatherer carved an image of a salmon on the soft limestone of a cave ceiling. It must have taken many hours to create the exquisitely detailed, metre-long image with hundreds of tiny marks on the salmon's tail, fin and gill. Its upturned jaw and gasping mouth show a fish fighting against the current, exhausted and on a mission to return home to spawn. Sur-rounding the ancient carving are a set of altogether different markings: straight, deep lines, most definitely not pre-historic. In 1912, someone had unsuccessfully tried to carve the fish out of the rock and take it away from its home – a metaphor for what humans have done to this fish for millennia.

More evidence of salmon's importance to early settlements around the Atlantic has been found not in art, but in soil. Archaeologists have discovered one of the earliest of Neolithic settlements in Ireland, close to Seamus Heaney's favourite river, the Bann. Nine thousand years ago, equipped with harpoons and fish traps made of wicker and clay, hunter-gatherers here survived on salmon. The fish was also important to the Sami, the nomadic people who live in the north of Scandinavia and parts of Russia. Four thousand years ago, along the Tana River that runs through Norway and Finland, Sami fishers used wooden boats to go from pool to pool, baiting salmon. On the rivers Tywi, Teifi and Taf in Wales, salmon were traditionally netted from a coracle, a round boat guided by a paddle, just big enough for a single fisher to sit in. In Cumbria they still practise haaf netting which involves walking through shallow waters and catching fish in something that looks like a football net. On the other side of the Atlantic, ancestors of the Penobscot people used spears and birch-bark canoes to catch salmon as they ran up the rivers of New Brunswick and Nova Scotia each spring. In these cool climates, it wasn't possible to use salt to preserve the fish (not enough sunlight for evaporation). Instead, the

salmon were buried underground and left to ferment (creating a food
with the same levels of funkiness as Faroese *skerpikjøt*). Later, in the
first century, Pliny mentioned Gauls living by the rivers of Aquitania
in south-west France who preferred salmon 'to all the fish that swim
in the sea'. It was around this time the fish got its name. Roman
legions watched in amazement as salmon moved upriver in the Rhine
Valley, pushing on through rapids and up waterfalls, and named the
fish *salar*, 'leaper', contributing to its scientific name, *Salmo salar*.

On the east coast of Scotland, there were people equally in awe of
the fish; in the seventh century, the Picts, before they vanished as a
culture, erected standing stones with carved images of leaping salmon.
One shows a fish hovering between a viper and a mirror; its symbolism
is another salmon mystery archaeologists are still trying to solve.

Other evidence points to wild salmon being a high-status food. One
thousand years ago – at the height of the fish event horizon – inside
the medieval Abbaye de Cluny in Saône-et-Loire, central France,
monks left behind an unusual record. They spent much of their lives
in enforced silence, depending largely on sign language to commu-
nicate. A guidebook to that language, written in 1090, shows the
symbol for 'fish' was made by placing the palms of both hands together
and wiggling them in front of your chest. The salmon, however, had
its own symbol, made by placing the thumbs under the chin. This
was understood to show only 'the very proud and rich are accustomed
to have such fish'.

Because of its high value, in thirteenth-century Ireland, each catch,
sale and purchase of a salmon was strictly recorded. As the biggest
landowners, monasteries had control over most rivers and much of
the trade. This was a lucrative business in which tonnes of Irish salmon
were salted, packed in barrels and shipped to ports in France, Spain
and Italy. By the seventeenth century, according to accounts, these
cargoes were so big, the sight of them 'would startle the common
people'.

It's also from Ireland that some of the most detailed accounts of
the salmon's decline were made. At the end of the nineteenth century
a writer named Augustus Grimble travelled the country researching
salmon. The salmon suffering the most, Grimble said, were those in
the River Bann, in the north. 'Poor Bann!' he wrote. 'We have never
come across a river so unfortunate as this one. Others suffer from one

or two, or perhaps several of the evils ... but for the unhappy Bann there exist in their strongest form every conceivable evil that is deadly to salmon life.' These 'evils' included pollution from the linen industry that had built up along the river. Waste from the factories, including lime, bleach and dyes, was poured into the river and 'destroyed all vestige of fish life'. Laws had been introduced, 'but the fines are small, and the disgrace is nil'. Meanwhile, the fish that did survive were being netted to excess. 'Heavy poaching', as Grimble described, was common and out at sea there were 'miles of nets illegally worked under the eyes of the coastguard'.

The Bann might have been an extreme case, but these pressures from the land and out at sea had an impact on salmon populations across Europe. Runs up and down rivers that had evolved over millions of years were being blocked by ever larger dams. The salmon, relentless as always, attempted leap after futile leap towards these giant concrete obstacles until they died. As fewer and fewer salmon got to complete their life cycle, their role in the lives of communities along rivers also declined. In 2016, in the Delana River in County Cork, where a dam was built after the Second World War, when a fisherman reported seeing two salmon swimming, it made newspaper headlines. It was the first sighting in more than fifty years.

Tougher environmental laws helped many of Europe's wild salmon rivers revive during the 1950s, but the decline seemed set, and the fish's numbers never fully recovered. In the rural communities of Ireland where wild salmon endured, it was a food to be savoured well into the 1960s. Richard Corrigan, a celebrated chef who grew up during this era, lived on the boglands of County Meath, west of Dublin, where the salmon appeared once a year. He'd hear the sound of the farm gate being opened in the early hours as a fisherman friend of the family left a hessian sack hanging at the back door. Inside the kitchen, out of the sack, came a flash of silver and a heavy thud as the salmon fell onto the table. His father would take an old carving knife, reserved for these rare gifts from the river, and cut the fish into thick steaks which he cooked in a cast-iron pan with a slab of butter. 'We longed for the smell of the oil of the salmon,' says Corrigan. Pieces of soda bread soaked up the fat and every mouthful was eaten slowly, in silence. 'We had no money, but on those mornings, we ate like kings.'

Despite its rarity and the precarious state of the fish, there was no let-up for the salmon. Humans kept hammering away at the population. Since the time of the Vikings, fishermen along the Irish coast have taken boats out from the shore to drop small seine nets in the water. Shaped like parachutes these nets could be pulled up out of the sea, hopefully with a catch. As a child in the 1960s, Ken Whelan, Ireland's foremost salmon scientist, watched fishermen huddled together by their boats in Kenmare Bay waiting for the arrival of 'the fish', as they described a big shoal. For weeks they had studied the water, looking for a V-shape to appear on its surface, the sign of salmon entering the bay. When it was sighted, a wave of excitement swept through the village. 'Most of the fishermen were in their sixties,' says Whelan, 'but they moved like lightning to get their nets in the water.'

One time the shoal was so big that when they tried to pull it up, the weight of it forced the net onto a rock and the fishermen lost most of the salmon. They seemed dejected when they came back on land, but one smiled and said to the onlookers, 'Ah well ... that one's for the river.' These fishermen understood the inefficiency of the way they were fishing. 'That's why it worked,' says Whelan, 'there was always plenty left for the river.'

But in the late 1960s, seine nets were being abandoned in favour of drift nets. With one end attached to a boat and the rest suspended by floats, drift nets could stretch for miles, and as they were made of fine-mesh nylon, they were invisible to the fish. Asdic sonar technology (one of the systems used during the war to hunt enemy submarines) was also used to locate the salmon. Two or three of these nets could cut off an entire bay, leaving nothing behind for the old boys with their seine nets and smaller boats. This became a boom industry, and for years fishing licences were handed out like confetti. 'Each net became a source of immense wealth,' says Whelan. By the late 1970s, with salmon numbers plummeting, attempts were made to put restrictions in place which resulted in the waters around Ireland's west coast becoming something of a war zone, with clashes between illegal drift-netters and fishery officials, including exchange of gunfire between naval patrol boats and nets-men. Eight miles of net could be confiscated in a single night. But there were worse problems for the Atlantic salmon further out to sea.

Their main feeding grounds off the west coast of Greenland, where salmon from thousands of different rivers converge in huge numbers, could now be targeted on an industrial scale. By the 1970s, fleets of large boats from Norway were catching between 2 and 3 million fish each year, more than the entire current population of the fish. It wasn't until the 1980s that an international treaty was put in place to stop the uncontrolled plunder. Today, most commercial salmon fishing is banned, and in Ireland only a handful of fishermen with historic licences get to work the estuaries. In Scotland, England and Norway, netting has also been severely reduced. And yet the salmon numbers keep falling. Something has gone badly wrong in our rivers and seas.

Ken Whelan points to changing ocean temperatures as one likely cause. 'In parts of the salmon's feeding grounds, the plankton have disappeared,' he says. At the same time, around the south coast of Ireland, new fish species have appeared. 'Trigger fish from the Caribbean and sea bream from the Mediterranean, brought in by warming waters and competing with the salmon for food. The oceans are changing and salmon are among the victims.'

Now the paradox. As their numbers in the wild head downwards, the total population of Atlantic salmon is experiencing a boom. At any one time, off the coast of Norway alone, it has been estimated that there are 400 million salmon swimming around in pens. Just ten of these enormous pens hold more salmon than the entire wild population in all the rivers, streams and seas in the Atlantic. As the wild fish declines, its farmed counterpart is thriving. Some people believe these two facts are connected.

Most of the world's farmed salmon is produced by a handful of Norwegian companies, including the Lerøy Seafood Group and Sal-Mar, but the biggest is Mowi. From its various operations based in the waters of Norway, Scotland, Canada, Ireland and the Faroe Islands, it produces nearly a quarter of all the salmon eaten around the world. Mowi's global reach has even allowed it to extend the natural range of the Atlantic salmon south of the equator as it also runs farms based around the Chilean coastline. I got to see Mowi's operation, from beginning to end, on Scotland's west coast. At the hatchery, I saw the tiny eyes of hatchlings pressing against the outer film of egg sacs, and then, at one of Mowi's twenty-five Scottish farms, I watched as hundreds of thousands of fish circled endlessly inside pens. Every now and then, an occasional salmon broke the surface of the water with a leap. 'I came into this business as a conservationist,' said Ian Roberts, the Mowi director who was showing me around. 'I want to prevent the last wild salmon being fished out of the ocean, I want to help provide an alternative.' Behind his thinking is the fact that most of the world's growing demand for fish in recent decades has been met by aquaculture. It's now the source of more than half of all seafood consumed by humans.

For the first seven months of their lives, inland from the Scottish west coast Mowi's salmon live inside a vast warehouse-like hatchery on an industrial estate in Lochailort. Every tiny detail of their existence is controlled and monitored twenty-four hours a day; by keeping stress levels low, rates of growth can be high. From the top of a metal staircase I watched as 150,000 fish swam in a clockwise circle around a large tank of sterile water. To trigger the physiological change in the salmon that turns them from a freshwater fish into an oceangoing one, a trickery of light is used. For several weeks the lights are kept very low, creating a 'false winter' for the fish, and then, by brightening the warehouse, spring arrives. When this happens, the fish start to circle the tank in the opposite direction and their gills and their skin begin to change. But instead of swimming down a river to head out to the sea, at the Lochailort site they're sucked through large pipes and into tanker trucks. All you can see is a flurry of dark shapes fighting the pull of the pump, the strongest swimmers catching the eye as they hold still inside the transparent pipe for a second. At the shore, a converted whale boat takes the fish to what will be their home for the next year and a half, a series of pens all held together by a cage inside a loch. After that, they're killed and processed. Half will be sold in British supermarkets, the rest will go overseas (farmed salmon is now one of the UK's biggest food exports).

One of the cages I saw was in Loch Leven, near Fort William, where Mowi produces 1,600 tonnes of salmon each year, a fraction of the company's global output of half a million tonnes. From the shore, the pens looked like a group of small islands in the centre of the loch. As the small boat brought me closer, I saw the metal poles holding the pens in place poking out of the water and the nets above that kept birds away from the fish. From the wooden deck that runs alongside the pens, every few minutes, there was a scattering sound, like shingle being kicked on a beach. This was an automatic spinner throwing protein pellets across the water. Below, hidden from view inside the sixteen pens twenty-two feet deep, half a million fish were feeding.

On current trends, the oceans will play a reduced role in feeding the world as catches decline, whereas aquaculture keeps on growing. An ancient practice which originated in China has really come of age. In the paddy system, fish provided pest control for rice plants and fertilised the crop with their waste. In the 1970s, aquaculture took a new and radical turn. Aware of the wild salmon's decline, two Norwegian brothers, Sivert and Ove Grøntvedt, started an experiment in growing these fish in captivity. They placed wild Atlantic salmon inside a net suspended in a fjord near their farm on the island of Hitra. The venture worked well enough for them to sell the fish and make a profit. Over the years, more Norwegian farmers picked up on the idea and copied the system. But they all began to realise something was holding back their productivity: the fish. Wild salmon grew too slowly, and the fish weren't that efficient at converting the feed they gave them into fat and muscle. What the farmers needed was the aquatic equivalent of the 'Chicken of Tomorrow' or the Large White pig. This is when a team of Norwegian animal breeders stepped in.

To help solve the problem, they had two hundred years of agricultural history to draw on. Robert Bakewell's eighteenth-century principles still held true, but they had also been advanced in 1940s America by the scientist Jay Lush who helped to transform America's meat industry. By applying the ideas of Bakewell and Lush, the Norwegian breeders managed to change the genetics of the wild salmon in a matter of years. Using fish selected from three different rivers, all with different traits, they bred a fish that would grow faster than the wild salmon and with less food. The first generation of fish grew 15 per cent faster than the previous generation; a decade later that had been doubled, and the breeders found themselves with a fish that was undeniably a salmon, but at a genetic level arguably a new breed. Some scientists see the differences between the farmed animal and the wild *Salmo salar* as so great, they refer to the new species as *Salmo domesticus*.

This was a significant breakthrough, for the Norwegian farmers and for the world. Green Revolution wheat and rice had filled empty bellies, livestock experts had created cheaper and more abundant supplies of meat. Farming salmon would enable more people to eat fish. The new fish, they believed, would provide a new source of protein while at the same time help tackle overfishing. As always, in reality, the trade-offs have been far more complicated.

Two weeks before I arrived at Mowi's fish farm on Loch Leven in February 2020, one of the company's pens further out to sea in Colonsay had been torn open. A battering from Storm Brendan had proved too much for the net and 74,000 farmed salmon had escaped into the wild. Placing pens further out in the more turbulent sea solves a problem experienced inland. Across the industry, waste – feed, faeces and chemicals – generated by pens, can have an impact on the marine life below and on a loch's ecology. In turn, the ecology of a loch can kill off an entire pen; thick algal blooms can overwhelm the salmon, damage their gills and suck oxygen out of the water. At this point, thousands of fish can be lost.

An equally distressing industry-wide problem is caused by the sea louse (*Lepeophtheirus salmonis*), a tiny crustacean, half a centimetre long. Because these parasites co-evolved with salmon in the wild, a fish might pick up a couple when they're out at sea, but as the lice can't survive in freshwater, they fall off on the salmon's return upriver. But a pen packed with tens of thousands of fish presents the lice with an unnatural opportunity, and once a pen is infested, they are able to multiply quickly. The lice move over the surface of the salmon in search of the softest tissue, around the face and gills, and once there, start to feed on the fish. If the damage is severe, the fish can die. These 'farmed' lice can spread out into the wider environment and pose a risk to the wild salmon population. Another concern for the long-term welfare of the wild Atlantic salmon are escaped farmed fish.

In the wild, there is more genetic variation between two salmon from different rivers than there is between one human and another. Over countless generations, each population of fish became adapted to its home: the length of the river, the strength of its current, the amount of food available, its temperature and the cocktail of tastes and smells in the water. These adaptations give each population of salmon in each river its own particular strengths and weaknesses, and provides it with its own unique and finely tuned life cycle. All of this is sustained by the wild salmon's homing instinct, its ability to get back to this same body of water and reproduce.

Farmed fish are different; they've been bred from a highly selected gene pool to do two specific things: eat a lot of food and grow quickly. They don't have the genetic toolkit needed for a life in the wild and the ability to make the journey between river and ocean and back again. When hundreds of thousands of domesticated fish escape from a pen, the risk is their genes will find a way into the wild population. It is possible for the farmed females to survive long enough to spawn, and their eggs can end up being fertilised in river systems. It's feared this introgression, the mixing of genes between wild fish and farm fish, could slowly change populations of wild salmon, making them more vulnerable to disease and predators.

Back in Ireland, after the wild Atlantic salmon fell into decline, so did a way of life. Sally Barnes runs the last smokehouse in the country that deals exclusively with the wild fish. She lives and works in the village of Castletownshend on the south-western tip of Ireland, five miles from the town of Skibbereen. Here, hundreds of smokehouses once received the fish from the spring and summer runs, and the buildings were busy with people skilled in the art of using salt and smoke to extract moisture out of the fish so that it could be preserved for hungrier days or longer voyages. Now, Sally Barnes and her one employee receive just over three hundred salmon a year, sold to her by the dwindling band of fishermen licensed to work the estuary.

Each one she cuts, guts and fillets by hand, and each fish will tell a unique story of the river it came from, its journey across thousands of miles of ocean and its struggle to return home. 'Something you don't get with the farmed fish,' Barnes says. Surgeon-like, she studies them to find out how to process each one; working out how much heat, how much smoke and salt and how much time is needed. She reads their bone and muscle structure and studies their layers of fat. Some-times the fish come in bruised from their travels, but these marks disappear as she gently massages the blood out of their muscles. Once they're resting inside the small smoking boxes, she moves flues and tinkers with draughts to get the smoulder of the beechwood shavings just right. To smoke a salmon takes Barnes between twelve hours and three days. 'It depends on the humidity,' she says, 'you read the world around you every time you smoke.' They come out a pale pink colour (and never bright orange) with a sweet and ever so gentle smoked flavour. After the smoke, armed with a pair of small tweezers, she goes through the fish to remove each tiny pin bone by hand. 'My work will come to an end soon,' she says. 'I could switch to smoking the farmed fish, but I don't want to make that compromise. I feel like I've become a wild salmon myself, a creature swimming against the tide.'

18

Imraguen Butarikh

Banc D'Arguin, Mauritania

For centuries, the Imraguen people survived as nomads on the coast of Mauritania in West Africa, living among the sand dunes and mudflats and fishing for their food and livelihoods. As the fish moved along the coast with the seasons, so did they. Now, the Imraguen, around 1,300 in number, are settled in nine villages in the Banc d'Arguin National Park, just below the Western Sahara, within reach of the richest waters off the coast of Mauritania. The park includes a vast open bay, the largest marine reserve in West Africa, which in 1989 was made a UNESCO World Heritage Site. Full of nutrients and thick with plankton, it is a perfect habitat for hundreds of fish species, migrating birds, monk seals and sea turtles. Traditionally, when shoals of fish arrived along the coast, the Imraguen waded out into the water, using long sticks to beat on the ocean surface, transmitting vibrations through the water and sending the fish towards nets arranged in a large circle. Some accounts describe pods of dolphins assisting the fishermen, lining up to push more fish towards the waiting nets. More recently, the fishers have used sail boats called lanches to reach deeper waters.

What the Imraguen caught and then processed was very special. The grey mullet (*Mugil cephalus*) is a 60cm-long, olive-green and silver fish. Around November, when the fish are ready to reproduce, they shoal in large numbers; the female fish get ready to release large clouds of eggs that the males then encircle and fertilise. If the Imraguen can catch a female before it has spawned, that's a real prize. Inside the fish's belly, they will find a pouch filled with around 20,000 bright yellow eggs held together by a delicate, paper-thin membrane. This is one of the most nutrient-rich and luxurious of all foods from the sea. After the men catch the mullet, back on shore the women carry out the meticulous procedure of removing the delicate 10cm-long pouches. Each pouch is hung on a wooden rack to dry in the wind and then pressed and salted until it becomes hard. By now, the egg sacs begin to look like curved pieces of smooth amber. These dry blocks of fat and protein are called *butarikh* in Arabic (meaning salt fish egg), and they can be stored for years. Caravans once carried the *butarikh* through the Western Sahara and on to North Africa. In the 1930s, French traders started buying the preserved egg sacs from the Imraguen to sell as an expensive delicacy in Europe.

Similar processing techniques are found in other parts of the world. Around the Mediterranean, preserved mullet eggs are known as bottarga or poutargue and in Japan, *karasumi*. In each of these cultures, dried egg sacs – known as roe – are a highly desirable food. Because they contain everything a baby fish needs, they are high in protein, vitamins, minerals and amino acids. Thinly sliced or grated, they add intense savoury flavours to food, with a taste ranging from Parmesan cheese to tropical fruit. For Imraguen people, *butarikh* has been a valuable product to trade and a form of medicine. 'It's an aphrodisiac,' one Imraguen woman whispered and then giggled, 'our version of Viagra.' But in recent decades a wide range of pressures from outside the Banc d'Arguin National Park have been bearing down on the Imraguen, pressures which have changed the way they fish, and, in turn, their way of life. Fleets of trawlers from Europe and Asia now operate along the West African coastline. This industrial-scale fishing activity has transformed the marine ecosystem of the region. How those industrial trawlers came to be in West African waters reveals much about the current state of our oceans.

From the time the first humans built boats and headed out into the ocean, the seas were a common resource for all. This changed in the second half of the twentieth century when, as tensions increased over access to fish and other natural resources out at sea, an international agreement was put in place. The United Nations Convention on the Law of the Sea, ratified in 1982, gave sovereign states control over the two hundred nautical miles of water from their coastlines, from the surface of the water to the seabed. This established Exclusive Economic Zones (EEZs) in which the right to fish was protected in international law. States without large fishing fleets could issue access agreements, allowing foreign boats to fish in their waters. Countries

which had overfished their own stocks could buy entry to more bountiful waters. This was the kind of arrangement the Mauritanian and
other West African governments started to enter into in the 1990s.
There was nothing new about this strategy. European boats fished off
the west coast of Africa in the early 1900s when stocks of pilchards
in the Bay of Biscay collapsed, and again in the 1950s when supplies
of albacore tuna fell into decline. Buying access to EEZs formalised
this strategy and paved the way for Europe's biggest boats to head to
some of the most diverse fisheries in the world.

Around two hundred trawlers, primarily from Spain, France,
Portugal, Italy and Greece, now fish along the African coast. These
boats are heavily subsidised by EU taxpayers under what are called
Sustainable Fisheries Partnership Agreements (SFPAs). Out of the
thirteen such deals in place in 2020, nine were with African states.
The EU pays Mauritania's government €60 million a year for an agreed
tonnage of tuna caught out at sea and smaller fish caught closer to
the shore (species such as sardinella, commonly used as fishmeal for
the aquaculture industry). Critics argue that the amount paid is only
a fraction of the real market value of fish caught (as little as 8 per
cent, according to calculations by the NGO Ecotrust Canada). For
European boats, this is a highly lucrative arrangement, and for European consumers it means a steady supply of fish in a continent where
overfishing has depleted domestic stocks. Almost half of the seafood
consumed in the EU now comes from outside European waters, and
the bulk of that fish comes from poorer countries.

Chinese boats, subsidised by government, are also estimated to
catch around 5 million tonnes of fish off the West African coast each
year. The word 'estimated' is important, as data on fishing activity
can be hard to come by: there's little monitoring, deals struck with
governments lack transparency and a large proportion of the fish
caught is unreported and potentially illegal. This is a global problem.
IUU fishing (illegal, unreported and unregulated) accounts for a fifth
of all the fish caught in the world and 40 per cent of the fish caught
off the coast of West Africa.

Most long-distance international fishing is only financially viable
because of the $35.4 billion per year spent by governments covering
everything from boatbuilding and fuel to ice and the cost of labour.
China pays the biggest amount of subsidy, $7.26 billion per year.

Without this funding it would be impossible for its fleet to fish thousands of miles away in Peruvian or Argentinian waters, or, for that matter, off the coastline of Mauritania. Africa's fishers have no way of competing with these subsidised industrial fleets and so don't get to fully exploit their own waters.

Much of the fish caught by the large trawlers along the West African coast is traded around the world, but some of it is landed and processed in Mauritania. Foreign-owned processing plants convert much of the smaller fish into meal for the aquaculture and livestock industries. Most of the factories in Mauritania are Chinese-owned and most of the fishmeal (and fish oil) is destined for China which, since the early 1990s, has been by far the single biggest producer of farmed fish on the planet. Its output is now greater than the rest of the world's aquaculture industries combined.

The trawlers aren't necessarily targeting the fish caught by the Imraguen, such as the grey mullet found closer to the coastline, but they can still have a powerful impact on a wider (and incredibly complex) food web. Fish spawn within protected zones, which act as nurseries, but the boundaries along these reserves are what marine biologists describe as 'leaky'. Fish move in and out as the seasons change, as do eggs and larvae, influencing fish stocks across a vast area.

In the 1990s as more trawlers arrived on the West African coast, grey mullet stocks started to fall and, along with them, a source of food and income for the Imraguen. Further along the coast, communities in Senegal had seen their own fish stocks decline and so fishermen in motorised pirogues headed into Mauritanian waters. With added pressure on the grey mullet and increased competition, the Imraguen started to use bigger and more powerful boats to reach further out to sea to target sharks and rays, both lucrative and also endangered. Fuelling this fishing effort was demand from consumers in Asia prepared to pay up to $500 a kilo for these species. Wholesalers from outside the Banc d'Arguin began to take greater control over the trade. When mullet stocks recovered, the Imraguen were no longer able to make a living through traditional fishing. They had become dependent on a global supply chain focused on other species. The people most affected in the Banc d'Arguin were Imraguen women who no longer had a regular supply of grey mullet to process and sell. Many were forced to leave the park, find work in the cities, or, like thousands of other West Africans from fishing communities, attempt precarious boat journeys to Europe. 'Industrial fishing by European boats creates more pressures on people in Africa to emigrate,' says Professor Daniel Pauly, a fisheries expert at the University of British Columbia, 'and when they arrive in Europe, people condemn them.'

The survival of the Imraguen fishing community is crucial to the future of the Banc d'Arguin. The park is their home, they depend on its biodiversity and are best placed to conserve the ecosystem. By law, they are now the only people allowed to live and fish inside the park. But the outside world keeps bearing down on their way of life, undermining more sustainable food traditions.

In an effort to counter this, in recent years, NGOs have stepped in with microfinance initiatives to enable the women to buy and process grey mullet that would otherwise be sold to wholesalers; other organisations have set up co-operatives and built workshops within the park. A town in northern Italy also contributed to this effort. Orbetello in Tuscany is one of the last places in Italy where traditional bottarga is made. With support from the Slow Food organisation the fishing community helped Imraguen women improve the quality of the *butarikh* and find customers in Europe. In 2015, more than two hundred Imraguen women were making *butarikh*. Since then, production has been in decline and the Banc d'Arguin remains under pressure. In 2020, the International Union for Conservation of Nature (IUCN) described the presence of the international fleets around the periphery of the Banc d'Arguin National Park as 'continuous and significant'. The assessment also described the park's conservation outlook as of 'significant concern' citing 'unsustainable fishing inside and outside' among the reasons. Efforts to revive the Imraguen *butarikh* mean an endangered food has been saved from extinction, but its future is fragile, just like the park itself.

19

Shio-Katsuo

Yasuhisa Serizawa is something of an endangered species. He lives in Nishiizu, a fishing town on Japan's south coast where he is the last surviving producer of one of Japan's oldest processed foods. Like the Imraguen, Serizawa uses salt, but the food he makes, called *shio-katsuo*, uses an entire fish, a skipjack tuna. As with *skerpikjøt* on the Faroe Islands, *shio-katsuo* is not a food for the faint-hearted and needs to be treated with great expertise and care. It's a leathery, savoury and super-salty product.

When I met him, Serizawa was holding an example of his craft, a half-metre-long tuna. Its silvery skin and white eyes were intact but its body was dry and coated in a fine dusting of salt. It was the most beautiful food I had ever set eyes on. Sprouting out of its mouth, through its gills and along its body, were golden bristles of rice stalks. The grass had been dried in the sun and softened with salt water so that the ends could be tied into large intricate knots. This artful threading of grass in and out of the animal's desiccated body had been done with such skill that every scale on the tuna's body remained pristine. Each fish takes Serizawa months to complete, and so he seemed as much an artist as a food producer.

The reason the fish is given such an elegant outfit in its afterlife is that as well as being food, it's also an offering to Shinto deities. At New Year, people in Nishiizu place the preserved fish in front of their homes and on public shrines. The woven rice grass represents a gift from the land to match the offering of the fish from the sea. 'At the shrines we offer prayers to keep the fishermen safe,' says Serizawa, 'and we ask for good harvests in coming years.' After the tributes have been paid, *shio-katsuo* becomes an ingredient; crumbled into a fine, savoury powder, it can transform the humblest of dishes.

Fishermen bring Serizawa tuna, usually caught in September when the fish are in peak condition, full of fat and muscle from months of feeding. The guts and the gills are removed immediately to avoid any 'off' flavours, but because of the fish's sacred status, the eyes are left untouched. The empty belly of the fish is then held open with bamboo skewers and salt is poured into the cavity and packed around the body, to slowly draw all of the moisture from the flesh. Two weeks later, the tuna is bathed in a special liquid prepared with juices saved from previous batches. This adds bacteria to the process and triggers fermentation, 'which makes it taste a little funky', says Serizawa. After the intense salting, pairs of fish are tied together and hung outdoors for several weeks under the shade of Serizawa's factory roof. It's then he'll begin knotting and plaiting rice straws, threading each one in and out of the fish, a daily ritual that goes on for weeks.

When *shio-katsuo* is disassembled from its ceremonial dressing, the flesh of the fish breaks into brown, yellow and silver flakes that glint. Added to rice and vegetable dishes, *shio-katsuo* adds big meaty flavours. Tiny pieces sprinkled onto a simple bowl of spinach can turn every mouthful into something unexpectedly complex. 'One plus one becomes three,' says Serizawa, describing the flavour transformation. And for more than one thousand years, just that sprinkle of *shio-katsuo* has helped turn 'poor' ingredients into noble ones.

A variation of *shio-katsuo*, better known and ubiquitous in Japanese cooking, is katsuobushi. Traditional versions of this rock-hard preserved fish can take six months to make and involve thirty individual steps. Like *shio-katsuo*, katsuobushi is made with skipjack tuna, but the process is more involved. First, the fish is smoked to dehydrate and harden its flesh which is then coated with spores of a fungus, *Aspergillus glaucus*. After the fish has been left to ferment for a week or so, it is dried in the sun and the mould is scraped off (the drying and scraping steps can be repeated multiple times). What is left is a light brown, hand-sized, curved object, supposedly the hardest food in the world. When shavings of it are added to kombu (the seaweed kelp) to make dashi stock, as with sprinkles of *shio-katsuo*, something magical happens. There's an explosion of flavour and a rush of umami caused by a chemical reaction involving enzymes, lactic and amino acids, peptides and nucleotides, all locked into the fish during the preservation process and now released.

Shio-katsuo is a far more ancient food, and one that has only survived as a local tradition around the town of Nishiizu. Now it is in the hands of Yasuhisa Serizawa, the last producer standing. I stared at the fish he was holding, still mystified by the straw that was sprouting out of its mouth and belly. 'How long would it take for me to learn how to make this?' I asked him, pointing at the fish. 'Fifteen years,' he said as he looked me up and down. And then, taking a closer look at my hands, 'Maybe twenty.'

The seeds of *shio-katsuo*'s decline were planted on 8 July 1853, when American Navy Commodore Matthew Perry reached the harbour at Edo (present-day Tokyo) and demanded an end to Japan's 220-year-long, self-imposed isolation. Until then, Japan's overseas trade had been kept to a minimum and had been tightly controlled; people weren't allowed to travel abroad or even build boats capable of ocean-going travel. Japan was mostly self-sufficient and, enforced by both Buddhism and Shintoism, mostly vegetarian. Stomachs were filled with rice, and flavour was provided by vegetables, pickles and soups, elevated by added ingredients such as *shio-katsuo*. Most animal protein came from the sea.

By the end of the 1850s, after Perry had issued America's demand, change was under way. Japan began trading again, exporting silk and tea and importing guns and cotton. Japanese intellectuals noted that the West was in ascendancy and that Asian nations were stagnating and heading towards decline. They also reasoned that Western power was fuelled on a diet of meat and dairy, whereas Japan was hampered by its vegetarian culture. A change in tastes was needed if Japan was to compete, they argued. In 1872, in what now looks like a PR campaign for animal protein, the government publicly announced to the nation that the new emperor had become a meat eater. Soldiers began to receive meat in their rations and new-style restaurants called *yoshokuya* opened where beef, pork and beer were served. Pigs were imported from Britain and introduced into Japanese cities, where they fed on urban food waste and helped to increase Japan's meat supply. The port of Kobe became an entry point for beef imports from America, gaining a reputation for meat that still endures.

This all added up to a seismic shift in Japanese food culture. Eating chicken had been taboo, and in most rural areas cows were considered to be a part of the family, even given burials. Shops that sold meat had often been regarded as places for social outcasts, frequented by 'heavily tattooed ruffians or Western-influenced students'. On the rare occasion people did eat meat, it was often for health reasons and treated as a medicine. By the early decades of the twentieth century, however, the only people shunning meat were the elderly who had been left behind by Japan's rapid transformation.

The food culture took another big shift when, after the Second World War and Japan's defeat, the American occupiers put a new plan in place to avert a food crisis. They imported wheat, skimmed milk powder and tinned ham (as happened on Okinawa). Rice consumption started to decline, from 170kg per person per year in 1962 to less than half that by 1986, just 71kg per person. Daily meat consumption, meanwhile, rose from 30g to 80g per person. This was when eating (now endangered) bluefin tuna became a Japanese 'tradition'. This fish is now one of the most desirable foods in Japan, and people assume it must be an ancient feature of Japanese cuisine. In fact, a century ago, bluefin tuna was seen as an oily, bloody, fatty and inferior fish, while the most favoured sushi ingredients in Japan were white fish such as flounder and sea bream, and seafood, including clams and squid. 'People would have looked down on a sushi chef selling bluefin tuna,' says Trevor Corson, an expert on Japanese food history. 'It was a garbage fish.' What changed its status was the post-war arrival of lots of red meat. Bluefin tuna had the same look and texture as the tenderest beef, and so it became increasingly fashionable in 1970s Japan as the national taste shifted towards these different flavours and textures.

At this time, the country was also in the middle of its technology boom, exporting cameras, electronic gadgets and optical lenses in the cargo holds of aircraft to North America. Instead of flying these expensive planes home empty, a logistics team at Japan Airlines looked for products to bring back and sell. One of the team, Akira Okazaki, discovered that sport fishermen along the North Atlantic coast were catching bluefin tuna and throwing them away. The airline created a refrigeration system to transport these enormous fish back to Japan. This supply chain helped make bluefin tuna the ultimate aspirational food, as well as one of the most endangered fish in the oceans. With appetites tuning in to new, meatier foods, who needed *shio-katsuo* or the modest bowl of vegetables it helped elevate?

Yasuhisa Serizawa hasn't given up on it though. He has vowed to continue his work as Japan's last *shio-katsuo* producer. Each year, he and a group of friends in Nishiizu enter a local cooking competition to remind people about this special ingredient. One year they made a dish of udon noodles with seaweed, spring onions and dashi sauce topped with a poached egg and the transformational sprinkle of powdered *shio-katsuo*. 'It was so tasty,' says Serizawa. 'We won the competition.' His big worry is that he doesn't have any children to follow in his footsteps and that the art of making *shio-katsuo* won't be carried on. 'I was born in this workshop and I refuse to let this tradition die.'

20

Flat Oyster

Limfjorden, Denmark

The Limfjorden isn't the most hospitable place to visit in late October; the ocean inlet on the west coast of Denmark is exposed, cold and grey, and as you look out across the shallow waters towards the horizon and the sea (usually obscured by rain), it would be generous to describe the place as alluring. This body of water, however, is among the most exceptional in Europe. Living on the sea floor, among the pebbles and sand, is one of the world's most endangered sea creatures, one that goes by various names: native oyster, European oyster, flat oyster and *Ostrea edulis*. In other European waters, populations of this bivalve are close to extinction. Ninety-five per cent of the oyster reef habitats where this species was once found have been destroyed. The additional pressure of two centuries of overfishing, disease, and attacks from parasites and predators have taken this species to the brink. The Limfjorden is one of the few places left where enough animals have survived in sufficient numbers for it to be harvested from the sea. Which is why I was here.

In the shelter of the trees along the shore, I put on a pair of thick rubber waders and eased myself into the sea until the cold winter water was around my waist. In my hand was a long, wooden pole with what resembled a kitchen colander at the end. 'The oysters will look like stones,' my guide, a local fisherman called Peter, explained, 'but stare a little longer and you might see a flash of green from their shell in the water.' I pointed the colander down towards the seabed, scooped and lifted back up, and among the gravel and seaweed were three grey-green discs. Taking one in the palm of my hand, its flat surface looked like slate, ever so slightly flecked with browns, yellows and gold, like autumn leaves. On the other side, a pattern fanned out in a spiral, running from the tip of the shell to its outer rim. It could have been an ancient fossil. Peter lifted an oyster from the sieve and tapped. 'Heavy. There's a lot of meat in this one.'

No one knows for sure why these oysters have survived in the Limfjorden when they've disappeared elsewhere. One idea is that the water in the inlet is so cold that oysters can exist here – just – while the usual oyster parasites and diseases can't. It's also shallow enough for the summer sun to attract enough phytoplankton (microscopic algae) for the oysters to feed on. In this way, the Limfjorden is an extremely rare ecosystem for the oyster, its very own sweet spot.

Even if you don't eat oysters, you should still care about their fate. It is a keystone species and supports other life in the oceans. Each day, an individual oyster will filter and clean 200 litres of seawater and, as they build up in numbers, they create a safe haven for other sea animals: about a hundred or more different species can live on and among oyster beds. When oysters accumulate in the millions (and even billions), they construct buffer zones that can help protect coastlines from erosion. The oyster is also one of the most delectable and healthy foods on the planet. When a character in a Saki story spoke of 'the sympathetic unselfishness of an oyster', he was completely right.

As a food, oysters have the amazing power of being able to transport their eater to a particular place and time. It is one of the few animals we eat when it's still alive, and one of the very few we eat every bit of (except its shell): its muscle, its belly and digestive tract, its heart, its gills and its blood. All of it in a single mouthful. Each of these parts has its own distinct flavour and texture. Whereas the muscle is chewy and sweet, the belly contains the flavours of the plant life the oyster had lived on. One oyster might taste grassy, another of olives or cooked greens. The oyster's 'blood' (or, at least, the fluid that makes up its circulatory system) is mostly seawater, another great variable that will influence its flavour. Some live in highly salty seawater, while others come from brackish water where freshwater rivers meet the ocean, giving the oyster less of a briny bite.

And then there's the time of year. Before the depths of winter, when oysters go into a state of hibernation, they gorge and fatten. This is when they are at their most plump and taste sweetest. In the spring, when the sea comes back to life and the oyster starts to feed again, their flavour changes once more. Summer, however, is when the oyster goes into its reproductive phase and more gamey flavours arrive as the oysters fill with eggs and sperm. By the time it has finished spawning in August, it will have used up most of its resources and be at its skinniest (the reason why we're told to eat oysters when there's an 'R' in the month). Other variables will be at work when you taste an oyster. Was it warm or cold when the oyster was harvested? Was it raining? Were streams bringing lots of nutrients into the sea? An oyster can be a reflection of time, place, climate and genetics. Some expert eaters claim they can shuck open a shell, chew the animal, drink in its salty liquor and identify the part of the coastline where it was harvested. Tasted this way, oysters are the closest thing to wine the sea has to offer.

Back on the shore of the Limfjorden, Peter took a knife and prised open an oyster. The animal sat phlegmatic against the iridescent inner shell of mother-of-pearl. I tipped it into my mouth and slurped in the sweet-salty taste of the sea that day. A metallic tingle filled my mouth. Peter the fisherman had grown up in one of the villages nearby. He was in his twenties and an oyster fan, but his parents and grandparents were not. Although they lived with millions of oysters all around them, none of the older generation had eaten a single one. 'They thought they were disgusting and used them as fishing bait.' Now these oysters had become one of the most endangered and sought-after foods in the world. Which is odd, because from the time of the earliest humans through to just over a century ago, the oyster was one of the most common foods of all.

One noticeable feature of the Limfjorden are the occasional low-lying 'hills' that punctuate the flat landscape. These are human-made, millions of discarded oyster shells that built up over thousands of years. They're called middens (from the Old Danish *mødding*, meaning a waste heap) or *køkkenmøddinger* ('kitchen midden'). Both terms were coined in the nineteenth century by a biologist called Japetus Steenstrup, who realised many of the bumps on the northern Danish landscape were the remains of an ancient diet.

Middens show up along coastlines all over the world. They can be as long as a kilometre and as old as 40,000 years, and big enough to dwarf Stonehenge. Each midden tells a story. Some ancient shell mounds were used as shelters, a protective barrier both against the elements and invaders (the sharp and noisy shells acting as a deterrent). One ancient Japanese midden is formed into the shape of a horseshoe with hearths and cooking pits in the middle, as if people had slowly built a living space around them as they consumed and then discarded the shells of hundreds of thousands of oysters. In Australia, indigenous people who lived on the coast performed rituals within the mounds, the shells seen as a physical legacy of their ancestors. In Gabon, West Africa, giant middens four metres high, spanning 2,500 acres, have been found around Iguela Lagoon. Here, one million enslaved Africans were held before they were sent on ships across the Atlantic, and as oysters were the only food available they became their last meal before the gruelling and often fatal crossing.

In Denmark, pottery and tombs filled with human bones have been found buried inside 7,000-year-old middens. Within the Limfjorden, the Krabbesholm middens run for a kilometre along the coastline, formed of millions of shells of *Ostrea edulis*. These middens, which are twenty metres wide, are among the earliest evidence of human settlement in Neolithic Denmark. Hunter-gatherers would have congregated here in the spring. Without knives to shuck the oysters, they used fire and heat to open the shells. Even after they became farmers, this location and these feasts remained important. At the end of the winter, when reserves of grain ran out, the farmers moved to the shoreline and survived on oysters during the 'hungry gap'. These giant and communal oyster binges would have lasted weeks and this seasonal migration would have endured for thousands of years.

It's possible none of us would be alive today without the oyster. Around 160,000 years ago, a long period of climate change triggered drought conditions so severe that deserts expanded and much of the African continent, the only place where humans could be found at that time, became almost uninhabitable to them. It's thought the human population plummeted from 10,000 people to just a few hundred. Close to extinction, we were saved by oysters. The remaining few moved to the coast, including the Cape of South Africa, where, according to the fossil record and excavations of middens, they survived on shellfish. This dietary shift changed us. Oysters contain zinc, iodine and amino acids, all of which would have improved our brain function. From that point in our evolutionary history, *Homo sapiens* continued to evolve and adapt along with the oyster, and for the modern humans who settled along the coastlines of Western Europe, in the Atlantic and across the Mediterranean basin, the species of oyster they ate would have been *Ostrea edulis*. It's only in the last century that the oyster retreated to the margins of European lives.

In Victorian Britain, oysters were so versatile that cooks wrote down more recipes for the bivalves than for eggs. They could be used as stuffing, made into steak and oyster pies and baked into oyster loaves. London of the 1850s had 3,500 oyster sellers and a street-food subculture with its own language: oysters could be served 'hockley' (open shell) or 'curdley' (with eggs). Victorian brewers nonchalantly poured hundreds of oysters into their copper brewing kettles to add a saline bite (and a preservative effect) to sweet dark stouts and porters. In South Wales into the early part of the twentieth century, beer and oysters was a combination served up in pubs to both rich and poor. In Scotland, the oyster was so abundant their shells can be seen in the stonework of buildings, used to give strength to the mortar.

In the 1840s, Henry Mayhew documented the lives of the traders at London's Billingsgate market and visited 'Oyster Street', the long row of boats moored alongside a wharf, a bewildering line of tangled ropes, masts, oysters and people. 'It seems as though the little boats would sink with the crowds of men and women thronged together on their decks,' he wrote. Each boat had holds filled with oysters, 'a grey mass of sand and shell … the *"natives"*'. As Mayhew scribbled his notes in all the chaos, he heard the cries of the oyster traders and boatmen, 'Fish alive! alive! alive O.'

Not long after Mayhew recorded this scene, something dramatic happened. In 1850, 500 million oysters were sold through Billingsgate market; by 1870, this had dropped to 7 million. A decade later, it was less than a tenth of that and in the early twentieth century, stocks of oysters kept falling. As with the decline of the salmon, we understand some features of the oyster's disappearance, but there is much we're still trying to work out. Among the factors at play were the arrival of invasive species (such as the slipper limpet, which arrived with oysters imported from America to stock farms) and diseases which killed off bed after bed of oysters. Climate also played a part; unusually hard winters can create a 'thermal shock' capable of wiping out vast numbers of oysters (one happened in the 1960s). But there is one single factor that explains most of the disappearance of the native oyster: human greed.

Two centuries of overfishing brought *Ostrea edulis* to the brink of extinction. Overexploitation was widespread; the expansion of railways in the nineteenth century led to millions of oysters being taken from the coast to expanding cities. Oysters flowed into towns and cities from coastal communities around the British Isles, from Strangford Lough in Northern Ireland to the Firth of Forth in Scotland, from the Mumbles in Wales to the Thames Estuary in the south of England. But by the middle of the twentieth century, the oyster beds in all of these places, and elsewhere in Europe, were almost empty. At this point the oyster started to make a comeback as a familiar food in Europe, but this involved a strange sequence of events, and a completely different species to the native.

In eighteenth-century France, oyster farming had been a boom industry. Napoleon Bonaparte encouraged the practice, believing it would provide food and help the French economy, and so oyster beds were given as gifts to retiring soldiers, creating an army of oyster growers. Because the native, *Ostrea edulis*, was already in short supply, other oyster species were introduced to these farms. First came the Portuguese oyster (*Crassostrea angulata*). In the 1860s, a ship laden with these oysters destined for Arcachon Bay near Bordeaux was caught in a storm and forced to offload its cargo into a nearby estuary. The oysters survived and settled along the coast, eventually providing the stock for what became France's modern oyster industry. In the 1950s, it was the Portuguese oyster's turn to be hit by disease, which is how the now common Pacific oyster, *Crassostrea gigas* (meaning giant), came to be introduced in 1966. If you eat an oyster in Europe today – or, in fact, in most of the world – the chances are that this is the species you will be eating. It was introduced in the United States from Japan in the early 1900s for commercial harvesting, and its population rapidly overtook native oyster species such as the Olympia or Oly (*Ostrea conchaphila*).

The Pacific had been cultivated in Asia for centuries. It's faster-growing and bigger than *Ostrea edulis*, as well as hardier and less vulnerable to disease. Unlike the smooth, flat, pebbly European native, the Pacific is made of sharp, jagged, overlapping layers (which is why it is also called the rock oyster). In the twentieth century, it spread right across the world. If *Ostrea edulis* was Victorian street food, then *Crassostrea gigas* is McDonald's. Five million tonnes of Pacific oysters are grown in oyster farms and traded each year in every continent on Earth, with the exception of Antarctica. Most of this spread has been intentional, but many populations of the Pacific started out as escapees from oyster farms, and have even proliferated in waters once thought to have been too cold for them.

From the Limfjorden, I drove two hours south along the Danish coast and waded three kilometres through the waist-high water of the Wadden Sea. This is an immense and open stretch of shallow water with rows of dark silhouettes on the horizon, ominous black shapes like the humps of giant whales. These are in fact mounds of Pacific oysters, billions of them all piled on top of each other. 'Mound' is an understatement. As I got closer, I saw these were islands formed from living oysters, a land mass so big it was possible to climb up and walk across them. Believed to be the offspring of escaped oysters from the French farming industry further south, these invaders have become so abundant the giant structures grow bigger each year. These rock oyster mounds are now a destination for food tourists. For a small entry fee, you can have a 'pick your own' seafood experience. 'Usually, oysters are a real luxury, something you only eat in small amounts,' said Klaus Melbye of the Wadden Sea National Park, as we stood on one of the oyster islands. 'Here you get to eat as many as you physically can. And when you're full, you can take more home.' This was one way of tackling an invasive species: eat through the population. The quantity of oysters was overwhelming. They crunched underfoot and turned every surface shiny black. Sitting on upturned buckets, we started to eat the biggest, creamiest oysters, some so plump just one could almost fill my mouth.

The Pacific oysters are also spreading further north and have appeared in the inlets of the Limfjorden, the last safe haven of Europe's native variety. 'One day, they might even overwhelm the natives,' said Melbye. If this happens it will change the entire ecosystem of the Limfjorden. Different oyster species (and subspecies within each) aren't just unique because of size, shape, colour and taste. Each oyster species plays a unique role in the ecological balance of a coastline. An equilibrium exists between it and thousands of other species in that part of the ocean. We don't know what will happen to this ecosystem if the native oyster is eventually outcompeted by the Pacific. 'Invasive species often end up dominating habitats,' says Professor Jens Kjerulf Petersen, the lead scientist at Denmark's National Institute of Aquatic Resources, who has monitored the Pacific's move northwards (it has even arrived on the Swedish coast). 'It's too simple to say they're not wanted or not welcome, but when a new species arrives in an environment, it doesn't always work out well for the existing ones.' In this situation, it's not competition for food between the two oyster species, but competition for space; Pacific oysters are great at building reefs and this can crowd out other species.

This is another example of an environmental change created by human activity; we plundered one wild species and mass-produced another. It's a surprising twist that has parallels with changes we have made on land, from the homogenisation of dairy cattle with the Holstein-Friesian cow to the spread of the genetics of the Large White pig. We humans are – much like the Pacific oyster – in new, unfamiliar waters. We don't know where this will lead us. But oysters have been on Earth for half a billion years: they are older than grass and much older than us. They will probably still be filtering the oceans of this world long after we've gone. Let's hope there will be plenty of diverse species left, including the native.

Sanctuary

The loss of biodiversity in the oceans might seem a hopeless, insurmountable problem. The global fishing industry has become dependent on the billions paid out by governments in subsidies. Quota systems also appear resistant to change. But the marine biologist Callum Roberts has a solution. As a PhD student in the 1980s, Roberts was given the task of counting fish that lived around a reef off the coast of Jeddah in the Red Sea. On his first dive, he saw a firework explosion of animal life bursting around towering castles of coral, as thousands of fish flitted through the water; flashes of bright yellows, greens, blues and greys. It was the most beautiful thing he had ever experienced, and he realised then his life's work was waiting for him in this magical underwater world.

All over the shallow reef, standing out against the coral, Roberts saw bright green algal lawns, which were fuzzy like the surface of billiard tables. For the foot-long surgeonfish, this was food; they patrolled the lawns to drive away any competitors, all except the damselfish, a tenth of their size, which hovered under the belly of the surgeonfish. Together, the two different fish species protected the algae that were food for both. This was one of many examples that helped Roberts realise the sea was a far more ordered and interconnected place than we had realised and that when these finely tuned systems are disrupted, it impacts on the entire ecosystem. One of the biggest disruptions of all, he saw, was the overfishing of larger fish species, the reproductive engines of the oceans.

Roberts set out to understand the extent to which humans had changed the oceans. The problem was, no one alive had any direct experience of what a more abundant, more bountiful ocean looked like. He started examining classic European paintings, looking for clues in the artwork of how much more diverse and bigger fish landings might have been. Other historical sources, including journals written by seafarers and dispatches sent by colonists exploring the New World, helped him build up a picture of what had been lost. Some of the most detailed accounts of fish stocks had been made on eighteenth-century ships which recorded the locations and size of fish catches (their lives at sea depended on it). What they describe is astonishing. On the east coast of the USA, streams appeared to be more full of fish than water, while others report boats at sea unable to move forward because of the numbers of giant cod that surrounded them. The stories might test the limits of credibility for a modern audience. 'But they just kept coming up in documents, over and over again,' says Roberts, 'and from different parts of the ocean.'

In the nineteenth century, off the southern coast of England were shoals of pilchards, sardines and anchovies so thick they darkened entire bays; banks of oysters so colossal that captains of ships needed to navigate with care; and scallops as big as dinner plates. The fisheries of the world seemed plentiful and limitless. But this was also the time when Britain's newly industrialised fishing fleet went out to sea, equipped with bottom trawls that were dropped on the ocean floor. Back then, they landed five times more fish into the UK than the modern fleet does in the twenty-first century. When you factor in the amount of technology and the fishing power with which we attack the oceans now, the decline in fish seems even more stark; we caught seventeen times more fish in the 1880s per unit of fishing power compared with today. There are simply far fewer fish in the sea.

During the 1990s, Roberts worked in the Caribbean, counting fish stocks and measuring the effects of newly created Marine Protected Areas (MPAs). These are large zones either near the coast or in the open seas which are protected by governments and where commercial fishing has been reduced or even banned. The idea is that MPAs work like a boost of vitamin C taken at the onset of a cold – they might not provide an instant cure, but they could help with a bounce back. Many scientists were sceptical, however, and the fishing industry was suspicious. But when Roberts dived into an MPA in Belize, a place that had been previously overfished, he found huge walls of fish, glinting like armour, including big groupers, barracudas as long as his arm and snappers. Roberts had the evidence he needed to show that life could return to the sea.

MPAs, Roberts says, are like fountains of marine life. As in the Banc d'Arguin, they are 'leaky'; they spread biodiversity to surrounding areas. Fish don't just remain inside the protected areas; eggs, larvae and mature fish flow out into neighbouring unprotected zones. As fish stocks build up, the animals live longer, grow bigger, become more numerous and produce hundreds of times more offspring. Fishermen who had assumed they were having something taken away when MPAs were created, started to realise they were being given something back. It was a win–win situation. The evidence for MPAs protecting the seas has been repeated again and again across the globe, including in Cabo Pulmo on the west coast of Mexico, which had been emptied of fish during the 1980s and was revived after local fishing communities decided to stop fishing and create a protected zone. Within a decade, the biomass of fish increased by nearly 500 per cent, close to what it would have been like if it had never been fished in the first place. The United States has one of the world's biggest MPAs, the Papahānaumokuākea Marine National Monument in the Hawaiian archipelago. More than twice the size of Texas, it contains an estimated 7,000 different species – 'an astonishing area', says Roberts. The industrial fleets that had once targeted tuna in those waters were convinced they'd be ruined. 'They're now catching more fish with less effort outside the zone', he says.

So far, less than 6 per cent of the world's oceans have been protected. Although many areas have been designated as MPAs, many of them haven't been enforced and commercial fishing has continued. They're a pointless network of 'paper parks', as Roberts describes them, protected in name only. Better policing can revive the marine life in these areas, but to make a real impact a greater proportion of the world's oceans need to be protected, at least 30 per cent, says Roberts. In January 2021, President Biden set this as a target for the US to meet by 2030. MPAs do provide cause for optimism and have shown that life in the oceans can recover more quickly than life on land. The damage we have caused is reversible, endangered species can be saved and ecosystems can be repaired. The science exists; all that is needed now is the political will.

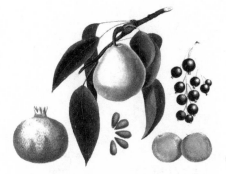

Part Six
Fruit

Varieties are the footprints of a journey through a fruit's history.

Joan Morgan, *The Book of Pears*

When humans domesticated cereal crops – the likes of wheat, rice and maize – it marked the birth of agriculture and enabled humans to settle. A great diversity of animals and vegetables followed. But when they started planting fruit trees, farming came of age. The fruits we eat today were domesticated long after the Neolithic Revolution, mostly between 6000 and 3000 BCE, in different regions around the world. In Central and East Asia, there was citrus, apple and pear, along with stone fruits – apricot, cherry, peach and plum. The 'Mediterranean fruits' were date, olive, grape, fig and pomegranate. Much later, from the Americas, came strawberry, pineapple, avocado and papaya.

But why did farmers turn to fruit so much later than cereals? A clue lies on the surface of an ancient work of art, the 5,000-year-old Warka Vase, one metre tall and covered from top to bottom in images linked to agriculture. The vase was excavated in 1934 near the Euphrates, just north of Basra, present-day Iraq. When the archaeologists pieced together the fragments, they saw depictions of barley, sesame, sheep and cattle along with a procession of workers and slaves. But at the very top was the image of a woman (the goddess Inanna) being offered a bowl filled with what appears to be dates, pomegranates and figs. This image, from 3000 BCE, is the oldest depiction so far discovered of a fruit culture (a civilisation in which fruit was grown rather than it being gathered from the wild). In the case of the vase and its makers, that culture was Sumerian, based in the ancient city of Uruk, one of the first great urban centres, the birthplace of writing and literacy and home to around 50,000 people. Here, canals transported food from large farms on the outskirts (watered by sophisticated irrigation systems) and into the city; all essential features for large-scale fruit growing. What the image on the Warka Vase shows us is that cultivating fruit was mostly an urban phenomenon. A date, olive or fig tree won't produce fruit worth eating for several years, and once it does, the tree can remain productive for centuries. Fruit involves a long-term commitment to a particular place. Orchards also need irrigation, which itself requires social organisation, long-term planning and a centralised power to make it happen. Where we find early evidence of fruit growing, we also find the rise of city-states and, ultimately, the origins of nationhood.

From a plant's point of view, producing seeds covered in sweet-tasting flesh is a sure-fire strategy for having its genes scattered far and wide by birds and mammals. A central feature of this evolutionary master-stroke is the ripening process. Fruit containing immature seeds is full of bitter tannins and poisonous alkaloids; this protects the fruit from being eaten too soon. But when the seeds are ready to go, a magical transformation takes place; chemicals are released that soften the fruit's flesh, reduce acidity and increase sweetness. Powerful aroma molecules signal to the world there's food available, a message reinforced by a change in a fruit's skin colour, from shades of green that act as disguise, to eye-catching bright yellows, reds and oranges. From our earliest times, we humans have been eager participants in this strategy. Way back in our evolutionary history something of a metabolic mistake was fixed into our DNA. Whereas other mammals can manufacture their own supply of vitamin C, we can't. Eating fruit is a solution to this problem, and for millions of years, humans foraged fruit from the wild to fill this nutritional gap. By the time the Warka Vase was made, we had worked out how to grow our own supply on a massive scale.

Growing fruit is a different proposition to farming cereals and pulses. It requires pruning and training branches and vines to make harvesting easier, and to keep a particular variety going involves grafting, effect-ively cloning (one approach is to take buds or small twigs from one tree and fuse them onto the roots or stems of another). Storing fruit is also far trickier than storing cereals. Immediately after harvest, decay sets in quickly. Preservation techniques are limited; you can dry apricots and apples in the sun, turn grapes into wine and apples into cider, but nothing as simple as storing grains of wheat or kernels of maize for when they are needed. And it can't be done on the same

magnitude. Some fruit growers made use of naturally cool environments including cave systems (which is still done, for example, in
Cappadocia in central Turkey, where harvested lemons are kept at a
steady 12.8°C). But in most fruit cultures, and for most of our fruit-
growing history, fruit was consumed in the place where it grew. This
is how many distinctive fruit varieties were created. As with other
crops, chance genetic mutations and human selections added up to a
bounty of diversity. Some fruit varieties were serendipitous discoveries.
Granny Smith and Golden Delicious apples, for instance, attracted
notice as chance seedlings, each found growing on a single tree by
one observant grower, while, we saw earlier, a mutant mandarin in
nineteenth-century Algeria gave the world the clementine. All in all,
botanists have been able to identify 3,000 different varieties (or
cultivars) of pear, more than 1,000 each of citrus and bananas, and an
incredible 7,000 of apple. And these are just the cultivated varieties
they've managed to record. This is a level of diversity few of us will
ever get to experience, but not because the fruit changed – the supply
chain did.

The first refrigerated ships set out to sea in the 1870s, opening up the
possibility of fruit being transported across the oceans. Then, in the
1920s, scientists discovered they could extend the shelf life of fruit by
modifying the atmosphere it was stored in (oxygen was lowered,
carbon dioxide was increased). This 'controlled atmosphere' slowed
down the ripening process, making it possible to store apples and
pears for more than a year (with bananas it's less than two months).
In the 1940s, trucks started to be equipped with new refrigeration
technology that quickly transferred to planes, trains and boats. This
completed what's called 'the cold chain' (the transportation of food
from farms to our fridges chilled and without interruption). Then, in
the 1960s, the first shipping containers appeared, which meant that
instead of it taking weeks to load a ship with thousands of individual
items, products could be placed inside corrugated steel boxes, eight
feet tall and twenty feet deep, and be loaded and offloaded within
hours. Within two decades, countries that had adopted containers saw
an almost ninefold increase in trade. Globalisation of the fruit trade
didn't just depend on free trade agreements and political deals it also
depended on the invention of a big metal box.

With the unbroken cold chain in place, fresh fruit grown on one side of the world could now be eaten on the other. The influence of the seasons on the availability of fruit (and other food) was lessened, and diets, potentially at least, diversified. But because not all fruit could meet the demands of the new global supply chain, homogenisation crept in. The varieties of fruit that could tolerate the rigours of international trade were planted in huge monocultures. In the second half of the twentieth century, just a handful of fruit varieties came to dominate the world's plantations, orchards and fruit bowls. For apples, this included the Red Delicious; for pears it was the Bartlett; for bananas, it was the Cavendish; and for citrus, the Valencia and Navel oranges.

During this time, fruit breeding came under the control of fewer and fewer companies. Until close to the end of the twentieth century this was usually a public endeavour, funded by governments and supported by universities. Increasingly, it is now in private hands, led by 'marketing groups' and 'clubs' which develop and own the top varieties in the global fruit market: the Jazz apple, Driscoll's strawberries, the Super Sweet pineapple and the Cotton Candy grape are all examples of this.

Breeding a new fruit variety can take years and millions of pounds of investment before it arrives inside a supermarket. Little is left to chance and these new fruit varieties have to be grown on a massive scale to turn a profit. To reach a global audience they also need to have a long shelf life and be able to meet the conditions of the cold chain as well as the specifications set out by supermarkets (from the fruit's size and colour to its sugar level and water content). This is why uniformity has been winning and diversity is in decline. But as the following stories show us, this system is changing – because it needs to.

21

Sievers Apple

Tian Shan, Kazakhstan

Eat an apple and wherever you are in the world, whatever its shape, size, colour or taste, its origin can be traced back to the Tian Shan, the snow-tipped 'heavenly mountains' that separate China and Central Asia. The wild trees that cover its slopes are a living gene bank. As the birthplace of the apple, the biodiversity of the Tian Shan holds the past, present and future of one of our most popular fruits. But in the last century, the human impact on the fruit forests of the Tian Shan has been so severe that the wild diversity there is at risk. We need to save those forests.

Think of the Tian Shan as the world's biggest orchard, except it is wild and the variety here is dizzying. Each tree is unique and so is the fruit; some apples are the size of tennis balls, others as small as cherries. Some are eye-piercingly lime green, others soft pastel pinks and purples. Eating from these wild apple trees is like playing a fruit version of Russian roulette. One might be sweet and honeyed; another spicy with hints of aniseed or liquorice; others so mouth-puckeringly sharp and astringent you'll want to spit them straight out. Across these wild fruit forests, the apples on each tree mature at their own particular pace, so the heavy scent of ripening fruit mingles with the heady esters of fallen apples fermenting on the forest floor.

Some parts of the forests are so dense that the apple trees are unreachable. One of the world's biggest known apple trees, at least three hundred years old and a trunk three feet in diameter, grows here, and other giants are still waiting to be discovered. The forest is rich in other wild fruits too: pears, quinces, hawthorn, apricots and plums.

Seeds of sweet wild apples (*Malus sieversii*) made it out of this isolated, ancient place and evolved to become the domesticated apple

(*Malus domestica*). How the apple radiated out from here involved three different animal species: bears, horses and humans. The theory is that over thousands, possibly millions, of years, bears selected the largest and sweetest fruits they could find in the forests. And because the hard, teardrop-shaped apple pips pass through the animals intact, it was the largest and sweetest apples that were spread most widely around the Tian Shan, scattered in their own portion of fertilising scat (bear poo). But it was horses who sent these apples further afield and towards domestication. Like the bears, the wild horses of the Tian Shan fed on the largest and sweetest apples but took the seeds greater distances, inadvertently pushing them into the soil with their hooves as they went. Humans first domesticated the horse in Kazakhstan and, once that happened, both the animal and the fruit set out on a long journey.

Apple pips travelled west along the Silk Road into Persia and then north to the Balkans and Greece, where the fruit took its place in mythology (golden apples were given to the goddess Hera on her marriage to Zeus). The Romans planted orchards across their empire, under the watchful eye of Pomona, the goddess protector of fruit trees. In more recent centuries, the apple was spread further in waves of colonisation and taken from England, Germany, France and the Netherlands to North America. As settlers moved west, the fruit took on a legal function as well as a dietary one. In some states, for a homestead to receive legal recognition pioneers had to plant fifty apple trees and twenty peach trees. In the early nineteenth century, spotting an opportunity, a man named John Chapman (also known as Johnny Appleseed) became a prolific planter of orchards, travelling ahead of the settlers with bags full of pips, planting apple trees in the wilderness and selling saplings and seeds to the incomers. The reason Chapman planted his orchards from seed was linked to his membership of a religious organisation, the Swedenborgian Church, which explicitly forbade grafting (they believed cutting of buds and twigs caused plants to suffer). Because each seed could potentially result in a new variety, the real legacy of Johnny Appleseed was a new wave of apple diversity, so much so that some botanists argue the fruit underwent a second domestication in America, as farmers had to select new eating apples from Chapman's unpredictable trees.

Around the same time as Johnny Appleseed was helping to spread the fruit across America, the Dutch and the English were planting the seeds of today's more globalised apple industry by establishing orchards in South Africa's Western Cape and in southern Australia and New Zealand (the area around Hawke's Bay became known as the 'Apple Bowl'). After the arrival of refrigerated ships and then containers in the twentieth century, these countries became big players in the international fruit trade. And yet, all of these apples could be traced back to those original fruit forests of the Tian Shan and *Malus sieversii*. These wild apples were named after German plant collector Johann Sievers who made it into Kazakhstan's fruit forests in 1793. Sievers had a hunch the Tian Shan was the birthplace of the apple but died before he could develop his theory further. His observations were credible enough, however, for the wild apples to be given his name and they're sometimes referred to as the Sievers apple.

Nikolai Vavilov pursued this theory when, in 1929, on a gruelling journey by mule caravan, he crossed Kyrgyzstan into Kazakhstan: 'the path turned out to be more difficult than we expected and in fact we happened to lose two of the horses ... ' he later wrote. 'Stiff with cold and with our teeth chattering, border guards looked at the arrival of our caravan with amazement.' Seeing the city of Alma-Ata (now Almaty – which translates into 'Father of the Apple') he described how 'thickets of wild apples stretch out through an extensive area around the city and along the slopes of the mountains, here and there forming a real forest ... large fruited varieties, not differing much from cultivated species'. In Almaty, Vavilov met a young student and future botanist, Aimak Dzangaliev. In remembering a visit to the countryside they made together, Dzangaliev said Vavilov, 'reviewed everything around Almaty in just one day ... Given his genius, his mind figured out just about everything.' Vavilov concluded that the Tian Shan was the centre of origin of apples. Dzangaliev went on to spend seventy years mapping the diversity within the apple forests. He was in a race against time. The Soviet Union had started a massive deforestation programme in the 1950s; thousands of acres of apple trees were cut down to allow for cotton-growing experiments that ended in failure. By the end of the Soviet era, Dzangaliev calculated that more than half of the wild apple diversity around Almaty had been lost through deforestation. In the 1960s, he planted orchards where some of the unique apples he had rescued from the forest could grow and be studied. Even this wasn't safe. In 1977, the Soviet authorities ordered that the collection be uprooted. 'That day, they brought me to my knees,' Dzangaliev said in an interview shortly before he died.

More damage was inflicted on the forests in the 1990s, when the break-up of the USSR brought a decade of chaos to Kazakhstan. Fuel supplies were disrupted and coal subsidies ended. To keep warm, people chopped down more wild apple trees. Large sections of forest were also cleared to make way for cattle and sheep, and uncontrolled housebuilding became endemic. Even the wild trees that survived faced risks, as the Soviets established large commercial orchards of domesticated apples nearby, diluting the wild gene pool. In 2007, *Malus sieversii* was placed on the IUCN Red List, a catalogue of endangered species, and described as 'vulnerable' and its population 'decreasing'. Today, only parts of the forests remain intact – including Krutoe and Tauturgen, to the east of Almaty.

One of the first Western scientists to visit the forests after the collapse of the Soviet Union was the Oxford plant scientist Barrie Juniper. In the early 1990s, he made a series of trips to the Tian Shan. Accompanied by two armed guards and living on a diet of mutton, rice and apples, he had to pay his way past Kazakh army officers to get inside the forests. 'Vast areas had been devastated by wholesale environmental destruction,' he said. Over the next fifteen years, he went back and forth between the Tian Shan and Oxford, documenting as many of the wild apples as he could. Using new DNA techniques, Juniper was the first scientist to confirm what Johann Sievers and Nikolai Vavilov had suspected through observation: all domesticated apples originate from the Tian Shan. No other apple species had played a role; it really was the gene bank for all the world's apples.

Juniper went to extraordinary lengths to prove this point, not only risking his life in the chaos of post-Soviet Kazakhstan, but also spending years planting an orchard in Oxford which would act as his own reference library of apple DNA. Gradually, he assembled a collection of as many old species of apple as he could find from different parts of the world to compare these with the genetics of the wild apples from the Tian Shan.

On a sunny autumn morning, I met Juniper at his orchard in Wytham, a picture-book Oxfordshire village with an abbey, thatched cottages and a 600-year-old pub. Completely hidden behind tall walls was a secret garden of one hundred apple trees, some fifteen feet tall, others more like thick untamed bushes. As we moved from tree to tree, picking fruit, Juniper introduced each one: the Newton Wonder, a chance seedling that had been discovered growing alongside a Derbyshire pub in the 1870s that went on to become a popular cooking apple; thin, conical apples named Lady's Fingers; and Brownlee's Russet, an apple from the 1840s with an intense acid flesh that tasted of fruit drops, all hidden beneath a scaly, rough skin. 'Wonderful apple,' said Juniper, rubbing one clean against his jacket. 'The perfect balance of sweet and sour and with a skin so thick it kept until Christmas.' We ate apples that tasted of pineapple (Ananas Reinette) and bit into small russeted varieties that are mentioned in Shakespeare's *Henry IV, Part 2*. '"There's a dish of leather-coats for you,"' Juniper quoted as he picked out one of the apples. 'Ugly and rough it might be, but in the sixteenth century this apple was sold from every barrow in London.'

While some varieties became popular because of a chance discovery of a single tree, others were the creation of skilled nurserymen, masters in the art of cross-pollination. By the end of the nineteenth century, people in Britain could eat or drink from a different kind of dessert, cooking or cider apple every day for more than four years and never have the same one twice.

The apples in Juniper's walled orchard capture a big part of the fruit's great appeal: its diversity and seasonality. In the 1920s, the nurseryman and fruit expert Edward Bunyard wrote *The Anatomy of Dessert*, providing an eater's guide to the tastiest varieties, from the strawberry flavour of a Worcester Pearmain to the 'melting, almost marrow flesh, abundant juice and fragrant aroma' of the James Grieve. And then there was the Blenheim Orange, an eighteenth-century apple grown from the pip of a discarded apple core that had grown next to the drystone wall of Blenheim Palace in Oxfordshire. Luckily, the tree and its fruit were discovered by a tailor named George Kempster (which is why the variety is also called the 'Kempster'). This apple, said Bunyard, has 'a nutty warm aroma ... and in this noble fruit [there's] a mellow austerity as of a great Port in its prime'.

Bunyard's descriptions provide a glimpse into a wealth of diversity that no longer exists. By the 1970s, apple eaters in different parts of the world had the nagging feeling something was missing. 'Apples, apples everywhere and hardly one to eat,' declared a newspaper article that went on to say, 'The big red and yellow plastic spheres, waiting in the market for the unsuspecting, are so suspiciously, so blatantly, thick skinned and shiny, it is easy to pass on by. What we must live on is the memory of what good apples taste like.'

The globalised cold chain and shipping containers wiped out most of the delicious diversity Bunyard had tasted. Ninety per cent of all apples are now sold by supermarkets, which guarantee year-round supply from countries including Spain, Italy, France and New Zealand. Unable to compete, two-thirds of Britain's orchards were gone by the 1980s, 'grubbed up' to plant more cereal crops or to free up land for building on. Some of these orchards had been planted by monasteries one thousand years before. Refrigeration and containerisation had made the world smaller and, in this globalised market, scale and specialisation were the keys to success. Many British apple growers gave up or went broke. And so today, the majority of apples eaten in Britain are imported. We benefitted from all-year-round apples, but we neglected our inheritance. When you destroy an orchard, you lose not only trees but also a way of life and biodiversity. Apples and apple orchards used to have the same symbolic importance for the British landscape and culture as citrus groves for Sicilians or vineyards for the French. Swayed by arguments of economics and convenience, we overlooked the cultural and ecological impact and the long view.

What most countries around the world now have are apple varieties with very specific qualities: they need to be sweet, crunchy and long-lasting. Varieties which fitted these criteria quickly colonised the supermarket aisles of the world. The Red Delicious (discovered by a farmer in Iowa in the 1870s) spent a century as America's most popular apple and has only recently been overtaken by the Gala. 'People wanted a sweeter apple, with a bigger crunch,' says Mark Seetin of the USA Apple Association. 'The industry loves the Gala. You can place it in nitrogen storage, take it out nine months later and it'll still taste like it just came off the tree.'

The Gala has also become the leading variety sold in the UK, with runners-up including Golden Delicious, Granny Smith and Braeburn.

More recent additions include Pink Lady, Jazz and Fuji. All three are products of twentieth-century breeding programmes (in Australia, New Zealand and Japan); all were created with long-distance travel in mind; and all came from a small group of 'elite' parent varieties. Breeding is a lengthy, complicated and expensive business, so the industry tends to play safe by tweaking the most successful apples. Golden Delicious, for example, was cross-bred to create the Gala, which in turn was cross-bred with the Braeburn to create the Jazz apple. The Red Delicious was crossed to give us the Fuji. These are all bred to be high-yielding, picked early, stored for long periods and grown in as many different countries as possible. Of great importance to the supermarkets, they also need to be easy on the eye and consistent. We know exactly what we will taste when we buy these apples; they hold no surprises, little deviation in flavour or texture whatever the season, or wherever in the world you happen to eat them. The tannin-rich Brownlee's Russet and the port-like Blenheim Orange offer greater complexity.

Creating these new commercial varieties is big business and varieties such as Jazz and Pink Lady are licensed as exclusive property of the 'marketing clubs' that bring together the whole supply chain of breeders, fruit growers and exporters. These clubs decide who is allowed to grow, distribute and promote a particular 'branded' variety of apple in different parts of the world. For the supermarkets, this works well; it means they only need to deal with a small number of suppliers.

A recent addition to the club system is the Cosmic Crisp, released in December 2019. A little larger than the average apple, tiny star-like flecks over its red skin explain its name, and the sound when you bite into it is supposed to out-crunch any rival. We might not think too deeply about it if we were to see it on display, but this fruit is the product of tens of millions of dollars of investment, two decades of planning, breeding and the sorting through and tasting of fruit from hundreds of experimental trees. An essential quality, as far as the industry is concerned, is that these apples last for more than a year in cold storage. Washington State owns the rights to the Cosmic Crisp patent, so farmers agree to pay royalties on every tree they buy and every box they sell. The scale of the investment has been huge, with 13 million new trees planted at a cost of $500 million. The Cosmic

Crisp may well be too big to fail. For that reason alone, it is likely to dominate apple sales for years, possibly even decades to come.

Despite there being many indigenous Asian varieties of apple, more and more Chinese consumers are buying America's Red Delicious. To the new and growing middle classes in China, this apple is seen as an aspirational food from the West. China has also planted millions of Gala trees in the east of the country, as well as Fuji, an apple that came out of a 1930s Japanese breeding programme. Meanwhile, a completely different kind of variety is proving popular in the United States. The genetically modified Arctic apple has been engineered to be a 'non-browning' apple, designed to be ready sliced and sold in plastic bags. There is a diversity, of sorts, in the twenty-first-century apple world.

22

Kayinja Banana

Uganda

The world's largest collection of banana diversity isn't in one of the regions where most bananas grow – in South East Asia, Africa or Latin America. It's in Belgium. The University of Leuven is home of the International Musa Germplasm Collection ('Musa' being the genus the banana belongs to). This is a living treasury of more than 1,500 types of banana with a bewildering array of sizes, colours and flavours. The Blue Java from Indonesia has a soft, unctuous texture and tastes of vanilla ice cream, while the Ele Ele banana, one of the plants introduced to Hawaii by South Pacific settlers, is picked green and cooked as a vegetable. Some types of banana taste like strawberries or apples; some have fuzzy skins; and one Chinese banana is so aromatic it's been given the name Go San Heong, meaning 'you can smell it from the next mountain'. Yet despite all its diversity, the banana is the fruit example par excellence of crop monoculture (crops of single variety).

Half of all the bananas in the world are globally traded and grown with the sole purpose of crossing the world in shipping containers. In 2019, this added up to more than 20 billion tonnes, £14.7 billion worth, and helped to make the banana the world's favourite fruit. The international trade is based entirely around just one variety: the Cavendish, a low-price, ubiquitous and super-specialised fruit. The Cavendish dominates the global fruit trade not just because of its taste but because of its biology, its size and shape, the thickness of its skin and the way it ripens. All of these things mean it can be grown, picked and shipped to every port in the world, transported to the biggest cities and the smallest villages. Despite the distances involved, when it arrives on supermarket shelves, it still manages to be one of the cheapest foods on offer.

What makes it the unrivalled superstar of monocultures is that every single Cavendish is a clone. This plant can't reproduce itself from seed (unlike wild bananas). Instead, some of the suckers the Cavendish grows underground are cut from the main stem and replanted (botanically speaking, the banana is a giant herb and not a tree). This makes it a highly prolific plant, but its clonal existence has drawbacks. The Cavendish has no way of evolving and its immune system can't adapt to new threats. In plantations filled with genetically identical bananas, if a pathogen can get to one plant, it can get to them all. And this is exactly what is happening.

On several continents the Cavendish is dying, entire plantations being killed off by an incurable disease, tropical race 4 (also known as TR4, Panama disease or Fusarium wilt). The global food system is now so interconnected the disease has spread between farms on different sides of the world. India, Australia, Africa and Asia have all been affected, including China. Recently, the disease was discovered for the first time in the biggest banana-growing region of all, Latin America. A few spores carried on a plant, a spade or on the clothing of a worker is all it takes to contaminate a plantation, and once it starts to spread through the soil, growing the Cavendish on that land is no longer an option. Although the crops most affected are the vast monocultures of Cavendish, the disease is so aggressive it can spread from these plantations and infect other varieties grown by small-scale farmers. If TR4 spreads further it will severely disrupt supplies of a favourite food in the West, but for half a billion people in Africa, Asia and Latin America, the consequences will be far more serious. In these parts of the world, bananas are a major source of calories, an important part of food security, a way of making a living and a food of great cultural importance.

It's worth knowing how the Cavendish came to dominate the world not only because it's such an extraordinary example of food colonialism on a grand scale, but also because it shows how we changed the global food system (and if we can do that once, we can do it again). Its global story begins in 1826 when an Irish botanist called Charles Telfair chanced across a banana plant growing in a family garden in southern China. Impressed by what he saw and the fruit he tasted, he took the plant on the next leg of his journey, which was to

Mauritius. From there, the banana came to the attention of Britain's foremost collector of tropical plants, the 6th Duke of Devonshire, William Cavendish, who planted it in the greenhouse on his Chatsworth estate in Derbyshire (where the 'Cavendish', as the variety became known, is still grown to this day). Word spread quickly about 'this highly interesting and most valuable plant ... a native of China', and when the English missionary John Williams travelled to islands in the South Pacific in the 1830s, he took some of the Chatsworth banana plants with him, along with their new name, the Cavendish. Only one of the plants survived the journey, and from its suckers came every banana grown on Samoa, Tonga, Fiji and Tahiti for the next one hundred years.

But this banana wasn't destined to become the world's number one fruit straight away. At the same time as the Cavendish was being taken from China to England and the South Pacific, another variety of banana was making its way around the world. This was the Gros Michel, aka the 'Big Mike' (a half-sibling of the Cavendish). It had been discovered by a botanist in southern China and taken to a garden in the French colony of Martinique. From there, it spread across the Caribbean and into Central America. When faster steamships started to cross the Atlantic and Pacific oceans in the 1860s, the banana trade was born. In 1866, the very first shipment of bananas arrived in New York City from Colombia. The person who realised the full potential of this relatively unknown and exotic fruit was a sea captain from Cape Cod named Lorenzo Dow Baker. In 1870, Baker took on a commission to transport gold miners to the Orinoco River in Venezuela. On the return journey, he landed in Jamaica for repairs, and in the local markets tasted the Gros Michel. He was so impressed, he decided to take a chance by buying 160 bunches to take back to New Jersey to sell. The skin of the Gros Michel was thick enough to preserve it for the two-week journey and by the time they arrived in the US, the bananas had ripened to perfection. They caused a sensation and made Dow Baker a profit. The rise of the Gros Michel as the top banana was under way.

At this point, a 25-year-old wholesaler enters the story. Andrew Preston convinced Dow Baker he could make the obscure banana more popular than apples. The company they founded in 1885 (later called the United Fruit Company and now called Chiquita) purchased land in Latin America and established banana plantations, using a workforce of indigenous labourers. Because the cold chain was also taking shape around this time, the bananas started to be sold around the world. By the 1940s, tens of millions of hectares of the Gros Michel had been planted across Central and South America. This single variety of banana transformed not only landscapes but also entire economies. In Latin America, the United Fruit Company became so powerful it was known as *el pulpo*, the octopus, because of the long reach of its tentacles. In the 1930s and 40s, under the Guatemalan President Jorge Ubico, the company gained control of the majority of Guatemala's cultivated land, which brought the promise of cheap labour. As well as dominating the country's banana production, it built railways, laid down telegraph lines and constructed seaports, all essential to the running of the banana trade. The fruit company effectively functioned as a state within a state.

In the early 1950s, a reformer Jacobo Arbenz Guzmán won office and attempted to confiscate unused land from the United Fruit Company and redistribute it to local families. Soon after, he was overthrown in a coup planned by the American CIA and forced into exile. Under the succession of military rulers and three decades of vicious civil war, nearly a quarter of a million people died, many of them peasant farmers. This remains one of the starkest illustrations of how a food commodity, and its control by a corporation, can help shape a nation's fate. Meanwhile, as ever larger monocultures of the Gros Michel were being planted, the conditions for its downfall were being put in place.

In the centre of origin of the banana, the jungles of South East Asia, wild bananas co-evolved with fungal diseases (including the ancient ancestors of TR4). As these diseases changed over time, so did the plant; an ongoing process in which the host (the banana) and the pathogens (the fungi) keep trying to outmanoeuvre each other. However, a sterile, cloned banana (such as the Gros Michel, and later the Cavendish), having lost the ability to adapt and change, can't take part in this evolutionary process. This means the diseases (which do continue to evolve) eventually win. When bananas were grown on small, isolated farms, the problem was easily contained, but when the first large-scale monocultures were established towards the end of the nineteenth century, these fungal diseases gained the power to devastate. Millions of plants were affected, entire businesses wiped out.

The response of the early plantation owners was to close down infected plantations and start again on virgin (uninfected) land. This is partly why fruit companies found land in Latin America so attractive. The first deadly Fusarium species to spread around the world was race 1. When infected with this, leaves begin to yellow and become mottled, and the plant starts rotting from within. By the 1950s, race 1 had spread through so many plantations with monocultures of Gros Michel, the variety had become uneconomical to grow. The industry needed a replacement variety with resistance to this disease, one that could slot into the global supply chain that had been built up around the 'Big Mike'. Enter the Cavendish, which took over where the Gros Michel left off. And for most of the second half of the twentieth century, growing the Cavendish and making it the world's banana of choice, worked. But history is now repeating itself. Like race 1, TR4 began to spread across the world's banana plantations, a type of disease for which the Cavendish had no resistance. The first significant outbreak was in China in the 1990s, and then it went global. To defend against it, strict biosecurity measures were put in place in Latin America, turning plantations into no-go areas for outsiders. It didn't work. In August 2019, Colombia's agriculture authority, the ICA, confirmed they had discovered TR4 in the country's banana plantations. We're still waiting to find out what the consequences will be.

One solution for the future of global banana production is to stick with the Cavendish and the monoculture model but genetically engineer or edit the plant's DNA to find a fix against the disease. The alternative is to look to genetic diversity, to move away from planting vast monocultures filled with clones and instead make use of the hundreds of varieties of banana that exist. The case of Uganda is helpful here, because in this Central African country both paths are being explored. For Ugandans, the banana is far more than a sweet fruit to be eaten raw; it's a staple food, the main source of carbohydrate for two-thirds of the population. Millions of people's livelihoods depend on the fruit; in rural areas, three-quarters of Ugandan farmers grow bananas, and diversity is key. More than forty different varieties are grown.

Africa is considered to be a secondary centre of domestication for the banana. The fruit arrived on the continent from South East Asia at least 2,000 years ago and, with further adaptation and selection by farmers, a new diverse group, collectively known as East African Highland bananas, emerged. Each cultivated variety has its own culinary uses and a different cultural role. There is the Nakitembe, a black-and-red-coloured banana which is steamed, mashed and served with vegetables or meat. The Ndibwabalangira is a bright green, intensely sweet banana once reserved for chiefs and leaders of Buganda, the largest of Uganda's ancient kingdoms. The Musakala has an ivory-coloured flesh and a slippery texture and smells like a cucumber when you cut it. The Mbidde has a whitish-grey pulp and bitter taste and is often used to make juice. And there's Namwezi, a medicinal banana; its name means 'lady moon banana' and it is some-times eaten by women when they are menstruating. The Bogoya is carbohydrate-rich and intensely flavoured and can be eaten raw or cooked into stews (Bogoya, by the way, is the Ugandan name for the Gros Michel). But one of the most versatile bananas is the Kayinja, grown in central Uganda. In traditional marriage ceremonies, the groom presents the bride's family with a beer brewed from the juice of the Kayinja. 'It takes a lot of hard work and effort,' says Edie Mukiibi, an agronomist and banana farmer and the leader of Slow Food Uganda. 'This gift of beer is seen as a sign of commitment to your life partner and shows that you will be a good provider for your future family.'

Food markets in this part of Uganda have entire sections dedicated to bananas. Some are sold at the entrance, a display of every shade of yellow imaginable, bananas at different stages of ripening and suiting all preferences. Walk deeper into the market, and you start to see piles of a variety called Matoke; a staple food cooked throughout the day, an ingredient in most meals. Head even further into the market and you'll come to areas filled with the aroma of sweet, ripening bananas where people gather to eat, relax and drink. Here, when it gets late, fires are lit, Matoke bananas are roasted, people dance, make music and sip Kayinja banana beer. But this traditional banana culture is changing. In 2014, the Ugandan government, with funding from the Bill and Melinda Gates Foundation, launched a 'banana improvement programme' with the aim of producing new, higher-yielding, more disease-resistant hybrids. Uganda has also been one of the main testing areas for genetically modified and gene-edited bananas.

Based at Queensland University of Technology in north-east Australia, James Dale's numerous titles include Banana Biotechnology Program Leader and molecular farmer. As a geneticist, he has spent forty years trying to redesign the banana. So far this has mostly been through transgenics: adding extra DNA from different species. Dale's biggest breakthroughs include finding TR4-resistant genes in wild bananas sourced from the jungles of Papua New Guinea, the plant's centre of diversity. In a trial carried out in northern Australia, Dale planted GM Cavendish plants in TR4-infected soil along with non-GM plants. The ordinary bananas in the plot became infected and died, but the plants with the inserted wild gene survived. In Uganda, he developed GM bananas supplemented with vitamin A (to tackle nutrient deficiency). More recently, he has turned his attention to genome editing. By switching on a TR4-resistant gene made dormant during the banana's domestication he believes he can save the variety. 'More diseases are on their way. To build resilience, we're going to need this new technology.'

Some Ugandan farmers fear that new science and breeding pro-grammes will result in traditional crops becoming endangered. One such farmer is Edie Mukiibi. 'We'll end up with patented "super-bananas" and one or two varieties replacing our rich diversity and thousands of years of history.' He worries about a 'one-size-fits-all' approach. 'The number of banana varieties in Uganda is already getting smaller. We farmers are the custodians of biodiversity, it's our respon-sibility to protect it,' says Mukiibi.

Dr Fernando García-Bastidas agrees. Something of a star in the fruit world, his social media followers refer to him as 'Bananaman', some-times even 'Super-bananaman'. Based in the Netherlands, after years of banana research at Wageningen University, he is a leading expert on TR4 and one of the scientists responsible for tracking the progress of the disease. In his lab, García showed me what a Cavendish plant looks like after it has been infected by TR4. From a high-security cold store, he pulled out a collection of plants that had been inoculated and were now slowly dying, turning into a black mass of decaying stems and leaves. Inside a locked refrigerator were tiny samples of the fungus. Inside one bottle was enough TR4 to wipe out every plantation in Latin America. Because of his research, when he visits banana plantations, he travels with very few possessions – when he arrives in a country, he kits himself out with new clothes and new shoes. 'I have to make sure I'm not the one who introduces the disease to a plantation,' he says. 'I'm supposed to be the scientist trying to stop it.'

At his workplace is a giant glass house which contains a forest of different wild banana plants, some tall, some dwarves, producing different-coloured fruits, some red, others tinged with blue. These have been sourced from the South East Asian jungles, where both the banana and the TR4 fungus originated. Garcia is drawing on millions of years of co-evolution. His plan is to breed some ancient and lost traits back into a new Cavendish-like plant, mixing the best of the past with the best of the present.

This work, known as reconstructive breeding, involves finding ancestors of the Cavendish and evaluating hundreds of wild and cultivated bananas, including varieties from Uganda (some of which have resistance). He thinks it might take him a decade of work, maybe two. 'Hidden away in jungles and on small farms are plants with traits we will need for the future,' he says. 'We can't afford to lose any of these plants.' But even if he helps to save the Cavendish, he believes we will also need to change how we farm. On this, García and James Dale are in agreement. Their scientific approaches might differ but both are convinced saving banana diversity, wild and cultivated, is essential and growing monocultures now looks too risky an option. The Cavendish is the canary in the coal mine, a warning against monocultures and reason enough to increase the pool of genetic diversity in all our crops. We cannot depend on single varieties for the future of our food. The consequences are clear to see in the crisis of the Cavendish as well as the Gros Michel before it. If we fail to acknowledge this, we remain at risk of history repeating itself again and again. There's a reason why monocultures do not exist in nature.

23

Vanilla Orange

My father, Liborio 'Bobo' Saladino, was born in south-western Sicily in a small town called Ribera. This is where I spent the summers of my childhood. Ribera was my introduction to farming, to crops and to harvests, and it shaped my thinking about food. Not far from Ribera is Agrigento, where tourists travel to see ancient ruins, and Sciacca, where they can lie on beaches, visit fishing ports with narrow cobbled streets and choose from a rainbow of colours in ice-cream parlours. Further inland from the sea and smaller than its more exuberant neighbours, Ribera rarely sees tourists. For much of its history, it has been a place of agriculture. On its outskirts, a towering, brightly painted sign proclaims: *Ribera: Città delle arance* – 'city of oranges'. The summer sun here is as intense as anywhere on the island, but Ribera has the advantage of being near one of Sicily's longest rivers, the Platani, and so oranges from Ribera became famous. Today in the food markets of the capital Palermo, the town's name is still associated with some of the island's best fruit.

For me, arriving in Ribera as a child was like that moment in *The Wizard of Oz* when Dorothy first realises she's not in Kansas any more. Coming from the black-and-white food world of 1970s Britain I was dazzled by the MGM Technicolor of Sicilian food, especially its citrus. A short drive from the concrete of downtown Ribera, with its shuttered houses and coffee bars, dusty tracks led to miles of orange and lemon groves. Rusty metal gates and tall, black, fabric windbreaks divided one family's citrus grove from another. In summer, I'd step out of the car into an oven-like heat and kick through crumbly, sun-baked soil to a soundtrack of crickets. Everything was slower in this heat. Earlier in the year, on visits around Easter, I could reach up, twist an orange off a branch and eat segments that filled my mouth with sweet juice gently warmed by the sunshine of spring. At the end of every meal, in the cool, marble-floored kitchen of my nonna's house, we all ate oranges. My uncle, a farmer who made his living by selling fruit, would prove to me that oranges possessed hidden magical powers by taking a piece of peel and bending it over a lit match, each squeeze creating a burst of miniature fireworks.

All life in Ribera seemed to revolve around oranges; even relatives who weren't farmers – uncles who were teachers or pharmacists and cousins who earned their money as traffic cops or bar owners – all, without exception, spent their weekends working their citrus groves. No one had a garden in Ribera, but with their orange trees on the outskirts of town, they had their *giardini*, their own private pieces of paradise. If they had told me that juice ran through their veins, I would have believed them.

The island's global reputation for citrus came from further north, from the 'Conca d'oro', the farmland surrounding Palermo. For centuries the sheer quantity of citrus trees grown here gave it this name, the 'Golden Shell' or 'Golden Bowl'. In the eighteenth century the Conca d'oro was the source of citrus for the British Navy, the solution for preventing scurvy that otherwise afflicted sailors on long voyages. The abundant supply of fruit from the rich, volcanic soils and the increasing demand for it turned Sicily into the most important fruit-growing region in the world. By the 1850s, more than a million cases of oranges and lemons were being shipped every year around Europe from Messina (more than 300 million individual pieces of fruit). Towards the end of the nineteenth century, customers across the Atlantic were driving the demand, and 8 million cases were exported to America each year. In the space of a few generations, the Conca d'oro had become the most profitable agricultural land in Europe. Citrus also helped give rise to the most successful criminal organisation the world had seen: the Mafia, or Cosa Nostra.

The extent of the Mafia's involvement in Sicily's citrus industry was first uncovered by a 29-year-old Tuscan journalist called Leopoldo Franchetti. Sicily had joined the new Italian Republic in 1861 and just over a decade after unification Franchetti travelled to the island to better understand this mysterious and, to observers in the north, troubled addition. Sicily was seen as an island of peasants and poverty, made famous by Greek mythology but largely unknown, partly because of its Arabic-infused dialect, unfathomable to many Italians. With a friend called Sidney Sonnino and armed with a repeating rifle to deter bandits, Franchetti travelled on horseback across the island. He learned that the citrus boom was a high-stakes business for all involved. Trees had to be bought, irrigation channels built and young trees diligently pruned, fertilised and watered. Money had to be invested upfront, with the potential for high returns in the future if things went well. But bad things can happen on citrus farms. Crops can be stolen, irrigation systems damaged, trees vandalised and fruit buyers intimidated. A network of criminals, the mafiosi, could both instigate and ameliorate all of these problems. It was in the fertile basin of the Conca d'oro that the Mafia perfected the art of the protection racket.

'Someone who had just arrived might well believe ... that Sicily was the easiest and most pleasant place in the world. But if [the traveller] stays a while, begins to read the newspapers and listens carefully,' Franchetti wrote, 'bit by bit everything changes around him.' A deadly rifle shot, for instance, might swiftly indicate displeasure caused when a farmer hired the 'wrong' person. 'Just over there, an owner who wanted to rent his groves as he saw fit heard a bullet whistle past his head in friendly warning and afterwards gave in ... The violence and murders take the strangest forms ... After a certain number of these stories, the perfume of orange and lemon blossoms starts to smell of corpses.'

Even the Mafia's initiation ritual featured citrus. Recruits had a finger pricked to allow a drop of blood to fall onto an image of a saint which was then set on fire. In some accounts, the blood was drawn with a thorn taken from a bitter orange tree. In the twentieth century, the Mafia became more interested in other businesses, mostly heroin (which was sometimes processed on remote citrus groves on the outskirts of Palermo). But citrus was never far from the psyche of the mafiosi. After notorious Mafia boss and killer Michele Greco, known as 'the Pope', was arrested, he protested his innocence to a newspaper reporter saying, 'Look, this is my Mafia: work and faith in God,' as he pointed to the mandarin oranges he grew on his country estate. So what exactly was Sicily's citrus bounty? What kind of oranges filled those lucrative (and sometimes dangerous) citrus groves?

*

In the 1920s and 30s, Domenico Casella, an agricultural researcher, attempted to catalogue the fruits grown across the island. The Nikolai Vavilov of Sicilian citrus, Casella's writing shows how in each region of Sicily farmers had selected different varieties of oranges. Some were the result of chance mutations that a farmer had noticed, others were carefully grafted from trees that had been prized for generations for their exceptional fruit. In the west of the island, Casella found 'blonde' varieties, descendants of the first sweet oranges introduced to Sicily by the Portuguese in the sixteenth century. There were also heavy and juicy *arancio barile* ('barrel' oranges) and seedy *biondi di spina o di arridu* (their thorns a legacy of more wild forms of citrus). To the east, around Etna, Casella noticed that the flesh of the fruit changed from being blonde to red – blood oranges. We now know that this is caused by a genetic mutation. The daily fluctuation in temperature around Etna, from intense heat during the day to the cool of the night, triggers these oranges to produce anthocyanin (the compound that makes pomegranates red and blueberries blue). The result is fruit with crimson-coloured flesh and reddish-coloured skin, and Casella listed the varieties, each with their own degree of 'bloodiness': *sanguigno zuccherino* (sugary blood orange), *ovaletto sanguino* and the later ripening *sanguino doppio*, along with *tarroco*, *moro* and *sanguinello*. In Ribera, Casella came across a real outlier. Although it looked like an orange, it didn't taste like one. There was sweetness but not even a hint of sour. 'Juicy, sweet and acid-free,' he said, of the *dolce o vaniglia* – the sweet or vanilla orange – 'a variety grown in Sicily for a very long time' and a local delicacy. The fruit could fetch twice the price of a sweet, sour orange.

Some of the oranges in Casella's catalogue are still grown in Sicily, but most are not. They flourished in their particular part of the island for most of the eighteenth and nineteenth centuries but disappeared towards the middle of the twentieth. A section in Palermo's Botanic Garden is now dedicated to lost varieties, including the earliest mandarins to have arrived in Europe (so fragrant, it's said, that if you peeled one in the morning, your hands would still carry its aroma when you went to bed); strange citrus hybrids with the core of a citron but outer layers of sour orange; fruits with skins that resemble the surface of a cauliflower; and lemons that look like pears. Across the island, in the small plots of land tended by thousands of farmers, the hybrids and the mutations that nature had thrown up became part of a cultural landscape. By the 1970s, most of this diversity was gone. The age of the container ship had arrived and Sicily's farmers were now having to compete with large-scale growers on the other side of the world (with the disadvantage of first having to get the fruit off the island). To survive, they had to find a new type of orange.

Every now and again, a plant can produce something so remarkable that, given the chance, it can change the course of history. In the 1860s, in the state of Bahia in Brazil, a farmer noticed, growing on a single branch of an orange tree, a big orange which appeared to have what looked like a belly button, as if the orange was giving birth to a tiny, second orange at its base. This mutant orange tasted sweet and delicious, it was seedless and its segments pulled apart easily. After the tree was grafted and more oranges produced, this fruit came to the attention of an American missionary who was so impressed that in 1869 she wrote to the United States Department of Agriculture about it. The letter reached the head of Experimental Gardens and Grounds, a Scotsman called William Saunders, who ordered some cuttings from the orange tree which, because of its strange belly button feature, had become known as the 'Navel'.

At this time, American seed collectors were exploring the world finding new crops and new varieties to grow. The west coast was opening up and the government was keen to provide farmers with seeds and plants that could feed future generations. Perhaps, Saunders thought, the orange trees in Brazil had potential. After the plants arrived, he sent three to a new settler in California, Eliza Tibbets. One was trampled by Tibbets's cow, but the remaining two grew in the front yard, watered with dishwater, and produced fruit. The oranges became a local sensation, and Tibbets sold budwood for grafting to hundreds of fellow Californians. By the 1890s, California had an orange industry, and it was based around the two trees Tibbets had nurtured. Today, California produces enough citrus to fill 50 million crates each year bringing in around $2 billion for the state's economy. The Washington Navel (taking the first part of its name from the role of Saunders and USDA) remains the most important orange in California. Its fruit is harvested between October and June, however, so to cover the rest of the year, fruit breeders had to find an orange that ripened between

June and October. This was the Valencia, now mostly grown in Florida. Because of their sweetness, their size and the absence of seeds, the Navel and Valencia varieties also caught the attention of Sicilians.

In 1906, an Italian diplomat described eating a 'Navel' that was 'bigger than the biggest oranges found in Palermo'. It was so juicy, he said, 'it would splatter all over the place'. Back then, only a small number of Californian trees had arrived in Sicily. By the 1970s, when Italy was facing more competition, agronomists saw the Navel as the fruit of the future, and it quickly replaced most of the older Sicilian varieties. But the problem with growing a globalised variety of citrus is that you have to compete in a globalised market. As the cold chain advanced and containerisation increased, Sicilian farmers found themselves in direct competition with enormous monocultures of Navels and Valencia oranges planted in Spain, Morocco, Egypt, South Africa and Brazil. And in recent years the island has really struggled. By the beginning of this century even supermarkets on mainland Italy were importing more oranges from outside Europe rather than from the little island at its foot. Local fruit markets in Sicily closed and farmers who used to be able to make a decent living working a small, ten-hectare citrus grove now found this impossible; bigger operators now dominate the island's citrus trade. Between 2000 and 2010, Sicily lost a quarter of its small farms; it became common to see deserted citrus groves, fruit hanging on trees, left unpicked. One old farmer I met during that period, Concetto Ferrero, had spent his pension trying to keep farming his terraces filled with oranges. I was there to watch his last harvest, listening to the noise of a gentle 'thud, thud, rumble, thud', as workers high up ladders used small finger scissors to cut oranges from the branches of the trees, dropping them into buckets hooked over their backs. 'Agriculture is on its knees; the land is being abandoned,' Ferrero said, 'centuries of tradition are over.' In Ribera, most of my cousins who had grown up in the town left Sicily to find work on the mainland. They are the first in twenty generations for whom the *giardini* (the orange groves) play no role in their lives. Their families had become fragmented, and their community changed for ever by the global supply chain.

Among Sicily's citrus groves I did find hope, and it came (indirectly) from an unexpected source: the Mafia. In the town of San Giuseppe

Jato, twenty miles south of Palermo, is the headquarters of Libera Terra ('Free Land'). This organisation runs farms on land seized from convicted mafiosi and operates them as a network of food businesses. Its office is on the first floor of an anonymous-looking building. Even after years of anti-Mafia investigations and thousands of arrests, for reasons of safety, I'm not able to identify the man I met that day (it's the organisation's policy, he politely explained). Over the last three decades, Libera Terra has allocated thousands of hectares of land once owned by criminals to a new generation of Sicilians. These wheat fields, olive groves and vineyards in different parts of Sicily now produce pasta, oil and wine, all branded as Libera Terra products. The project is also growing traditional varieties of oranges, so helping to protect Sicily's citrus and its biodiversity. On the outskirts of Lentini, near the island's east coast, a team of young Sicilians are growing varieties of blood oranges on ancient terraces that Domenico Casella would have visited on his 1930s travels. The Beppe Montana cooperative, like many Libera Terra projects, takes its name from a fallen anti-Mafia hero. Montana was a policeman who investigated a Mafia family in nearby Catania and paid with his life, shot down close to orange groves.

Mafia land is being used to cultivate hope. 'Lentini had a population of 40,000,' one of Libera Terra's directors told me, 'now it's less than 20,000. Young people could see no future, and the citrus groves were left abandoned.' A decade before, he had stood in the courtroom and watched as the local mafioso who owned the citrus grove was given a life sentence. 'He was a killer,' the director said. Since then, men and women from Lentini, many in their twenties, have taken on the citrus grove and, under the Libera Terra umbrella, have managed to sell the oranges abroad. It's a flicker of optimism for young Sicilians and their country's citrus varieties. But things are not looking so hopeful for Eliza Tibbets's legacy.

In the town of Riverside, California, in the spring of 2019, workers from the Parks Department cordoned off a solitary orange tree at the corner of Magnolia and Arlington avenues. 'We're going to install a kind of Plexiglas around it,' explained Georgios Vidalakis, a professor of plant pathology at the University of California. 'We can't be the generation to lose this tree.' The tree in question was the last surviving Washington

Navel planted by Eliza Tibbets. The worry was that it would be killed by HLB (huanglongbing), the incurable disease that has swept through most parts of the citrus-growing world (it thrives in monocultures). If Tibbets's last tree was to become infected, the leaves would turn mottled and the fruit misshapen, bitter and inedible. Eventually, the tree would die. HLB was detected in Florida in 2005 where it reduced the citrus crop by 75 per cent, causing the lowest production since the Second World War. Jobs in the citrus industry have declined by 60 per cent in the past decade, and Brazil has taken over as the world's leading producer of orange juice. HLB has now arrived in California. By January 2020, a quarantine zone covering a thousand square miles had been created around Riverside, San Bernardino, Los Angeles and Orange County, and the movement of fruit and citrus plants inside the zone had been banned. Residents were even given the number of an emergency hotline in case they spotted any signs of disease on trees in their neighbourhoods. 'If we don't act quickly, we could lose all fresh citrus within ten to fifteen years,' predicted Carolyn Slupsky, a professor of nutrition at the University of California, Davis. 'That would be devastating to people's health and livelihoods.' And another sobering example of why just one variety of orange should not be considered the only fruit.

The Lorax

When Rachel Carson's *Silent Spring* was published in 1962, she woke the world up with a powerful but simple message: when humans harm nature, it eventually backfires on us. 'Our heedless and destructive acts enter into the vast cycles of the earth and in time return to bring hazards to ourselves,' she said. In *Silent Spring*, the public learned that since the 1940s two hundred new chemicals had been created, 'for use in killing insects, weeds, rodents and other organisms, described in the modern vernacular as pests'. Just as the muscles of the Green Revolution were being fully flexed, she placed her spotlight firmly on the chemical component of modern food production, laying bare the war humans were waging against nature. In trying to alter nature, she argued, we had poisoned the land with indiscriminate use of pesticides, the birds were dying, and the eerie quiet that was left was a warning to us all.

Carson was dying of cancer towards the end of writing *Silent Spring*, but she lived long enough to see President Kennedy act on her arguments by setting up a committee to investigate pesticide use. Eventually, DDT, the chemical she singled out for causing the most destruction to wildlife, was banned. In the 1940s, it had been used by apple growers to kill off the moth larvae in their orchards. Carson found it to be a bird killer and carcinogenic to humans. *Silent Spring* changed the world, not only because of Carson's scientific expertise but because of her brilliant storytelling.

A decade later, another American storyteller also succeeded in getting millions of people to think about the destruction of nature and the loss of biodiversity. Like Carson's book, *The Lorax*, by Theodor Geisel (aka Dr Seuss), opens in a mythical town in the heart of

America, where Grickle-grass grows and there's no birdsong except
for the noise of old crows. It goes on to tell the story of how a
beautiful, fantastical forest full of Truffula trees is chopped down to
supply factories making pointless garments called Thneeds. Despite
the efforts of the tree-loving Lorax, the very last Truffula tree is
eventually chopped down. The Onceler, the greedy businessman who
destroyed the Truffula trees, finds himself alone and out of business,
surrounded by a wasteland of his own making. Dr Seuss was dealing
with urgent issues still outside of mainstream news coverage: pollution, greed and deforestation. *The Lorax* was *Silent Spring* for
children.

Someone who grew up reading *The Lorax* was scientist Gayle Volk,
a plant researcher at USDA and a world authority on apples. Today
when she remembers the story of *The Lorax*, it makes her think of
the thousands of hectares of forest cleared in the Tian Shan, the
birthplace of the apple. Volk's research involves finding answers to
future problems expected to become more common in the global
crop. 'We've taken a big risk by reducing the fruit's genetic base,' Volk
says, 'and one of the most valuable resources we have to protect the
apple's future is the diversity within the Tian Shan.' Volk's colleagues
from USDA made it into the forests in the early 1990s, shortly after
Barrie Juniper's first expeditions. They travelled through Kazakhstan
collecting apple seeds and material for grafting. Sometimes, when fuel
supplies allowed, helicopters took them into the most remote areas
of forest.

What they gathered was then planted in America's national apple
collection in Geneva, New York State. For thirty years, the trees that
grew out of the wild apple seeds from Kazakhstan were used as a
gene pool by the fruit industry. 'They bred in some of the wild ancestor
because that's where they found novel resistance to disease,' says Volk,
who looked after the collection. Now, the world's apples, along with
all other fruits, face even greater perils. 'The winters are becoming
milder, insects and diseases aren't being killed off, growers all around
the world are seeing more risks of pests and disease.' In the spring
of 2018, Volk and a few other USDA colleagues went back into the
Tian Shan to revisit the locations their colleagues had explored in the
early 1990s. 'Places where they had collected seeds no longer had trees;

in the space of twenty-five years, huge numbers of trees had vanished. Once all that diversity is lost, there's no going back.' This is what makes her think of *The Lorax*. 'People don't realise the treasure we have within our midst,' she says. 'And you don't miss something until it's gone.'

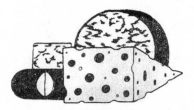

Part Seven
Cheese

If you don't like bacteria, you're on the wrong planet.

J. Craig Venter

It's 10,500 years since we first domesticated cattle and a watershed moment is approaching: the world's dairy farmers will soon be producing more than one billion tonnes of milk each year. The sharp increases in world milk production seen in recent years are striking (from 690 million tonnes in 2009 to 850 million tonnes in 2019), but what is more extraordinary are the countries driving most of that growth. Traditionally, milk and cheese were part of Western diets, but industrial-scale dairy farming is now booming in China, and Asia overall is becoming 'milkier'. This trend is allowing us to watch a phase of human evolution in real time. As a species, we're unique in consuming the milk of other animals. But we didn't start out this way. Our ancestors were lactose-intolerant (as are two-thirds of the world's population today, including most of Asia's). For us to drink animal milk, and on the scale we do now, required firstly ingenuity and secondly biological change.

During infancy, the cells that line our small intestine produce an enzyme called lactase. This makes milk digestible by breaking down the sugar molecules it contains (lactose). For most of our evolutionary history, this enzyme switched off after children were weaned, so drinking milk would have made adult humans sick. However, after we domesticated cattle, sheep and goats, a mutation in the human genome started to find its way into the population. Those who had the mutation kept on producing lactase into adulthood (we call this 'lactase persistence'). It is likely this gave them an evolutionary advantage as milk contains calcium, carbohydrate and micronutrients and is available all year round. Stored inside the udders of animals it was portable, too. So advantageous was lactase persistence that in Northern and Central Europe, and parts of Africa and the Middle

East, the trait became fixed within a few thousand years (in evolutionary terms, the blink of an eye). Even so, between the start of animal domestication and the rise of the mutation, there was a gap of thousands of years. One solution to this problem of lactose intolerance was to convert milk into cheese.

When liquid milk is transformed into solid cheese, its entire chemistry is changed through two main processes: fermentation and coagulation. One, fermentation, happens when bacteria naturally present in the milk – or added as a starter culture – begin to digest the milk sugars (the lactose) and release lactic acid. The acidification creates an environment hostile to harmful bacteria, which helps to preserve the milk. The longer fermentation continues, the more lactose levels will fall (in aged hard cheeses such as Parmesan these levels can be extremely low). The other process, coagulation, might have been discovered when our ancestors butchered young ruminants, opened their stomachs and found clots of fermented and coagulated milk inside. When they ate this clotted milk, they discovered it was tasty and easy to digest. We now know this coagulation is caused by the action of rennet, a package of enzymes which are secreted by the fourth stomach of any infant ruminant animal such as calves, lambs and kid goats. On contact with milk, these enzymes knit together proteins within it to form curd. This set 'cheese' curd can then be manipulated (cut, stirred and drained) which allows even more liquid (containing lactose) to be removed from the milk. Without any understanding of the science at work, Neolithic farmers solved the problem of milk intolerance by making cheese.

The first real evidence of these techniques being used comes from central Europe. When archaeologists excavated the banks of the Vistula River in central Poland in the 1970s, they discovered hundreds of strange-looking clay fragments, dated back to 5000 BCE, pitted with tiny holes. The find puzzled them; they couldn't work out what this pottery would have been used for. A decade later, an American archaeologist suggested they might be pieces of a bowl used to separate curds and whey (he had seen similar-looking patterns in an antique collection of sieves once owned by Victorian cheesemakers). It wasn't until 2012 that new scientific techniques confirmed his suspicions when microscopic particles of fat (lipids), 7,000 years old, were found absorbed within the clay. This pottery is the earliest evidence of cheese-making anywhere in the world (younger milk-infused pottery has been found in Croatia, dated to 5200 BCE). The cheese made with it, scientists concluded, would have looked like a clumpy version of mozzarella (though in reality the prehistoric cheese would have been closer to ricotta).

Over millennia, milk processing became increasingly widespread and more sophisticated. In the ruins of the ancient city of Ur, temples dedicated to milk and cattle contain friezes depicting people making butter by rocking clay urns. At Memphis in Egypt, a 5,000-year-old jar of cheese was found inside the tomb of the ruler Ptahmes. Made with a blend of sheep's, cow's and goat's milk, this was food stored away for the afterlife. Meanwhile, to the east the Sumerians had become such sophisticated cheesemakers they had descriptions of twenty different types of cheese (categorised according to their colour, levels of freshness and taste). In the Roman Empire, hard cheeses were produced on an industrial scale (the likely origins of Parmigiano-Reggiano), food for armies to march on. Picking up techniques from one conquered people and passing them on to another, the Romans became great transmitters of cheese-making knowledge and skill.

Cheese changed the world, enabling humans to extend their reach and settle in some of the most inhospitable places on Earth, among mountain ranges and in highland areas. By turning milk into cheese, the life-giving energy of the sun could be captured and stored. The goodness of the grasses and wild flowers which grew during spring and summer was transformed into food eaten in the depths of winter.

From one ingredient, milk, humans in different parts of the world created an incalculable array of unique cheeses. Wherever it was made, what it looked like and how it tasted depended entirely on the environment it was produced in: the type of soil and pasture; the species and breeds of animals being farmed; the resources people had access to such as salt and firewood; and, crucially, the microbes present within the milk and in the air (bacteria, moulds and yeasts). More than any other food, cheese had an intimate connection to a specific place and to a particular season.

Historically, France best illustrated the wide diversity of possible cheese styles. Charles de Gaulle might or might not have said, 'How can you govern a country that has 246 varieties of cheese?', but the sentiment rings true. Each region of France had its own particular ways of doing things, including how it processed milk. This makes it possible to navigate the history and geography of France through a cheeseboard. Hard styles such as Comté, Abondance and Beaufort all speak of tough lives in remote Alpine places where cooperation between farmers became essential. During the summer, people left their villages to take animals high up into the mountains in search of the best pasture. At high altitudes, working in groups, they milked their animals and made huge wheels of cheeses firm enough to be transported back to their communities for the winter. Further south, in the warmer Auvergne and Occitanie regions, cheeses such as Roquefort, Fourme d'Ambert and Bleu d'Auvergne were kept inside limestone caves. Microbes flourished within these cool and humid natural stores and left the cheeses marked with (now famous) vivid veins of blue mould.

In Burgundy, in the centre of the country, cheese-making was for centuries the preserve of monasteries. Here, dark, humid cellars (places where moulds flourish) could be used for maturing cheese. Monks washed these cheeses clean using alcohol and brine, which is how strong-smelling, 'washed-rind', meaty cheeses, such as Époisses, were created. In the Île-de-France and Normandy, in the north, people lived and farmed on more silty and sandy soil, where building cellars to store cheese in was less practical. Instead, cheeses were matured in barns, where the flow of air introduced microbes that coated them in a fine, velvety mould. Because these farmers also lived closer to towns and cities, their cheeses didn't need to be hard and long-lasting. The results were soft, mould-coated cheeses, including Brie and Camembert. Meanwhile, in the Loire Valley in western France, one of the legacies of the Arab conquest of the eighth century had been the introduction of goat farming. Here, cheeses such as Chabichou du Poitou and Sainte-Maure de Touraine evolved, all made with goats' milk. Bite into a traditional piece of cheese and you will be eating into history, culture and an ecosystem.

It's impossible to put a number on exactly how many different cheeses there are in the world; there are as many potential cheeses as there are ecosystems. And within each ecosystem an individual cheesemaker will add their own unique twist to the process. In the UK in the nineteenth century there were several hundred Lancashire cheesemakers, all helping to create an incredible range of textures and flavours for just one style of cheese. By the end of the twentieth century only one of these traditional farmhouse cheeses remained. This decline in cheese diversity happened in most parts of the cheese-making world, to lesser or greater degrees.

Urbanisation, war, science and technology all help to explain this decline, along with a whole host of regional causes, but there are some common factors driving the loss of many of the world's cheeses. Chief among these is the transformation of milk (the most perishable of all agricultural products) into a globally traded product. Fewer than twenty multinational companies now control a third of the world's milk supply (worth around $83 billion a year). To make this possible, the world's milk has become increasingly standardised, a process set in motion by the Industrial Revolution. In the early 1800s, countries producing greater quantities of milk than their populations could consume began sending dairy products around the world. For instance, Irish milk was turned into heavily salted butter and sold through the powerful Cork Butter Exchange to places as far afield as Brazil, the West Indies, South Africa and India. By the 1860s, clothbound cheddar made in North America was being exported by boat to England. In the 1870s, with the arrival of refrigerated ships, the infant global dairy trade expanded (by the 1880s New Zealand butter was being transported to Britain).

As towns and cities grew in size, drinking fresh milk became more common among urban populations since rail networks could bring in fresh supplies of the liquid from rural areas. Dairies within cities also proliferated. This movement of milk, together with more industrial production and mass consumption, triggered an increase in disease, particularly bovine tuberculosis.

To combat this, in the early twentieth century, pasteurisation (heating up milk in short bursts to destroy microbes) became a legal requirement in most of Europe and North America. This killed off the bacteria in milk, the good along with the bad. To replace the missing microbes needed to make cheese (the lactic-acid-producing bacteria) 'cultures' were developed by businesses specialising in the manufacture of microorganisms. Nature, geography and climate no longer determined the character of a cheese – science did. You could now make a Cheddar-, Camembert- or Gorgonzola-style cheese wherever you were in the world, whatever the season – all you needed was a sachet of bacteria ordered from a catalogue. The connection between place and product was fundamentally broken and the complex array of microbes derived from the pasture, the animals and the farm (before, essential components of cheese-making) were increasingly viewed with suspicion. Only now, as the science of our gut microbiomes is better understood, are we realising that missing out on these microbes might be detrimental to our health as well as depriving us of exciting flavours.

The amount of milk traded internationally increased fivefold between 1960 and 2010. During the same period, milk consumption in China saw an estimated fifteenfold increase, led in part by sales of infant formula and dairy products made popular with the arrival of Western-style coffee bars, takeaway pizzas and ice cream. As milk became globalised, incomes for dairy farmers became more volatile. In the UK, between 2010 and 2015, the average price of milk sold in supermarkets fell by one-third (making a litre of milk cheaper than a bottle of water). Downward pressure on prices led many dairy farmers to operate on a larger scale. In the US, for example, until the 1990s, most farms had fewer than two hundred cows; today, the largest corporate dairies can house more than 9,000 cows. This is when, in pursuit of ever greater efficiency, the industry focused increasingly on one breed: Holsteins. Between the 1960s and early 2000s, the genetics of these animals was altered to such an extent that their milk yields doubled. Much of the cheese we eat today, wherever we are in the world, is made from milk processed by a smaller number of companies, sourced from the same breed of cattle, using bacteria created in a handful of labs. We are at risk of losing the diversity created by thousands of years of cheese-making.

Most cheese is no longer an expression of a place but a carbon copy of food that could be produced anywhere. By preserving diverse cheeses, we can save living diversity from the ground up; soil, grasses, animal breeds and microbes. This is better for biodiversity, as well as giving us more interesting flavours. It would be foolish to lose dairying and cheese-making skills too. This knowledge of how to turn landscapes into food in different environments, in some cases built up over millennia, might be part of a toolkit we need to call upon in future. The cheeses you are about to meet also represent another kind of diversity, that of human experience.

24

Salers

Auvergne, Central France

Of all our relationships with other species, perhaps the most troubling and mysterious is the one we have with microbes. On the one hand, most of our favourite foods and drinks depend on them (chocolate, coffee, wine and beer involve fermentation as much as cheese-making). Our own bodies also play host to trillions of them; without the bacteria and yeasts in and on our bodies, we couldn't survive. Yet science has taught us microbes can also be dangerous, that some bacteria can kill. In the twentieth century, the view of microbes being deadly organisms took precedence. As a result, we waged a war on them, and cleansed and sterilised our homes and our food without discretion – all in the name of safety. Only recently have we learned that, from a health point of view, we have lost something in this process. The latest science is clear: having a diet rich in microbial life – one that features fermented foods such as kraut, kimchi and traditionally made cheese – is good for us. These living foods help feed our gut microbiomes, the trillions of bacteria and yeasts we all host and which are intricately linked to our health. But these are the very foods much of the world turned away from and became suspicious of in the last century. We exterminated as much microbial life from our diets as we could and opted for industrialised and ultra-processed foods instead. In the last fifty years, we have lost one-third of the diversity in our gut microbiome, a change more profound than many of us realise. For this reason, eating a raw milk cheese can be seen as a positive way of bringing microbes back into our lives and into our stomachs. And perhaps one cheese above all can help demonstrate the power of good bacteria at work: Salers.

*

Salers is the name of a village and a breed of cow as well as a cheese. All three can be found high up in the Massif Central in the Auvergne region of southern France. This is where one of Europe's most uncompromising foods is made, part of a farming tradition that stretches back at least a thousand years. It is one of the oldest surviving cheeses and also one of the most gruelling to make. In April, as spring approaches and the pasture on the mountains becomes thick and fertile, the farmers and their cattle move away from the village, in some cases travelling twenty miles, to go higher up the mountain. For six months, they live in small stone cottages called *burons* and follow an almost monastic existence of work and isolation, each day beginning and ending with milking. A day's work can start at four in the morning and finish at ten o'clock in the evening, during which time they can produce one large 40kg wheel of cheese from the milk collected that day. In the past, these would have been taken back down to the village by cart at the end of the season. Fewer than ten producers are left making Salers this way, and this endangered craft is dependent on the milk of an endangered dairy animal.

With long curved horns and a thick, curly, mahogany coat, the Salers cow has the look of an ancient animal. And it is. It resembles the images of the cattle captured in rock art inside the Lascaux cave, just fifty miles away from the village of Salers. These cows are perfectly adapted to the rough and rocky Auvergne, a panorama of mountains and plateaus formed by hundreds of extinct volcanoes. For the people who settled this region, growing wheat was never an option. Instead, survival mostly depended on converting pasture into milk and then into cheese. The Salers cow made this possible because it's a perfect mountain forager, light and nimble enough to reach the wild grasses, herbs and flowers that cloak the high-altitude pasture. The technique used to milk these animals is also ancient. In modern farming systems, calves are taken away from their mothers within days of being born so that every drop of milk from that point can be dedicated to human consumption. In the Salers system, calves get to suckle their mother, and 'take a quarter' from one of the teats. This not only gets the milk flowing but also helps clean the teats. After being pulled away from the udder, the calf is tied to its mother's foreleg and salt is sprinkled on its back, encouraging the mother to lick and soothe her infant.

The close physical contact between the animals is seen as important in keeping the milk flowing. The cheesemaker, with his head nestled against the body of the warm animal, starts milking. What he is collecting is the product of a wild mountain landscape, biodiversity in liquid form. The cattle graze on clover, gentian and anise, arnica, harebell and fennel, and much more. This plant diversity is expressed through the cow's milk – a rich creamy and complex microbial soup, which in turn creates distinctive flavours in the cheese. When you eat this food, you are eating from mountains and consuming a landscape.

Science can now explain why cheeses made on mountain pastures such as the Auvergne taste so distinctive. The greater the level of biodiversity in the pasture a dairy animal feeds on, the more its milk will be filled with aromatic compounds called terpenes (these are part of the plant's defence system). Animals fed on pasture absorb these compounds which are carried over into their milk (terpenes don't feature in milk from cows given commercial feed). As a cheese matures, terpenes come into their own, helping to create layers and layers of flavour. What might have started out in the summer as a low-key bite of cheese is transformed into a truly memorable one. But in a Salers cheese, another set of invisible characters are given the opportunity to express themselves too. After milking, the warm milk is poured into waist-high, wooden vats called *gerles*. When the liquid comes into contact with the wood it's true to say the cheese is on its way.

For health inspectors used to seeing clinical-looking equipment inside white-walled dairies, the sight of this set-up would be terrifying. The decades-old barrels never come into contact with cleaning chemicals; instead they're rinsed out with liquid whey left over from cheesemaking. This is because Salers cheesemakers aren't simply processing milk, they're farming microbes. The bacteria that live on and in the wooden *gerles* are so diverse and vigorous that, unlike with most other cheeses, no starter culture is needed to sour the milk and kick-start fermentation. When microbiologists analysed what happens inside the vats, they found that, within seconds of being poured inside a *gerle*, milk is inoculated with huge amounts of beneficial bacteria. Levels of lactic acid bacteria were so high that it would be almost impossible for dangerous pathogens to survive in this environment – any that are present are simply overwhelmed by the healthy (desirable) microbes, a phenomenon referred to in science as 'competitive exclusion'.

When the cheese is left to mature, the lactic acid bacteria continue to deter any unwanted microbial threats. Seen from the microbe's point of view, the job of a cheesemaker is to make the best possible home for good bacteria. To prove this point, scientists even tried experiments in which they spiked a *gerle* with a dose of the pathogenic bacteria *Listeria monocytogenes*. Weeks later, when they tested the cheese made in the contaminated vat, the pathogen was gone; the *gerle* was too hostile an environment for the potentially lethal bugs.

Cut open a wheel of Salers after it has been matured for a year and you'll see a grainy, mottled, rich yellow paste. Each wheel has its own particular flavour. At its best, Salers can taste meaty, brothy, buttery and grassy. At its worst, it can be 'wild and obnoxious', according to Bronwen Percival, a cheese expert who has watched the mountain farmers at work. This surely is one of the beauties of diversity; food that's complex, just a little unpredictable and most definitely not dull.

25

Stichelton

Nottinghamshire, England

At six o'clock one morning, I stepped into a warm, white-walled dairy on the edge of Sherwood Forest to watch England's 'King of Cheeses' being made, a Stilton in all but name. Joe Schneider works to an old recipe for the blue-veined cheese, but because he uses unpasteurised milk, he's not allowed to call it Stilton. Rules passed in the 1990s mean the famous cheese can now only be made with pasteurised milk. To avoid prosecution, Schneider called his cheese Stichelton, Old English for the town that gave Stilton its name.

Schneider arrived in the UK from America in the late 1990s and began a love affair with cheese-making, a 'mix of hard science and alchemy' as he describes it. Two decades on, in his East Coast accent, he told me his mission. 'The cheese I make is part of British culture – it shouldn't be allowed to disappear. I'm not going to let it, although this isn't my heritage.' For Schneider, there's a lot more at stake here than just a name; he believes what he's making is the authentic version of England's greatest cheese. By saving it, he's protecting the very essence of what cheese had been for millennia; a food with a direct connection to place – a connection that comes from the microbes in a farm's milk.

Schneider grew up in 1970s New York. It was a time when processed food was in the ascendant and where 'cheese' meant Kraft Singles, Velveeta and Cheez Whiz sprayed out of a can. After training as an engineer, he took to travelling, eventually moving to Amsterdam with his then girlfriend, now wife. There, he fell into a job making feta cheese for a Turkish dairy owner he met at a party. But his destiny was sealed when he walked into the now legendary cheesemongers, Neal's Yard Dairy in London. He stood in the middle of the shop open-mouthed. 'There were these giant truckles of cheese, some weighed thirty pounds,' he remembers, 'each one beautiful, round, cloth-bound and mottled.' It was an intense, multi-sensory experience filled with extraordinary and beguiling colours, shapes, textures and smells. It changed his life. 'I said to myself, I'm going to make a cheese that belongs in this shop.'

Stilton's origins are one of the great mysteries of British food. Its story is filled with claims and counterclaims of its provenance and the source of the recipe. The cheese's name, however, is more easily traced. In 1722, the antiquarian William Stukeley (best known for his research into Stonehenge) wrote that the Cambridgeshire town 'is famous for cheese, which ... would be thought equal to Parmesan were it not so near us'. Two years later, Daniel Defoe made the same comparison in his *Tour Thro' the Whole Island of Great Britain* but added an unappetising twist: 'Stilton is famous for cheese, which is called our English Parmesan, and is brought to Table so full of mites or maggots, that they use a spoon to eat them.' In fact, Stilton was never made in Stilton. Its makers were based further north, in the heart of England, in the counties of Derbyshire, Leicestershire and Notting-hamshire (where Schneider makes his Stichelton). Stilton was the place where the cheese was sold.

It started life as a farmhouse cheese but what Stukeley and Defoe tasted was a food of the Enlightenment. Wool, coal and iron had transformed Britain into an industrial power and the agricultural revolution was in full swing; this was the time when the livestock breeder Robert Bakewell (based in Stilton country) was applying his new methods to increase Britain's supplies of meat and milk. Transport links were being improved, among them the Great North Road, which connected London, Leeds, Sheffield and Edinburgh. A crucial stopping point along the route was the town of Stilton, which is why cheeses sold by merchants in the town became so widely known. By the end of the eighteenth century, cheese had become an important British export, with thousands of tonnes shipped each year from docks in London and Liverpool. Stilton, like all of the renowned British cheeses, was a product of this age of trade, scientific discovery and urbanisation. The expansion of the road networks, railways and canals in the mid-nineteenth century shaped a quintessentially British cheese style: low moisture, high acid and firm texture. As well as Stilton, this included

Cheddar, Caerphilly, Cheshire, Gloucester, Lancashire and Leicester. All were suited to being transported. And as cities across Britain grew in size, so did the scale of cheese production.

By this time, Stilton had evolved into a creamy blue-veined cheese. The milk ladled by hand, the curds not pressed, just salted (giving it a crumbly texture), it was shaped like a cylinder and matured for at least a year, during which time it developed a thick, golden, pitted crust. What made it such a celebrated cheese was the time and attention required to make it. According to a nineteenth-century cheesemaker, 'Stilton, with the exception it makes no noise, is more trouble than babies.' Each one had to be turned daily so that it drained under its own weight and then rubbed by hand to form the crust. Perhaps because of this, it was seen as a cheese for gastronomes, a food for feast days and celebrations, including Christmas.

By the early twentieth century, farms had given way to factories as Britain's main source of cheese, and Stilton was no exception. The last truckle of Stilton made in a farmhouse dairy went on sale in 1935. But a decade later, there was no Stilton at all. The Second World War resulted in the government taking control of dairy production and factories were ordered to stop making Stilton and switch to Cheddar (seen as a more efficient use of milk). It wasn't until the 1950s people got to taste Stilton again. Even then, the traditional features of the cheese remained intact; it was still made in the same three counties, involved a slow, long and laborious process, and most significant of all for this story, it was made with raw (unpasteurised) milk. But history was on the side of pasteurisation.

The use of heat to kill off microbes and reduce spoilage had been pioneered by Louis Pasteur in the 1860s as part of experiments to help the wine industry. The technique of applying a short burst of heat to liquid milk followed in the 1880s. But it wasn't until after the First World War that the process became more widespread. Used on supplies of fresh milk, pasteurisation was an unmitigated public health success. Between the 1850s and the 1940s, when milk drinking became more common in towns and cities, tuberculosis killed more than half a million Britons. Pasteurisation helped bring an end to these large-scale fatalities, but there were opponents to it. Campaigning 'vitalists' argued the case for unpasteurised milk, saying heat would destroy the 'life' in milk and so affect the nation's health and vigour. But heat treatment won the day and in 1922, with the passing of the Milk and Dairies Act, pasteurisation of milk became a legal requirement. For the cheese industry, pasteurisation of milk had been less of a public health issue as the build-up of lactic acid bacteria during the cheese-making process reduced risk from pathogens. But pasteurisation did have commercial appeal and so cheesemakers started to embrace it. By killing off bacteria (both good and bad), milk became a blank canvas onto which manufactured starter cultures could be added. This offered a greater level of control over the process and removed unpredictability. This way, whatever the time of year, and even working with milk pooled from a number of different farms, a consistent cheese could be produced week after week, year after year. Stilton makers followed the trend and switched to pasteurisation. All except one, Colston Bassett, which first started making the cheese in 1913. But in the Christmas of 1988, an outbreak of food poisoning was blamed on its unpasteurised cheese. Although the link was never proven, this rattled the industry, and the final batch of raw milk Colston Bassett Stilton was made soon after. In 1996, the transformation of the Stilton recipe became official when the cheese was added to the list of the European Union's Protected Designation of Origin (PDO) foods. This legal status (which covers thousands of foods across Europe) acts as a guarantee a product has been made in a specific region using traditional methods. The application (made by the Stilton Cheesemakers' Association) specified the cheese could only be made with pasteurised milk. In effect, under European rules, the most traditional form of Stilton (the one made with raw milk) became extinct. Few people in Britain would have noticed, but to a small group of cheese enthusiasts, what had taken place was nothing less than an act of cultural vandalism and an agricultural tragedy.

Neal's Yard Dairy, the cheesemongers that so inspired Joe Schneider, was founded by Randolph Hodgson in the late 1970s. The shop was partly a commercial venture and partly an act of countercultural radicalism, born in the spirit of the punk age. Hodgson had studied dairy science for a career in the food industry but ended up wanting to challenge homogenisation and corporate control as it spread through British food and farming, and he did this by saving endangered cheese. A dwindling band of farmhouse dairies had survived this far into the twentieth century, and these were joined by a handful of maverick new cheesemakers hoping to revive lost traditions. Hodgson and Neal's Yard Dairy proved crucial to both. As a cheesemonger, Hodgson provided an outlet for producers who stood no chance (and had no interest) in selling their cheese through supermarkets. But he was also a champion of their work and an adviser. He spent much of the 1980s visiting cheesemakers on their farms, tasting, giving feedback and helping to solve problems. As a result, he helped save many British cheeses from going extinct and helped preserve knowledge and farming skills that were fast disappearing. Chief among his priorities was his desire to protect the few raw milk cheeses left in Britain, including Colston Bassett. 'When they started to pasteurise, Randolph went through a kind of grieving process,' says Schneider. 'Something he really cared about and believed in was gone.' Hodgson even pleaded with Colston Bassett to make small batches of their Stilton with raw milk to sell through Neal's Yard Dairy just to keep production going, but they said they couldn't. And then the PDO happened. 'That's when Randolph said, "Screw it, if no one else is going to make the cheese, I will."' It would take a decade for the idea to become reality, by which time he and Schneider had become friends. In October 2006, at the Nottinghamshire dairy I would later visit, they made the first batch of Stichelton.

In Britain today, experienced cheesemongers are likely to agree on just a handful of truly great farmhouse cheeses, including the likes of Montgomery's Cheddar and Kirkham's Lancashire, cheeses that have generations of history and experience behind them. Schneider added Stichelton to that list within a decade and from a standing start. Yet this cheese, based on the most traditional of Stilton recipes and in demand around the world, still can't be called a Stilton. 'The PDO will allow me to make a cheese with pasteurised milk, fill it with cranberries and stick a banana in it and call it a Stilton,' says Schneider. 'But if I call my raw milk cheese a Stilton, I'd be prosecuted.'

From the large windows of the Stichelton dairy, I could see the cows returning to their field. A layer of yellow cream glinted across the surface of the morning's milk as it settled in a long, rectangular stainless steel vat. This was the first step in the twenty-four-hour 'make' (farm-house Cheddar can take as little as six hours). People have tried to speed up Stilton recipes, but it can't be done; making Stichelton is a long and physical process. Just a minuscule (Schneider says 'homeopathic') amount of starter culture is added, to encourage the acidity to develop gradually, ensuring each step of the make (something of a slow-motion high-wire act) can be taken ever so gently. This is not a consistent cheese. Most often it is outstanding, but sometimes Schneider will make a Stichelton which is incomparable, up there among the world's best.

To create the blue veins that run through the cheese, Schneider adds spores of the fungus *Penicillium roqueforti* at the start of the make. Later, when the cheeses are maturing, holes are pierced into the centre, letting air in and activating the mould. This causes further breakdown of fats and proteins, adding sharper, more piquant flavours, making the texture softer and creamier and giving parts of the ivory coloured cheese its distinctive indigo blue veins. Before it became possible to manufacture *Penicillium roqueforti*, Stilton makers were said to have used old pieces of leather which they left hanging outside their dairies until they became coated in a delicate layer of mould. They then draped these through the vats to inoculate their milk.

Five hours into that day's make, the milk had coagulated, and the whey drained away. Schneider now had to move the warm curds from the vat and onto a long cooling table. Most Stilton makers now do this mechanically, but Schneider insists that it has to be done by hand, one ladle at a time. In a single motion he took a scoop from the vat on his right and swung it across to the cooling table on his left. For an hour, I watched him bend, turn and twist, heaving the curds from one side to the other. The room was silent except for the trance-like slip-slapping sound of moist curds falling onto the table. 'Do it any other way and you'll damage the curds and change the texture of the cheese,' he said. I felt I was witnessing the last fragile link in a chain that had been forged centuries before, one that connected humans, animals, pasture and microbes; a beautiful and natural synchronicity. Science had changed that, casting nature as the enemy and giving the laboratory the status of saviour. In this dairy, I could still feel the sense of wonder for that other lost world. 'To think,' I said, as I watched the firm curds pile up, 'a few hours ago it was milk.'

'And just two days ago,' Schneider said, 'it was grass.'

26

Mishavinë

Accursed Mountains, Albania

Running along the northern border of Albania is a mountain range called Bjeshkët e Namuna, the 'Accursed Mountains'. Tucked among its 3,000-metre-high spires are villages and hamlets which after a few days of heavy snow can be cut off for weeks at a time. Even after the spring, the outside world is still a faraway place. Until recently, major roads didn't extend this far, leaving this one of the most isolated and (in monetary terms) poorest parts of Europe. Many settlements can still only be reached by bumping along rough tracks cut into thick forests. This mountain region was home to Albania's ancient tribes, the Skreli, Gruda, Kelmendi, Kastrati and Hoti, ethnic groups for whom blood feuds spanned generations. Life in the Accursed Mountains could be hard, ruthless and desolate. But without cheese-making, it would have been impossible.

Because they are so isolated, Albania's northern highlands remained a mystery to the outside world until a British traveller named Edith Durham explored the region in 1900. Exhausted by years of nursing her sick mother, she had been advised by her doctor to travel and to get a course of mountain air. She headed first to Montenegro, and then crossed into Albania and the Bjeshkët e Namuna. Wearing a waterproof Burberry skirt and equipped with a diary and sketchpad, she recorded tribal life among the mountains. Over the years she returned again and again and in Albania today she is referred to as *Mbretëresha e Malësoreve*, 'Queen of the Highlanders'. Her account of this place was so detailed that when foreign correspondents were sent to report on the war in Kosovo just over the border in 1998 many were issued with Durham's book, *High Albania*, for orientation. In it, she describes a brutal world in which 'blood vengeance' had spread throughout the land. 'All else is subservient to it,' she wrote. 'Blood can be wiped out only with blood.' She believed tribal allegiances in the Albanian Highlands had remained unchanged for generations and that the same was true of food. 'The afternoon passed in dark dwellings,' she wrote, 'drinking to people's health in rakia, chewing sheep-cheese, and firing rifles and revolvers indoors ... The sofra, a low round table, was brought and a large salt sheep-cheese, cut in chunks, put in the middle, to help down the rakia (a strong fruit spirit) ... bowls of kos (sheep's yoghurt) were so sour that it drew the mouth.' At large communal meals, Durham was often guest of honour and chief witness to a culinary spectacle. She described a whole sheep stuffed with herbs turned over a large fire, later eaten with maize bread dipped in melted cheese. A century after Durham, I followed her footsteps up into the Albanian Alps to find out what remained of that culture and the salty cheese that had helped down the rakia.

My guide was an Italian aid worker in his sixties, Pier Paolo Ambrosi. In the early 1990s, he had stood at a port on Italy's east coast and watched, mystified, as boat after boat brought thousands of Albanians across the Adriatic Sea. The Albania of Edith Durham's time had been cut off from the outside world by geography, but later that century the country was even more isolated, this time by politics. This small nation of around 3 million people, sandwiched between Greece and the remnants of Yugoslavia, withdrew into an extreme form of communism. For four decades, its Marxist dictator, Enver Hoxha, forced Albanians into a secretive and solitary state. No one could enter or leave; religion was banned. It was the only country in Europe where Christmas was forbidden, and even if it hadn't been Albanians would have been too poor to celebrate. To instil a sense of fear and paranoia, 700,000 machine-gun nests were built around the country, one for every four Albanians. The enemy was without, not within, Hoxha wanted people to believe. When he died in 1985, the Communist regime limped on, but the economy crumbled, and food supplies ran perilously low. The winter of 1990 was a tipping point and, by 20 February 1991, protesters in the capital Tirana felt empowered enough to pull down the seventeen-foot gold-leaf statue of Hoxha. The protest sealed the end of the Stalinist state. Chaos followed and thousands of people were killed. Those who could escape Albania did so. By the end of the 1990s, one fifth of the population had migrated, including the people Ambrosi watched arriving in Italy on overcrowded boats.

The Catholic charity he worked for sent him in the opposite direction. 'We wanted to find out where the people were coming from, who was left behind,' he says, 'and so my idea was to spend a few weeks exploring Albania.' He ended up staying for nearly thirty years.

The regime had controlled every detail of Albanian life, from the allocation of jobs to the provision of shoes and clothes. Everything was in short supply. 'In one region, the Ministry of Economy allocated 1.2 socks per person, in another 1.5,' Ambrosi said, realising the same bureaucratic madness had also been applied to food. A family might receive a ration of a kilo of pork one month, followed by three months of no meat at all. People could spend days outside shops waiting in line for milk to arrive. After the regime's collapse, things got worse before they got better. In the north, this resulted in massive depopulation. Ambrosi found deserted villages across the Albanian highlands as the exodus to the cities took place; within a decade, Tirana's population quadrupled. But in the most remote parts of the Accursed Mountains, a handful of self-sufficient communities survived, little changed since Edith Durham's time. Here, the old food ways could still be found. This was where we were headed.

The higher up into the highlands we travelled, the further back in time it all felt. 'This road is a link between the old world and the new,' said Ambrosi, referring to a track still under construction that eventually tapered off into gravel. We passed people guiding horse-driven carts stacked with sheaths of hay and were forced to stop and wait as shepherds moved their flocks along the path ahead, the bells around their necks ringing out as they headed towards the mountain pasture. 'They have right of way here,' Ambrosi said as the sheep surrounded the jeep. Our destination was Lepushe, a scattering of houses made of wood and stone at the top of a glorious plateau, close to the border with Montenegro. Around us were miles of ancient pasture; wild grasses and flowers filled the vast open space enclosed by snow-capped peaks in the distance. It was here, on one of his early expeditions, that Ambrosi discovered a cheese that Neolithic farmers would have recognised, Mishavinë, a food that harked back to the very beginnings of cheese-making and dairy animals. Elsewhere in Albania food traditions had been wiped out along with religion; under the dictatorship there had been just two state-approved cheeses, 'white cheese' and 'yellow cheese'. But in the highlands, Mishavinë hadn't changed for a thousand years. Just three farmers were left making this cheese and one of them lived in Lepushe, a man called Luigj Cekaj. There, in the Accursed Mountains, Cekaj and his wife Lumtumire were keeping one of Europe's most endangered food traditions alive.

To survive in the mountains, at the end of each spring Cekaj's ancestors had trekked high up into the Albanian Alps where they lived with their animals until the end of summer. This place has the lushest, most biodiverse and unspoilt pasture left in Europe. For months at a time, animals can graze on hundreds of different wild flowers, herbs and grasses, many of which are used as medicinal plants by the shepherds. The milk the sheep grazing here produce is exceptional; microbially rich and packed with nutrition (as well as those flavour compounds, terpenes). Traditionally, the shepherds made cheese while still up on the mountain pastures. Over fires, they gently warmed the milk. As with Salers, there was so much bacterial life in the milk, no starter culture needed to be added. Lactic acid fermentation happened naturally, acidifying the milk, making it sour and giving it its preservative powers. Rennet taken from the stomach of a lamb was used to coagulate the milk, and when the curds were cool enough, they were salted and stirred with wooden sticks until they broke down into pea-sized pieces. Handfuls of curds were then wrapped in cloth and pressed under the weight of rocks to drive out the whey. The less moisture the cheese contained, the longer it kept. Using washed skins from slaughtered sheep, the shepherds made sacks into which the cheese was stuffed, smearing butter over the skins to make them airtight. These sacks of cheese were hidden somewhere cool close to the villages – inside a cave or buried underground – and left for months. As spring turns to summer, the pasture changes, and with it the milk and in turn the cheese. When the grasses and herbs burst into life after the snows clear, 'the cheese tastes so spicy it can sting the back of your throat', says Luigj. 'But later it becomes mellow and its taste will make you think of forests and flowers.'

There are just a few cheeses left in the world that are still matured in animal skins. Collectively, these ancient cheeses are called Tulum (goat skin is most commonly used as it is tough). This method goes all the way back to the Fertile Crescent and the origins of animal domestication and cheese-making. As winter approached, the shepherds left the Albanian Alps to return to their homes with a cheese that would help them see out the long days of snow and ice. One evening, with Luigj, Lumtumire and Pier Paolo Ambrosi, I ate some Mishavinë. It was the colour of straw, dense and crumbly, and tasted so strong and sharp (with the faintest hint of the animal skin) it could be used like a condiment to add bite to other foods. This was the power of the pasture. The next day, we ate Mishavinë for breakfast, served with the fiery distilled spirit that Edith Durham had described. It worked; the salty cheese really did help down the rakia.

When Ambrosi first came to these mountain villages, he found some only had ten families living in them where there had once been a hundred. Perhaps more people could be encouraged to become makers of Mishavinë, Ambrosi thought, and bring much needed income to the villagers. 'The people had something unique to offer,' he says. 'If production could be increased, there was a chance they could stay and live in dignity.' Ambrosi called on the help of a woman called Drita Tanazi, one of the few young people left in her village in the highlands. In her mid-twenties, Tanazi had seen most of her generation go first to Tirana and then overseas. 'Too often we don't know what becomes of them,' she says, 'and each year another house is abandoned.' Together, Ambrosi and Tanazi recruited other farmers and started training courses so that more people could also become cheesemakers. From three producers, they soon had twenty. Next, they had to find people interested in buying the cheese. In finding a chef called Altin Prenga, they had a breakthrough.

Prenga, like half his fellow Albanians, had left the country in the early 1990s. With his brother he had escaped on a boat destined for Italy where they found work in hotels and restaurant kitchens. After a decade, they felt it was time to return home. With everything they had learned in Italy, they wanted to set up their own restaurant and, if they could make a success of it, help rebuild Albania. On their family farm fifty miles north of Tirana, they opened Mrizi i Zanave ('In the Shadow of the Fairies'). Set among sprawling wheat fields, vineyards and vegetable plots, this is more than a restaurant, it is a collection of kitchens and workshops where Albania's pre-Communist food history is being restored.

When you arrive here, there's no escaping memories of the Hoxha regime. Rows of concrete bunkers and machine-gun posts that look like giant mushrooms punctuate the landscape. A few have been left in their original stark concrete grey, but most have been painted in bright colours, graffiti-style, creating a startling juxtaposition for diners to contemplate while eating at the outdoor tables. A much bigger example of Hoxha's legacy can be found further up the gravel road that runs alongside the farm. Behind a tall, concrete wall lined with rusting barbed wire is a derelict prison.

'This is where protesters were sent?' I asked Prenga. He shook his head. There were no protesters under Hoxha, at least none who survived, he said as he put his hands in the shape of a pistol and fired an imaginary shot at his head to explain their fate. This prison had been a place for those caught committing misdemeanours such as worshipping at one of the clandestine churches or hoarding food supplies. We stood beside a small brick building, too low for anyone to stand in, too short to lie down in. 'People were shut in there as a punishment,' said Prenga. 'Once inside they had to crouch for days at a time.'

Prenga was turning the now abandoned prison buildings into small food factories, places where farmers could bring their produce, shepherds their milk, and foragers wild strawberries and mushrooms they had gathered from the forest. Here at the farm, millers, bakers, butchers and cooks were using these ingredients for the restaurant or turning them into products that could be sold in Tirana. The ambition of Mrizi i Zanave is to save the skills and knowledge that have survived in those villages that are still populated. Soon, Prenga told me, the old punishment block was going to reopen as a smokehouse and some of the cells were being turned into kitchens where wild berries would be made into sweet preserves. To find his suppliers, Prenga had embarked on a road trip to see who was tucked away in the highland settlements, which is where he came across Mishavinë and the efforts of Tanazi and Ambrosi to keep the cheese alive.

Near the old prison, I saw a row of thick bushes at the side of a road. These, it turned out, had been planted decades ago to conceal a path that led to a concrete tunnel. This was blocked by a heavy, barred gate. Like the bunkers, the tunnel had been built by the Hoxha regime as part of the self-defence system in case of invasion. Thousands of these secret tunnels dotted the country and were used to store guns and provide hideouts from enemy armies. 'Take a closer look,' said Prenga, and I peered through the iron bars into the darkness. Wafting towards me was the pungent smell of cheese, maturing away for the customers of Mrizi i Zanave. The tunnel was now a storeroom for Mishavinë. 'The dictator left behind a perfect cheese cave,' he said with a laugh.

In 1908, Edith Durham wrote, 'In the Balkan Peninsula, as elsewhere, the fittest survive in the struggle for existence. The next few years should be interesting.' Those were the closing words of her book *High Albania*. Wars and a dictatorship followed, but some of what she recorded on her travels survived, including the product of ancient pasture, a food of the Accursed Mountains.

Snow room

The factory that makes starter cultures for much of the world's cheese and yogurt is in an unprepossessing suburb of Copenhagen, in Denmark. The word 'factory' gives the wrong impression: it looks more like a giant chemistry lab in a sci-fi movie. Inside are bright, long corridors that branch out into 'research zones' and decontamination areas where, through windows, you can watch robotic arms move liquids and powders around some of the most sterile rooms ever created. It is so big that one of the company's 4,000 workers might whizz past you on an electronic scooter. Chr. Hansen is the largest producer of lactic acid bacteria in the world. From here, frozen pellets and vials of liquid bacterial cultures are dispatched around the globe to cheesemakers.

Want to make a mature-tasting Cheddar or a version of Monterey Jack? Chr. Hansen has a list of starter cultures in its catalogue to produce those styles. Or perhaps an Alpine cheese made with holes, such as Emmental? You can order a culture that will help you create it. The same goes for Camembert, Mozzarella, Pecorino or Feta-style cheeses. The company boasts the most extensive culture range in the dairy world. With these off-the-shelf microbes, a food manufacturer can have all the world's cheeses within their reach. All they need to do is select a type and a flavour profile from the company's catalogue and place an order. It's an impressive operation that has taken more than a century to build.

The 'Chr.' stands for Christian, from the founder's name, Christian Hansen. A pharmacist by training, he founded the company in the 1870s with the ambition of bringing cheese-making into the industrial age. With new science, an important but ancient food could be modernised and made with greater consistency and, he hoped, with added safety. Hansen's first breakthrough was to isolate the rennin, the enzymes cheesemakers used to coagulate their milk. Now, instead of having to rely on the linings of animal stomachs, dairies could buy manufactured rennet. Then he turned his attention to bacteria, and the starter cultures that produced the essential lactic acid. Until this point, most cheesemakers relied on the naturally occurring microbes in their milk (as with Mishavinë) or on their equipment (like the Salers *gerle*) or dosed their fresh milk with a portion of whey from a previous 'make' (as with traditional Icelandic skyr). Hansen found an alternative that left no room for error. He identified, isolated and then preserved different strains of lactic acid bacteria. As pasteurisation spread in the twentieth century and dairies became bigger, Hansen's products became essential tools for cheesemakers. Making cultures involves a highly technical process. To this day, only a small number of companies around the world can do this work, and Hansen was the first.

When I visited Chr. Hansen in 2018, the CEO was Cees de Jong, a former medical doctor. 'Cheese needs three things,' he told me, 'milk, a culture and a coagulant. The only thing we don't make here is the milk.' Along with the microbes and the enzymes, Chr. Hansen also provides cheesemakers with recipes and technical advice to help them adjust a flavour in any direction they want. 'We give them total control.'

The company's main asset is its collection of 40,000 different types of bacteria. When he started out in his previous profession as a doctor, de Jong said, the mantra had been that the only good bacteria were dead bacteria. 'Science is changing. The world is waking up to how important microbes are to our well-being.'

And the company is always on the lookout for new ones. A few years ago, one scientist had walked past de Jong's office holding a sealed box containing a couple of dead birds. 'He was checking their gastrointestinal tracts, looking for interesting microbes we don't have in our collection.'

But most of the research is less primal. Chr. Hansen sends microbe hunters out across the world to buy unique collections of bacteria. 'It could be from a starter culture from a cheesemaker in Bulgaria or bacteria from a yogurt producer in Greece,' de Jong said. Chr. Hansen then grows these traditional strains on a larger scale to sell to dairy companies around the world.

As we continued through the building, I saw big blow-up pictures on the walls, images of the company's bestselling bacteria, multicoloured, kaleidoscopic, psychedelic structures. We peered through windows into sealed rooms where lab-controlled ferments using skimmed milk powder were under way. 'Half of all the cheese and yogurt being made around the world today contains an ingredient we produce,' de Jong told me. 'Whether it's hard, soft, plain-looking or blue, when you next bite into a piece of cheese there's a fifty–fifty chance it has been made with our ingredients.' That ingredient could be one of Chr. Hansen's bacteria or enzymes.

Before being sent out to cheesemakers, the cultures are kept inside one of the world's biggest freezers, a vast storeroom kept at a steady −55°C. 'We can only stay inside for thirty seconds,' de Jong said, 'and take small steps and walk like a penguin to make sure you don't slip. You are about to enter a different world.'

As I entered, bursts of condensation funnelled out of my nose and mouth. To be heard we had to shout over the noise of the massive fans above blowing out cold air. The conditions in the room were so extreme it had its own weather system, and snow was falling from the ceiling and settling on my hair and jacket. Inside the freezer, a diversity of microbes had been captured, tamed and frozen. In a way, it's like a Svalbard for the world's microbes: a bacterial universe being saved.

But diversity needs to be preserved out in the world too. From the time of the earliest cheesemakers, humans harnessed the hidden power of nature, from pasture to cow, from milk into cheese. Cheese has been an important part of the human story, a food that not only ensured survival but helped forge cultures too. During the twentieth century, science promised more of everything: more food, more safety and more homogeneity. There was a lot to be said for this, but something irreplaceable is being lost because of it. Cheeses like Salers, Stichelton and Mishavinë are all more than just food. The making of them helps preserve and sustain a way of life, a special ecosystem, a connection to nature we can't afford to squander. They give us options as we head into our unknowable future. The cheesemakers in the Albanian Alps and on the Massif Central and people like the solitary Joe Schneider are becoming a rare breed. They don't just make delicious cheese, they are also curators of the precious species we rarely consider, but without which we all fail: microbes.

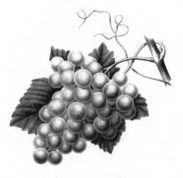

Part Eight
Alcohol

Like all good foods, wine, beer, and spirits nourish and satisfy the body. What sets them apart is the very direct way in which they touch the mind.

Harold McGee, *On Food and Cooking*

Fermentation, the transformational process orchestrated by microbes, is essential for making alcohol as well as cheese. But while milk is turned to cheese by lactic acid bacteria, alcohol is the product of fermentation by yeast. These single-celled members of the fungus family are everywhere, microscopic and hidden from the eye: floating in the air, on the surface of all plants, and in every inch of soil. In nature, when yeast comes into contact with ripe fruit, it starts to break down sugar molecules and excrete a form of alcohol called ethanol. This process protects the fruit from rival bacteria, slows down its decomposition and keeps pathogens at bay. It also releases a vapour trail which acts as a signal to insects and mammals (including humans) to come looking for food and so, ultimately, to disperse the fruit's seeds. The interconnectedness between plants, humans and yeast provides the best explanation for why drinking alcohol became a feature of so many cultures around the world. It also led to the wonderfully named 'drunken monkey hypothesis', proposed by biologist Robert Dudley, that we are drawn to drinking alcohol because our ancestors were exposed to low concentrations of alcohol in nature. As a species, we grew up on it.

Fruit filled an important nutritional gap for early humans, but to consume sufficient amounts their bodies had to adapt to be able to cope with ethanol. Ethanol is toxic or, as we usually say, 'intoxicating', and not all primates are able to process the chemical. Just as we evolved to be able to digest milk, a gene mutation in our past increased our ability to metabolise alcohol. This gave an evolutionary advantage as it meant humans could forage from the forest floor and across savannahs, eating up large quantities of fallen and fermented fruit without becoming ill. The ethanol within the fruit even increased the amount of fruit early humans could eat because of the 'apéritif effect'; alcohol not only makes us feel happier, it also stimulates appetite, so when we drink, we eat more food and therefore consume more energy, more quickly. For early humans who had followed a vapour trail to a nutritious patch of ripe fruit, being able to eat lots of it in a hurry before other animals arrived was a big gain.

Drinking booze, if this theory is right, is hardwired in our DNA. The mutation that helped us metabolise alcohol stayed with us and, millions of years later, our ancestors found ingenious methods of manufacturing drinks with greater levels of alcohol. When farmers started to domesticate cereals and fruits and used them to make alcohol, they were also inadvertently domesticating yeast strains too. In the case of brewing this happened because yeasts were saved from previous brews to make new ones. In evolutionary terms, this is called artificial selection. In the nineteenth century, Louis Pasteur found a way of isolating specific yeasts which helped turn brewing into a more exact science. Whatever form it took, over the course of thousands of years, alcohol became one of the most powerful influences on human culture. The history of our species is interlaced with alcohol. The ways we live, love, argue, create, socialise, philosophise and farm have all been shaped by it.

An alcoholic drink is as much the product of geography as a piece of cheese is. In regions blessed with plenty of sunshine, fruit provided the easiest source of fermentable sugars, which is why wine cultures emerged in the Caucasus Mountains of modern-day Georgia and the Zagros Mountains of Iran. In these hot and dry regions, water was often in short supply, but wild grape vines with their deep roots could access groundwater. Planting a vineyard and making wine from grapes was an elegant method of water extraction and as yeasts occur naturally on grape skins, the production of alcohol was unavoidable. In cooler regions, such as Northern Europe, where wheat and barley growing proliferated, brewing cultures developed instead. Because the brewing process involves boiling as well as fermentation, it produced a drink that was safer than water, full of energy and micronutrients as well as beneficial microbes. Herbs, spices and hops were used to add flavour and to have a preservative effect. Beer was 'liquid bread' (possibly even an offshoot of bread-making). In China, glutinous rice was fermented into alcoholic drinks such as mijiu, and in Japan it was turned into sake. In Africa, Ethiopian honey gatherers made tej (or mead) and in Central Africa, as we have seen, beer was brewed from bananas. In parts of South America, maize and potatoes were used to produce beer and spirits, and on the Central Asian Steppes, the Kumyk people found a way of making alcoholic drinks from fermented mare's milk.

Because of its mind-altering qualities, perhaps it was inevitable that alcohol should become intertwined with religion and embedded in belief systems. In Christianity, transubstantiation means that wine can become the blood of Christ. In Japan, sake is offered to deities at Shinto shrines. And as we saw in the Andes, shamans pour potato spirits over sacred stones in tribute to Pachamama, Mother Earth. For most of the beer-brewing techniques developed in the last thousand years, we have monks to thank. And although the Koran forbade the drinking of alcohol, it was Arab chemists in the ninth century who mastered the modern science of distillation. Beyond its medicinal applications, the technology later made possible the production of *aqua vitae*, the 'water of life', the basis of whisky, vodka, bourbon and brandy.

For millennia, the relationship between humans and alcohol was hyper-local; it depended on the variety of a grape, a type of landrace barley and the imagination and ingenuity of the makers who crafted their distinctive tipples. To really know the culture of a place, Ernest Hemingway famously advised not to bother with sightseeing but to spend time in its bars.

This 'local' quality started to be diluted during the Industrial Revolution, and as the drinks trade became more globalised in the twentieth century things changed completely. In parallel with milk's story, booze became a global commodity, increasingly controlled, produced and distributed by large corporations. Beer exemplifies this trend: one in four beers drunk around the world are now brewed by just one company, A-B InBev (ABI), which owns Budweiser, Stella Artois and Corona and produces more than 88 billion pints a year (it sells the equivalent of three Olympic-sized swimming pools of beer an hour – more than its three nearest rivals combined). The company's strategy of buying up breweries has seen it engulf big brands as well as seemingly independent 'craft breweries' (e.g. Camden Town Brewery in the UK and Goose Island in the US). The wine world is more fragmented and has fewer giants, but in 2019 it was estimated that by volume, three firms accounted for 60 per cent of all wine sales in the United States. One of them, Gallo, the largest privately-owned winery in the world, sells around 70 million cases each year.

Meanwhile, in vineyards across the globe, the story became one of increasing homogeneity and the loss of genetic diversity. More than 1,500 grape varieties have been recorded, many of which are indigenous, ancient and, like landrace crops, highly adapted to their local environments. It's estimated that around 80 per cent of all vineyards now grow just ten or so 'international' varieties – the likes of Chardonnay, Merlot and Syrah, which started to dominate winemaking in the 1960s. China, which in recent years has become one of the biggest winemaking nations on the planet (it has the world's fourth largest producer, Changyu), is also choosing to grow these international varieties. Instead of opting for those that are drought-tolerant or best suited to its soils or its short growing season, it has planted enormous vineyards filled with the globally ubiquitous Cabernet Sauvignon grape.

For decades, across the drink world, heritage and traditions were dying and biodiversity was in decline. This was true not just for wine and beer but for many other drinks, including perry, cider's sibling. Fortunately, alcohol has not only attracted the attention of big business, it has also inspired a new generation of producers all determined to make drinks that belong to a more diverse and deeper story.

27

Qvevri Wine

If there's one characteristic that unites the people I've met while researching this book, it is a refusal to compromise. Winemaker Ramaz Nikoladze is the supreme example of this. Before travelling to Georgia to meet him, people who knew him prepared me for three possible scenarios. The first was spending lots of time eating food and drinking copious amounts of his wine. The second involved Nikoladze busy at work in the vineyard or cellar making wine, most likely to a sound-track of deafening guitar music. The third scenario worried me the most: silence, lots of it. Nikoladze, I was warned, was a deep thinker, a serious person, a little reserved and not much of a talker. I figured this was understandable – he carried a great responsibility on his shoulders. While the origins of wheat and bread lay in the Fertile Crescent, and maize culture started in southern Mexico, the birth of winemaking was Georgia, the crossway between Europe and Asia. Nikoladze, as an endangered maker of an endangered wine, seemed to feel the weight of this ancient inheritance. Of the three possible scenarios awaiting me, I experienced them all.

His home is in a region of western Georgia called Imereti, known in the classical world as Cochis, home to the Golden Fleece and the destination of the Argonauts. Whereas eastern Georgia stretches out into vast open landscapes, the western side is a hillier place bordered by the foothills of the Caucasus Mountains; the greater range in the north, the lesser in the south. Georgia was at the epi-centre of grape domestication. It was in this region, Nikolai Vavilov argued in the 1920s, that humans first tamed wild vines and became winemakers, where wild grapes suitable for cultivation could still be found, and the fruit's diversity was at its greatest. Georgia's geology made it the perfect setting. The father of modern soil science, the nineteenth-century Russian geographer V.V. Dokuchaev, described Georgia as an 'open-air museum of soils' with nearly fifty different types (a huge amount of diversity for a country smaller than Ireland).

As well as the patchwork of wild grapes that still grow today, there's other evidence to show Georgia's long relationship with wine. At Neolithic sites in the east of the country, traces of pollen from grape cultivars 8,000 years old have been unearthed. And in 2017, south of the capital Tbilisi, equally old shards of clay were dug up, pottery once soaked in wine. But the most powerful proof of Georgia's ancient wine history comes from its people. Wine flows through the nation's history, through its art, religion, legends and songs. When two farmers meet, the first greeting will be 'How are you?' followed by a second, 'How is your vineyard?' Wine, they'll happily tell you, is in their blood.

This was the culture Ramaz Nikoladze was born into, someone with too many generations of winemakers behind him to count and 8,000 wine vintages to build on. Now in his late forties, he had grown up in the closing decades of the Soviet Union, a period of history that began for his family with the confiscation of his great-grandfather's vineyards by the Bolsheviks in the 1920s. By the time Georgia regained independence in 1991, the country was on its knees and its wine (produced for the USSR) was one of the most industrialised and adulterated in the world. In the less populated regions, including isolated pockets among the hills and beneath the mountains of the west, a more ancient form of winemaking for home consumption survived, along with a diversity of grape varieties lost in other parts of Georgia. On the family farm, aged sixteen, Nikoladze produced his first batch of wine, made in a way his great-grandfather would have recognised, a direct connection to a tradition that seemed destined soon to die. Three decades on, Nikoladze is at the vanguard of a movement to prevent that happening.

Inside his home and down some concrete steps, I was led into what I was told was a wine cellar. At first, there appeared to be no wine, just bare walls and a stone floor along which was a row of covered circles, each two metres apart, the size of dinner plates. Nikoladze removed one of the covers and I peered down into a black hole. Buried in the ground were four large, egg-shaped, terracotta vessels, each filled with fermenting grape juice. Qvevri (pronounced kwev-ri) are ancient winemaking pots that pre-date the invention of the barrel by several thousand years. Convection currents flow around the inside of these oval containers, allowing yeast to make contact with all of the liquid inside, resulting in evenly fermented juice. Below ground, temperatures remain constant and so the wine develops slowly whatever the season, insulated by the earth tightly packed around.

At the very bottom of the qvevri is a pointed cone, at which the lees (the dead yeast cells) collect after their life's work is done along with the seeds and stems of the grapes (containing bitter tannins), leaving the wine above pristine. After 8,000 years of winemaking, Georgians argue the qvevri still hasn't been bettered. Qvevri are also works of art. Built from a series of coils, one placed on top of another, over months, they are moulded and smoothed into these vast egg shapes. They are then fired and painted inside with hot beeswax to sterilise the microscopic clay pores (a final touch that helps prevent the wine spoiling). Some qvevri can be giants: three metres deep, large enough to hold 1,300 bottles of wine. But like the traditional wines made inside them, the making of qvevri has become an endangered craft. Few people are left with the skills (combined with the physical strength) to construct them.

From the storeroom next door Nikoladze collected some of the wine he'd already bottled. 'Are we tasting or are we drinking?' he asked. I thought for a few seconds. 'Drinking,' I replied. It felt the most respectful thing to say. Back above ground we gathered at a table. Nestan, Nikoladze's wife, had spent the day making *khinkali*, boiled dumplings filled with spiced lamb; *lobiani*, parcels of hot bread filled with beans; and *khachapuri*, warm, gooey cheese-stuffed bread. The scene was set for my immersion into Georgian qvevri wine. Nikoladze poured one made with a local white grape variety called Tsolikouri. The wine was gorgeous (fresh, crisp, full-bodied) but the colour was what intrigued me; not red or white, but a translucent orange, an amber wine.

Broadly speaking, red wine is given its colour because juice from red varieties is fermented in contact with the grape's skins (the pigment from these not only adds colour but also flavour because of tannins). White wine is typically made from the juice of white varieties fermented with the skins off. The amber wine Nikoladze had poured me was a hybrid of the two: white grape varieties fermented like a red wine. This approach is called 'skin contact'. Traditional Georgian winemakers might place stems inside the qvevri as well. These wines go beyond the grape as they are flavoured by the entire bunch.

Nikoladze poured from more bottles, including one made with Krakhuna grapes (the name means 'crispy' in local Imeretian dialect), another deep amber wine. Every now and then he disappeared into his storeroom to bring up more bottles. All the while, out of two tall speakers, the music of The Clash boomed louder and louder. We progressed to a bottle made from Tsitska grapes, another Imeretian variety. Its juice had been fermented inside the qvevri for eight months. When it was poured, it gave out a light golden glow. 'This wine is like my husband,' said Nestan. 'It can be one thing one day, different the next and different again the following day. I like this wine. No ... I love this wine. That's why I call it Ramaz.' Nine bottles in, I began probing Nikoladze for his winemaking secrets. What was he aiming for? I asked. 'Authenticity,' he said. 'Wine without compromise,' he added after a long pause, 'zero compromise.' The indigenous grape varieties, the qvevri, Nikoladze's winemaking skills, all were important ingredients of the wines we were drinking. But to my mind, his attitude trumped it all.

Nikoladze's 'zero compromise' approach started in the vineyard. Instead of regimented vines all planted in orderly rows, his vines were more like a forest. Nestled within them were birds' nests, while nettles and bean plants were growing among the grapes. No pesticides are used; nature is handed control. 'Perhaps I am a little lazy,' Nikoladze said, explaining how one year he had left the vineyard untended and the wine it produced was the best he had tasted. As the vineyard became more overgrown, had the wine changed? 'Wild,' he said, smiling, 'more and more wild.' His work growing grapes was obvious, but invisible to the eye was his role as a microbe farmer. Nikoladze relies on wild yeasts to ferment the juice into wine, strains which in turn depend on the biodiversity of his vineyard. And that's all he uses. The grapes he grows and the yeasts that grow on their skins and in the air – nothing else is added. To truly describe the wine that results is impossible; each glass is an experience, rather than a set of tasting notes. But a description by the wine writer and Georgian expert Carla

Capalbo can help. 'There's a vibrancy, an energy and a wildness I crave in these wines. It's like the horse that's running free instead of the one that's been taught to do dressage. It hasn't been subdued or brought down. It's unfettered.' That doesn't mean *sauvage* to the point of undrinkability, it's more like a different language, one we're forgetting to understand.

Georgia's position in the heart of Eurasia has given the country a long history of invasion. Pagan kings were dethroned by Mongols, then Persians and then Christian converts, who in turn were conquered by Muslim Ottomans. This was followed by a Russian invasion, annexation, collectivisation and the Cold War. Throughout this tempestuous history, wine was one of the few constants. Georgian warriors were said to have gone into battle with small cuttings from their vineyard, placed under their chainmail. Whatever its symbolism, there was a practical motivation for doing this. If these warriors returned home to find their villages destroyed and their farms burnt down or occupied, they carried with them a cutting from a vine that could eventually be replanted. Cuttings could have come from one of the five hundred or so indigenous varieties so far identified in Georgia, a large proportion of all the grape diversity in the world, including varieties found nowhere else. Without this wild and cultivated gene pool, Vavilov might argue, the likes of Pinot Noir, Nebbiolo and Syrah might never have existed.

Georgia's drinking rituals reflect the country's bloody past. When glasses (or sometimes drinking horns) are clinked, the toast is 'Gaumarjos!' which means 'to your victory!' Winemakers also describe a spiritual dimension to their work; wine is seen as a form of liquid sunlight and drinking a way of communing with God. In agrarian parts of the country, most homes were built around vineyards, cellars and qvevri, but nothing was bottled. Transported in animal skins and poured from jugs, these were drinks made for the home table (Ramaz Nikoladze didn't bottle a wine until he was in his late thirties). From this culture there arose a set of values, and these are as much about what wine is as what it isn't. According to the ethos of this world, you raise wine as you would a child. Even the term 'winemaker' can be frowned upon – humans don't make wine, nature does. The producer is nothing more than a guide for the grapes which are predestined to encounter wild yeasts and be fermented into wine. Placing grapes inside a qvevri is a low-intervention way of allowing a wine to develop and stand on its own feet. The Georgians describe the wine in the buried qvevri as being wrapped in the mother's embrace, with the earth as mother. If the farmer has done his job well in the vineyard and produced strong grapes, then nothing else is needed in the qvevri. 'Bad farming and poor winemaking are like children who have told lies,' said John Wurdeman, an American-born winemaker based in eastern Georgia, helping to explain this faith in nature. 'You need more and more lies to cover up the first, and on it goes.' And so, if the soil is healthy you don't need lots of fertilisers; if the plants are healthy and diverse, they won't need to be showered in pesticides; and in the winery, you won't need an industrial process to 'correct' the wine. But this ancient way of making (and thinking about) wine was to change in the twentieth century, directed by Russia, Georgia's giant neighbour to the north.

In 1918, following the fall of the tsar, Georgia declared independence but this status was short-lived. Just after the Red Army's invasion in 1921, the British journalist Henry Nevinson, who knew Georgia well, gave accounts of 'Russian domination'. The country was being 'taken over by the same "hooligans" who served as spies and secret police under the Tsar', he wrote, 'but now call themselves Bolshevik ... The officials mock at Georgian claims to nationality and independence [and] Russian soldiers roam from village to village devouring all that the peasants have produced; and Georgia besides being the most beautiful country I have seen, is by nature one of the most fertile.' A few years earlier, he had visited winemakers and watched as 'grapes [were] squeezed in primitive presses, cleaned with boughs of yew, and the juice run off into huge earthen-ware vats sunk into the ground ... big enough to hold a man'. In the seven decades that followed Nevinson's account, particularly under Stalin (a Georgian), the Soviet mission was to bring 'industrial efficiencies' to the countryside and eradicate much of what had gone before, including Georgia's way of producing wine. Small hillside vineyards were abandoned, deemed too inefficient, and workers moved to the flat expanse of Kakheti in the east. In newly planted vineyards, a selection of six main varieties – all selected by Communist central planners – were grown, resulting in many indigenous grape varieties facing extinction. In factories, wine devised by the state went into production. Flavour profiles, levels of alcohol, sugar and acidity were all set from above. No vineyards were identified on labels, only the banner of the state monopoly, Samtrest.

By the 1950s, the Alaverdi Monastery, which had produced wine since the seventh century, lay in ruins, turned into a tractor park for the Red Army. Its ancient qvevri were now used to store diesel, symbols of a heritage being vandalised. After the 1960s, things went from bad to very bad. Quotas were increased year on year regardless of how prolific or poor the harvest was. This resulted in 'fake' wines being sold, a concoction of grape concentrate, tannins, sugar and water. Then, in 1985, Mikhail Gorbachev announced a series of drastic anti-alcohol policies, including reducing production, so thousands of hectares of vineyards were grubbed up. After independence in 1991, chaos and conflict took hold in Georgia. The economy collapsed and the big wine cooperatives shut down. Large vineyards were turned into plots for growing much needed vegetables and fruit.

But not everything had been lost. In the more remote parts of the country, despite tight state control of the country's wine, backyard growers and family winemakers had saved many of the old grape varieties and made wines in the same old way using qvevri. During the decades when the quality of most wine went from bad to awful, a black market had grown up in Tblisi and other urban centres, a trade in secretive batches of traditional wine made in farm buildings and cellars free from state interference. One of the drinkers of these illicit wines was an academic called Soliko Tsaishvili. Inspired by historic accounts of Georgian wine and rare samples from the secret qvevri makers, in 1989 he set out to make his own traditional Georgian wine. From villages in Kakheti, he bought Rkatsiteli grapes (one of Georgia's old noble varieties) and made wine in a cellar in Tblisi. By 2003 he had moved east to Kakheti and bought his own vineyard. Here, he started his mission to revive the qvevri and plant more indigenous grape varieties. 'Truth is not found in other people's grapes,' he once said. 'You can't call that your wine. Truth is in growing your own grapes.'

Word of this mission spread to other winemakers, including Ramaz Nikoladze in the west. Eventually, a network of like-minded producers took shape. When Italian wine importer and Slow Food member Luca

Gargano came across their qvevri wine and took some back with him to Italy, the tiny Georgian project (called 'Our Wine') began to get recognition from the outside world. Gargano realised that as well as protecting the essence of Georgian traditions, Tsaishvili and Nikoladze represented an older, perhaps purer approach to winemaking that was being lost around the world.

At the same time as Georgia's wine tradition was being dismantled by communism, capitalism was transforming winemaking elsewhere. Up until the 1950s most of Europe's vineyards were still small-scale, worked by hand and home to a wide range of indigenous grape varieties. The quality of the wine was still heavily influenced by nature, with the vineyard's soil and the weather the main determinants of vintage. During the 1960s all of this was to change. Just as Borlaug and other scientists were transforming wheat and rice, and as the food system was becoming more industrialised, winemaking was about to experience its own revolution.

A key figure in this wine revolution was Émile Peynaud. Based at the University of Bordeaux's Institut d'Oenologie, this ingenious scientist, winemaker and teacher set out to improve the quality of French wine. To Peynaud it looked as if too much was being left to chance; too many wines were thin and tart and tainted by spoilage. He wanted to replace the vagaries of winemaking with hard science. This way he believed France could make not just more wine, but better ones. Some of his suggested improvements seemed obvious: pick only the best fruit and discard the rest; pick riper grapes for softer tannins; pay more attention to hygiene; get rid of dirty barrels. But Peynaud also bridged the gap between the laboratory and the cellar. Methods of testing a wine's pH, sugar levels and alcohol were introduced. This helped winemakers take greater control over what had been at best an instinctive practice, at worst a mystery. French wines became more consistent as producers now had specific parameters to aim for under Peynaud's guidance. Advances were also made in selecting and manufacturing a smaller number of yeast strains, so helping to reduce the unpredictability in viniculture. The cumulative effect was that by the end of the 1970s, France had increased its wine exports tenfold, out-producing Italy, Spain and Portugal combined. Peynaud is now regarded as the father of modern winemaking.

Although he valued diversity and believed there was no single formula for a great wine, after the 'Peynaudisation' of Bordeaux, a more homogeneous approach to winemaking began to spread around the world, along with a more global consensus about what a truly great wine should taste like.

Building on Peynaud's success and France's booming exports, a generation of consultants (many taught by Peynaud) travelled the world to share the secrets of Bordeaux's success. Among them was Michel Rolland, perhaps the most sought after wine consultant of all. Rolland had studied under Peynaud in the early 1970s and went on, in the 1980s, to advise wineries across five continents. What Rolland and his fellow consultants offered was success in the marketplace. Helping to shape the marketplace were even more influential wine critics, chief among them the Californian Robert Parker, whose scores, high or low on a scale of 100, could make or break a wine. This combination – greater technical control in winemaking, globetrotting consultants and powerful critics – created internationally favoured styles, making reds, for instance, bolder, riper, oakier and more alcoholic. Parker denies favouring a particular style and Rolland has said there isn't a recipe for great wines: plenty of wine experts disagree.

Helping in the rise of dominant styles were changes to labels on bottles. Until this point, wine had been identified by region – Burgundy, Barolo, Rioja and so on – but from the 1960s, grape varietals started to appear on more labels (beginning with the likes of Cabernet Sauvignon, Chardonnay and Merlot). This trend was established in the New World, started by a wine merchant called Frank Schoonmaker, but went mainstream under the inventive marketing of Californian winemaker Robert Mondavi (Mondavi wines are among the top five bestselling wine brands). The aim of the strategy was to make wine more accessible to consumers and it turned a small number of grape varieties into superstars (added to Cabernet Sauvignon, Chardonnay and Merlot were Chenin Blanc, Pinot Noir, Riesling, Sauvignon Blanc, Semillon and Syrah).

Around the world, thousands of winemakers keen to share in this success replanted their vineyards with these celebrity varieties. Bordeaux's Sauvignons and Merlot went global. From Argentina to Australia, vineyards – many centuries old – were replanted with these more fashionable varieties. Italy's number of indigenous grapes was halved during the 1970s, while the Douro region in Portugal is a good illustration of what was lost. Historically, vineyards there had been planted with a mix of indigenous grapes (in some cases a hundred different varieties), a type of planting called a 'field blend'. Just like a field of diverse landrace wheat will offer a farmer insurance against risk, these field blends protected against disaster; if some of the vines failed one season, others were sure to deliver. But in the 1970s, the region decided to focus on just five main varieties as part of a strategy to get a bigger share of the international market, a market which itself was seeing seismic change.

New methods of transportation made it possible to move wine around the world in greater volumes. Tens of thousands of litres could be pumped into colossal storage containers and onto ships, while plastic flexi-tanks (often referred to as bladders) were invented to store 30,000 bottles' worth of wine in one compartment. Industrially produced wines could cross continents for a few thousand dollars and then be bottled and labelled at their destination. They were mostly destined for the expanding wine shelves of supermarkets. Mass-market winemakers also chased the success of the new dominant styles and flavours. And so the Parker effect trickled through the world.

Technology allowed all wines to replicate the high-scoring styles, regardless of what had taken place in the vineyard. Colorants, sweeteners, enzymes and powdered tannins were added to the producer's toolkit, all helping to change the appearance and mouthfeel of a wine. Other innovations, such as nanofiltration, microfiltration, ultrafiltration and reverse osmosis, could make wines sparkle with clarity by removing the tiniest particulates; and micro-oxygenation was used to smooth out any flavours deemed too challenging. If these mass-market wines had started out with any sense of place, by the time they were bottled that connection had been broken. But for every action, there is a reaction, and in France, the techno-fix approach to wine led to a resistance movement.

Among the members of this movement was Jules Chauvet, a Beaujolais-based producer, trained chemist and renowned expert on fermentation. Chauvet clung on to the idea that the vineyard was a complex ecosystem within which lived a species massively undervalued by the wine industry, the wild and diverse yeast populations found on and around the grapes. He rejected the idea that commercial yeasts provided the only route to making excellent wines. He also believed that powerful doses of sulfites added during vinification were to be avoided as they killed off the very microbial life winemakers should instead be encouraging. Chauvet's approach wasn't about leaving things to chance. Like a traditional raw milk cheesemaker, he believed natural methods involved great skill and good science. In the case of wine, this started in the vineyard. Strong and healthy grapes grown without pesticides would foster desirable yeast populations which in turn would create magnificent wines, he reasoned. During vinification, production methods had to be slow, gentle and meticulous not only to avoid any contamination but to protect the microbial legacy gifted by the vineyard. If Émile Peynaud is the father of modern winemaking, Chauvet is the father of natural wine. His ideas have inspired producers in every wine-growing region of the world.

In 2020, the influential INAO (Institut National de l'Origine et de la Qualité) which administers French appellations issued an official definition of natural wine. The standard states, for example, that grapes have to be hand-picked and yeasts can only come from the environment of the vineyard or the winery. The definition 'Vin Méthode Nature' had been called for by natural winemakers themselves; the growing success of their wines led to fears that big producers were jumping on the bandwagon and marketing their wines as 'natural'.

Back in Georgia, without realising they were part of a global movement, qvevri revivalists Ramaz Nikoladze and Soliko Tsaishvili and their like-minded counterparts were becoming exemplars of natural winemaking. Because of their unique history – from the legacy of the ancients to the vacuum left behind by communism – these Georgian winemakers knew what wine had been and could still be.

The gulf between the two broad approaches – conventional and natural – has created the greatest division in the winemaking world for generations. Critics say that natural wines taste like 'flawed cider' or 'rotten sherry' or 'an acrid, grim burst of acid that makes you want to cry'. Worse still, the natural wine movement has been bundled together and labelled an 'undefined scam'. This is missing the point. For wine enthusiasts and for everyone else, it poses many of the biggest questions we are exploring in this book: What has our food and drink become? What impact are different farming systems having on our planet? Why does diversity matter? How is homogeneity spreading?

In Georgia, all wine leads to the supra, a communal experience where food, drink and music come together. On his travels through the Soviet Union after the war John Steinbeck portrays Georgians almost as supernatural beings, their every action performed with flair, infused with an independence of spirit that seemed unbreakable. They could, he decided, out-perform all other nationalities when it came to drinking, eating, dancing and singing. My supra experience backed his analysis; huge portions of food (more *khinkali* dumplings and more *khachapuri* bread), acrobatic traditional dancing (not by me) and polyphonic songs full of deep drones that pulsated through the room as jugs of wine were passed around the table. Orchestrating the feast from the head of the table was the *tamada* (our toastmaster) whose role was to elevate drinking and eating into an almost sacred act. He was a bearded giant called Luarsab Togonidze and as he held a big jug in his hand and broke into a toast the room went quiet. 'This is to love, love never goes out of fashion, love never gets old. I want us to drink for love in all of its dimensions. Every moment lived without love is wasted. With wine, food and music, we can express love freely.' As he poured the amber liquid into people's glasses, he raised his voice again. 'To love. To endless, unconditional, love!' Every time wine was poured or a song came to an end, Togonidze made another poetic toast. Some were two minutes long, others ten, all of them addressed the biggest themes in life: death, war, love, beauty, history, tradition – and wine.

Togonidze gave his first toast when he was nine years old. One of the roles of a good *tamada*, he told me, was to remind people wine was no ordinary drink. 'Georgia's past has been full of tragedy, too many invasions, too much war. People lived each day as if it was their last, they learned to celebrate, to embrace life, to see its beauty ... and cherish what they had. This included wine. It is something holy.' With him Togonidze had a collection of drinking vessels, intricate wooden cups and goblets made of precious stone and horns inlaid with silver. For the last toast of the supra, we drank from the plainest and most unassuming vessel of all, a 3,000-year-old cup made from clay. When it touched my lips, I imagined the people who had held it before me and raised toasts like these with Georgian wine. 'Let's drink to our traditions,' Togonidze said. 'They make us what we are today. *Gaumarjos!*'

28

Lambic Beer

The fight to save an endangered food or drink often comes down to a small cast of heroes and heroines prepared to dedicate their lives to the task. One such hero was Michael Jackson, 'the Beer Hunter', the first person to apply serious journalistic rigour to the world's diverse beer cultures. Jackson, who started out as a newspaper reporter, believed that beer (like any food that's been crafted with care) deserved to be treated with reverence. Wine was allowed serious critical attention—why not beer? Through his writing, Jackson went on a mission to correct that. Each beer, he realised, had its own history, its own intricate production methods and distinctive ingredients, from the subtle flavours of British cask-conditioned ales to black lagers, Baltic porters and aromatic Finnish sahti. But as he travelled through Europe in the 1970s and 80s, documenting and tasting drinks, his work acquired a sense of urgency; he saw he was witnessing a process of extinction. Beloved breweries centuries old, once part of the fabric of communities, were closing their doors, their unique drinks disappearing with them.

Jackson's books and broadcasts revel in the diversity and eccentricity of the brewing world, reading as love letters to the likes of Berliner weisse and Bohemian pilsners. But the drinks for which he developed the deepest passion and which he found most fascinating came from Belgium. It was here, Jackson believed, that drinkers could encounter the greatest variety of beer; some made with fruit, some seasoned with spices, farmhouse beers and beers made in monasteries. Each of these was served in a different-shaped glass. Many were not only presented like wine, they tasted and looked like wine.

Belgium's deep, unbroken brewing history made it a 'centre of diversity' for beer. It was the mothership of brewing, a place with the

most beguiling range of styles and flavours, where it had been made
for so long that, just as when a crop has existed somewhere for centuries or millennia, it had been able to adapt and diversify. So embedded
was brewing in Belgian culture that up until the 1970s low-alcohol
'table beer' was served to children in schools. In this small country
of around 10 million people, each district had its own ultra-local subculture of brewing, each small village and town its own interpretation
of what beer should be. In books and articles, Jackson, who passed
away in 2007, made sense of the near anarchy of techniques and
ingredients and drew up a map of styles. Among all of the diversity
Belgium had to offer, the drinks that intrigued him the most were the
lambic beers of Pajottenland, the farming region south-west of Brussels. He described these beers as the 'Champagne of Cereals' and the
'Burgundy of Belgium'. 'To sample lambic,' Jackson wrote in his *Beer
Companion*, 'is to encounter one of the world's most complex drinks;
it is also to experience a taste of life half a millennium ago. No other
commercially brewed beer can trace its history back so far. Nor, in its
production process, has any changed so little.'

What made these beers so compelling was that, although each
barrel was the product of years of meticulous work, much was left
to nature and therefore, from the brewer's point of view, to chance.
Lambic brewing is part of beer's wilder side. As with the most distinctive cheeses, yeasts and bacteria floating around in the environment
get to express themselves in the final product. Not that this beer's
untamed nature is evident at the outset. Brewing lambic begins, as
with all beers, by making a soup out of cereals, usually malted barley
(grain that has been allowed to germinate and then roasted to bring
germination to a halt, by which time more fermentable sugars will
have been produced for yeasts to convert into alcohol). The grains
are then milled into a rough powder called grist and infused in hot
water (a process called mashing). As the 'mash' is stirred, the grains
free up their natural sugars, sweetening the liquid and turning it into
'wort'. In a large copper vessel (the kettle), the wort is boiled for
several hours. About a thousand years ago, at this point in the process
some brewers started to add dried flowers picked from the vines of
a climbing plant we now call hops (*Humulus lupulus*, 'wolf plant').
Packed with bitter compounds, these flowers not only add flavour but
also act as a preservative. Broadly speaking, these are the initial steps

followed by most of the world's brewers. The lambic makers of Pajot-tenland follow the path to this point, with two variations. Firstly, they add wheat to their grist. This gives a tart, thirst-quenching taste to the finished beer. Also, while most brewers look for the freshest, most intensely aromatic hops (so balancing the sweetness of the wort with bitterness), in Pajottenland, lambic brewers use hops that are about three years old, so dehydrated they've lost most of their aroma and taste. All lambic brewers want from these dry flowers are their pre-servative powers.

The greatest point of departure for lambic beer, however, comes at the crucial microbial stage when ordinarily brewers will add (or, as they call it, 'pitch') yeast into their wort. As with starter cultures in cheese-making, these yeasts are now almost exclusively selected strains isolated under lab conditions. For a brewer to create a particular style of beer, they need a specific microbe to take over the fermentation process. As this yeast feasts away on the sugars in the wort, heady ethanol is released along with carbon dioxide (creating fizz). But the selected strain of yeast will also determine which flavours dominate and if the beer is to become an ale or a lager. Lambic brewers opt out of this opportunity to control fermentation. Instead, without pitching a single spore of yeast, they pour the wort into a large metal container that sits inside the brewhouse. This *koelschip* (coolship) looks like an oversized metal paddling pool. Here, the wort is left to cool down and to be exposed to a mysterious microbial world. Floating around in the atmosphere and living invisibly on every surface in the brewhouse are wild yeasts. Specially slatted windows let in air from the outside so even more wild yeasts and microorganisms settle on the wort. This triggers a spontaneous form of fermentation which most other brewers would find terrifying. Wild yeasts are usually seen as the enemy, an unpredictable source of trouble, creators of chaos and agents of spoilage. But over generations, lambic brewers have discovered ways of working in harmony with these microbes and exerting (a little) control over them, taming them (just enough, anyway).

One important feature of this method of brewing is that it is highly seasonal. It can only happen during the cooler months of the year, because desirable microbes get to dominate in cold temperatures as harmful pathogens lie dormant. After one night in the coolship, the wort is transferred into wooden barrels. A British cask ale might be left to ferment inside a maturation tank for around a week, a German lager for perhaps two months, but barrel fermentation for a lambic beer can take three years. During this time, waves of different yeasts and bacteria get a chance to work on the sugars in the brew, helping to develop more and more complex flavours. Some of this beer will be bottled straight from the barrel, but most will be blended. Like artists working with a range of paints, lambic brewers select beers from various barrels to create a semblance of harmony. By mixing and matching lambics of different ages and characters, a gueuze is made. The final result is entirely at the whim of the blender's palate. This is not a beer for unadventurous drinkers. It took generations of brewers to perfect the method, years of experience for some to learn how to blend it and it can take a lifetime for a drinker to figure out how to enjoy it. Lambic's wild character reaches across the entire flavour spectrum, from the zing of a sharp lemon to the floral sweetness of honey. A glass can have the pungency of spice and the mouth-puckering bitterness of dark chocolate. No other beer has provided as much fun or creative inspiration: 'old bookshop', 'horse blanket' and 'tobacco pouch' are just three of the ways Lambic beers have been described. These beers are enigmatic and hard to pin down, not just in terms of their flavour but in terms of their history too. Much of lambic's origins remain a mystery, nothing is really certain. But there are clues.

When Bruegel painted his masterpiece *The Harvesters* in 1565 he captured a group of Belgian labourers taking a break in a wheat field on a hot, dry day, lying down under the shade of a tree, cutting bread, eating from bowls and drinking from clay jugs. Some beer-loving art historians (or art-loving beer drinkers) think that the liquid inside the jugs is lambic. Their reasoning is sound. Back then, brewing lambic beer would have been part of the seasonal rhythm of farming in Pajottenland, a region of gently rolling hills between the Dender and Zenne rivers. Here, as summer turned to autumn and the fields of barley and wheat were being harvested, the perfect conditions for fermentation would approach; not so warm that brewing could easily run out of control, not so cool that too much microbial life had ground to a halt. At this point, farmers turned into brewers for a while, producing a refreshing drink that was safe and storable (one that could be drunk by labourers resting under a tree in the months and years to come).

From these agricultural beginnings, this rural, post-harvest brew became a drink for the growing urban population of nearby Brussels. Tax receipts from the end of the sixteenth century describe a beer that shares lambic's characteristics being traded around the city. As Brussels expanded, specialist cafes opened serving beers brewed on the hundreds of different farms across Pajottenland. Soon, a new profession emerged: barkeepers skilled not only at sourcing the most desirable barrels of lambic beers but also blending them to create distinctive drinks. The cafes serving these unique blends were (and still are) more like private sitting rooms than pubs.

Eventually, much of the brewing itself moved into the city, so by the end of the nineteenth century Brussels had hundreds of lambic producers right in its heart as well as on its outskirts. But less than a century later, lambic beer was nearly extinct. The First and Second World Wars caused some lambic breweries to close, as fuel, wood and manpower had to be diverted to the front lines and coolships and brewing kettles dismantled so their metal could go to the war effort. In the post-war era, wider changes in food and farming saw an end to most of the remaining breweries. Post-war recovery led by the Marshall Plan saw American food imports arriving in great quantities, transforming diets and palates and putting sour lambic in direct competition with Coca-Cola. New wheat and barley varieties ushered in by the Green Revolution changed the raw materials brewers had used for centuries. And then a new fashion started unfolding across Europe. It began in the 1960s and took greater hold in the 1970s: a taste for pilsner lager. This relatively young upstart in the drinks world quickly edged out much of the diversity Michael Jackson loved.

Clear and golden pilsner beers first began quenching European thirsts in the heat of the industrial age. First perfected in the city of Plzeň in Bohemia in the 1840s, an important trading centre near the German border, this pale drink with a frothy head made a big impact (up until then, most lagers were dark in colour). It also had the good fortune to have been developed during a scientific revolution in brewing, one that would propel pilsner to its current status as the world's most dominant beer style. Longevity was one reason for lager's popularity. Lagers were already suited to being kept longer than other beers (*Lagern* in German means to store) and refrigeration meant pilsners could be stored even longer. Later, in the 1870s, as we've seen, Louis Pasteur succeeded in isolating yeast strains. This allowed brewers greater control over 'off-flavours', and as pilsner was a more delicately flavoured beer (less forgiving than ales) this new clean taste made it even more desirable. Its rise came just as glassware was becoming more affordable; the look of this clear, golden pretty-looking beer must have mesmerised drinkers at the time. New rail networks spread the novel beer style far and wide. Further advances in the twentieth century sped up the process of brewing lager, making it possible to go from grain to glass in a matter of weeks. Despite all its long brewing history and diversity of styles, even Belgium submitted to the new taste for lager that took hold across Europe. By the 1980s, three-quarters of all beer drunk in Belgium was lager and most of this was being made by one company, Interbrew. Today, pilsners account for 95 per cent of all global beer sales.

For the few surviving lambic brewers, lager as well as ever larger breweries proved to be a near fatal blow. An online project, lambic. info, compiled by three young beer enthusiasts based in the USA, lists the lambic breweries that closed in the twentieth century. It includes Bécasse-Steppé, a cafe opened in 1877 which grew to become a famous gueuze brewer and blender, only to be bought out in the 1970s and then absorbed by Interbrew in the 1990s. Another, De Neve, set up to the west of Brussels in 1792, was first bought out by a competitor in the 1970s and also taken over by Interbrew in the 1990s, its building later converted into luxury apartments. Désiré Lamot, founded in 1837 and which presented lambic at the World's Fair in 1885, closed in 1991. And there are similar stories for the other 320 breweries on the list. When breweries disappeared, so did hundreds of irreplaceable beers and blends, never to be tasted again. By the mid-1990s, only ten lambic breweries remained in Pajottenland and just one had clung on in Brussels. This was Cantillon, which Michael Jackson described in the early 1990s as looking 'more like a garage, with an interior that was as much a working museum as a brewery'. Back then, it had weathered wooden beams, stone floors, dark spaces filled with copper equipment and dusty galleries in which steam-powered machines with flywheels sat beside lines of rugged barrels filled with beer. When I followed Jackson's footsteps and walked into Cantillon nearly three decades later, the only difference was the ownership had passed from the fourth to the fifth generation of Van Roys, the family who have owned the brewery for two hundred years.

My guide was Cantillon's in-house historian Alberto Cardoso, a fast-talking lambic evangelist. Three flights up a creaking flight of stairs at the top of the brewery is a claustrophobia-inducing attic space with a low ceiling and a floor taken up entirely by the coolship. Rectangular in shape, the container is about the quarter of a tennis court in size with knee-high edges. 'In this room everything is subcontracted to nature,' said Cardoso, 'and each day, nature gives us something different.' This is the coldest part of the building and so when hot wort is piped into the coolship from the kettle below, a wall of steam turns the room into a beer-infused sauna. Everything around us – the wood-panelled walls, the beams, the ceiling – is disturbed as little as possible. This is to keep the brewery's resident microbial community intact and uncompromised. When the building is cleaned, no chemicals are used and spiders are left alone (they keep insects away, carriers of other less friendly microbes). When a new roof was fitted, dusty tiles from the old one were nailed onto it, all to conserve the resident yeasts.

On the floors below the coolship, hundreds of barrels are lined up. Some are a century old, but all are fellow hosts of Cantillon's unique microbial population. Inside these barrels, wild yeast strains are joined by lactic acid bacteria in orchestrating the magic of fermentation. The dominant yeast strain is *Brettanomyces* (meaning British fungus), so named because in the nineteenth century its presence in English breweries was considered disastrous, a source of funky 'off' flavours. In the wilder microbial world of lambic brewing, *Brettanomyces* is embraced as the bringer of sharp, edgy, citric flavours.

The art of blending is also being practised and protected at Cantillon. Jean-Pierre Van Roy, the current head brewer, samples fermented flavours from hundreds of different barrels to create a drink that is recognisably 'Cantillon'. 'Nature proposes one thing,' said Cardoso, 'but Jean-Pierre creates another.' Young beers still fermenting away add energy and spritz to the more mellow three-year-olds; a case of maturity bequeathing subtlety on a wilder, sourer character. The result is not only an endangered beer but an endangered flavour. 'Sugar and sweetness, once a rare luxury, is everywhere now,' said Cardoso.

'Our beer is a reminder of something more complex: sourness and bitterness.'

West of Brussels, in Pajottenland, there are a small number of surviving lambic producers, among them Girardin, a fourth-generation brewery based on a family farm. Both the brewery and farm are run by the enigmatic Paul Girardin. In his *Guide to Belgian Beer*, the drinks writer Tim Webb figured, 'The [Girardin] family must know the high regard in which complete strangers around the world hold their beers and yet they remain reclusive, and the business continues much as it always has, catering just to locals.' Those who have managed to glimpse Paul Girardin at work say the magic starts with the wheat and barley on the farm. As harvest approaches, he wanders the fields, picking grains off stalks and nibbling away. When he finds an area of the field that he thinks tastes just right, he marks it out as the crop for that year's brew, selling the rest. The closest I made it to visiting the brewery was a brief conversation on the phone with Heidi, Mrs Girardin. Like the hundreds of other curious enthusiasts who enquired before me, I was politely told a visit wasn't possible; Paul was too busy, had important work to do and was a little shy. There is, however, a tiny bar in Pajottenland where you are guaranteed to find bottles of Girardin's lambic beers (and other rare bottles). This is an unchanged and traditional cafe in the village of Eizeringen called In de Verzekering tegen de Grote Dorst.

Translated from Flemish, this long name means 'In the Insurance Against Great Thirst'. Its owner, Kurt Panneels, rescued the cafe from closure when its landlady retired at the end of the 1990s. He now lives above it with his family, and in its tunnel-like cellar he has assembled a collection of the rarest lambic beers in Belgium. On the ground floor, the 1930s clock on the mantelpiece seems to be suggesting that time has stood still. Here, you can feel the history of Belgium's cafes, many of which were small, intimate spaces run by women in their own homes. These places were the crossroads of Belgium society, places where people from different walks of life – rich and poor, young and old – could mingle.

During the week, Panneels works as an architect, but every Sunday he opens the cafe at ten in the morning until eight at night. The only other time he opens is when there is a funeral in the village. It is one of the greatest bars in the world. Visitors travel from Japan, America and across Europe to drink here. 'They arrive as strangers,' says Panneels, 'but end up drinking together and sharing different lambics.'

Lambic, a drink that came dangerously close to extinction in the twentieth century, is now being sustained by the passion of its loyal twenty-first-century following. Many cite the books and television programmes of the 'Beer Hunter' Michael Jackson as having sign-posted their way into this captivating world. Cantillon has its own bar now, crowded with craft beer fans from around the world who drink lambics as they wait for guided tours in one of three languages. Perhaps they find something in this wild, spirited beer that is now missing from most other drinks: the taste of resistance, a vote for noncon-formity, a chance to try something different. As Jackson said, lambic 'has a taste of life from half a millennium ago'.

29

Perry

Three Counties, England

If lambic beer is the burgundy of Belgium, then perry is the champagne of England. This cousin of cider (made with pears not apples) is another drink that has teetered on the brink of extinction, kept alive by the knowledge and stubbornness of just a handful of people. Like Ramaz Nikoladze's qvevri wine, the story of perry is as much about ancient landscapes, tenacious trees and rare fruit as it is about recipes and craft. If we lose this drink, we will not only lose a source of pleasure but also more of the world's biodiversity.

A perry pear is less predictable than a table pear. Most are small, hard and inedible, although some can be soft, juicy and disintegrating. Like the apple, it originated on the slopes of the Tian Shan in Kazakhstan, eventually making its way to England with the Romans. The farmers who grew these pears must have been patient and forward-thinking because the fruit is exasperating, from start to finish. Firstly, they grow at a stubbornly slow pace; the seventeenth-century saying 'you plant pears for your heirs' applies to all types of pear, but especially so to the perry. A generation will pass before a tree produces a good harvest. Secondly, the trees often fruit one year and then give nothing the next (and possibly the one after that). When the fruit does come, the window of ripeness is fleeting; if the pears aren't gathered in time, they start to blet from the inside out. Things don't get any easier once the juice is pressed; the beautifully clear liquid is volatile and given the slightest excuse to spoil, it always will. In comparison, turning apples into cider is a straightforward process because, just as in winemaking, naturally occurring yeasts on the fruit happily get to work converting sugars into alcohol. But making perry requires much more attention, which explains another saying: 'Cider is a hard master but perry is a beautiful and fickle mistress.'

For the brave few prepared to face down these challenges, the rewards can be scintillating. Lighter than wine, more elegant than cider, a good perry might be honey-coloured with the lush, musky fragrance of a damp autumnal forest or an old-fashioned sweet shop. A sip will fill your mouth with the bitter-sweet taste of ripening orchard fruit, tinged with the acid of lemon drops, the bone-dry tannins of tea leaves and the sugar of candyfloss. This is all accompanied by a tickle of tiny bubbles, the result of conditioning in the bottle from the primary fermentation. In Georgian England, perry was an esteemed drink. Its producers, based in the west of England, pioneered techniques for creating fizz that were picked up by the vignerons of Champagne who in turn invented a sparkling wine and named it after their region.

Like champagne, perry captured the essence of a place: the three counties of Worcestershire, Gloucestershire and Herefordshire, once home to the largest and most diverse collection of orchards in the world. Here, during perry's heyday in the eighteenth and nineteenth centuries, the finest perry pears grew from giant trees and skilled perry makers worked their magic. Just a tiny number of producers are carrying on that tradition today. One of the best (or certainly most persistent) is Tom Oliver.

Oliver has spent most of his working life following two passions. As a music producer he is the tour manager for the band the Proclaimers, a job which has taken him around the world, mixing sound. When he isn't on the road, he lives and works on his Herefordshire farm, making cider and perry, blending flavours. When I visited him, it was late September and autumn had arrived. Oliver had invited me to spend a day with him collecting fruit and (if we found enough) making perry. My timing was good; after years of holding back, one of the rarest perry pear trees in England, a Coppy, had decided to bear fruit. 'This single tree is so rare it should be considered a living monument,' he said. 'For people in the know ... it's as important as Stonehenge or the pyramids.' To find it, we drove to an abandoned orchard, the location of which Oliver keeps a secret. In this rural part of Here-fordshire, all farmers once kept an orchard or, at the very least, a cluster of apple trees and maybe even a perry pear tree or two, to make their own cider and perry. Most of these orchards had been grubbed up by the 1970s as perry went out of fashion and cider became more industrialised. And so, for years, in his spare time Oliver has explored the county, wandering through fields, knocking on farmers' doors and checking out abandoned orchards, just in case something special had been left behind. In 2010, he made his 'once-in-a-lifetime discovery' in the abandoned orchard we were now standing in. At the end of the nineteenth century, there had been twelve acres of Coppy trees. By the middle of the twentieth, as Britain fell out of love with perry, all but one of these trees had disappeared from the landscape, along with thousands of other perry pear trees across the three counties. Maize, potatoes and strawberries were more profitable and so the giant trees were chopped down. Among perry makers Coppy had taken on a near mythical status (the drinks it once made no doubt getting more delicious at every telling). From a distance, I could see the last remaining Coppy in all its monstrous proportions – sixty feet in height and width. As we got closer, I noticed a red-and-yellow-coloured carpet of perry pears spread out on the ground around it. From the branches above there hung thousands of small, red, conker-sized fruit. 'Imagine the weight of all that,' Oliver said, looking up at the clusters of pears still on the 250-year-old tree. 'The only thing capable of killing this tree is itself. One year it'll produce a crop so big it'll fall.'

We started picking fruit off the ground. The fact that they had fallen from the branches above was proof enough the fruit was ripe for perry making. It smelt sweet and intoxicating under the canopy, a mix of burnt sugar and heady ethanol. 'That's bletting,' said Oliver, explaining how the sugars in the pears were already breaking down. Bletting is good, rotting is bad, he added, and we were just in time. We gathered the fruit to the steady beat of more ripening pears thudding to the ground from above, birdsong looping around us. It was a dewy morning and the fruit was glistening. An artist would have struggled to capture all the colours and shades. After filling five buckets, my back was aching. 'Don't worry,' Oliver said, 'it'll be worth it.'

If you were unwise enough to bite into a perry pear the experience would most likely begin with a brief burst of sweetness followed by overwhelmingly bitter acids and astringent tannins, as if all the moisture was being sucked out of your mouth, 'a bit like chewing a tea bag', as Oliver describes it. In skilled hands, however, the fruit can bestow something else entirely. The Coppy might be the star of the perry world, but there is a beguiling cast of supporting characters, other varieties (also endangered) and all with mesmeric names. There's the Arlingham Squash, the shape of a teardrop and identifiable by a petite bulge at the end of its stem. Like the Coppy, the variety was saved after the chance discovery of a single tree. Then there's the Blakeney Red, once so prolific its juice was used to dye the khaki uniforms of soldiers in the First World War. The Brown Bess is a leathery, rough-skinned variety; one of the few perry pears sweet enough to be used in the kitchen. Trees of the Green Roller used to line the banks of the River Severn and bore fruit that looked like miniature Conference pears. Only a small number of these trees have survived. The Holme Lacy, first found on the banks of the River Wye near a church, broke records when a single tree of it produced five tonnes of fruit in a single year. All that remains of that tree now are a cluster of rooted branches. Other varieties of perry were given their names (such as Merrylegs and Mumblehead) by drinkers who felt the full effects of their fermented juice.

Some of these varieties are old enough to have been used for perry making in medieval times which is when the first written accounts of the fruit and the drink appeared. In the fourteenth-century poem *Piers Plowman* is the line 'piriwhit ... poured together for labourers and poor folk', while a seventeenth-century description hinted at the perry pear's medicinal properties, 'a tonic for the kidneys, sure to bring longevity to its followers', wrote horticulturist Ralph Austen, adding that the fruit also makes 'excellent wine, not inferior to French wines, cheering and reviving the spirits'. Perry was a drink of kings as much as labourers. Popular pear varieties at the time included the Barland pear, so astringent it was said even pigs refused to eat it, but which made perry 'quick strong and heady high coloured'.

Perry began to travel further afield from the three counties in the 1630s. By then, the invention of powerful coal furnaces made it possible to make glass strong enough to withstand the pressure created by fermentation. Primary fermentation took place inside the barrel, the secondary fermentation inside the stronger bottles, allowing the legendary effervescence of *méthode traditionelle* (later adopted in

Champagne) to develop. Another boost for perry came with the Anglo-French war of the 1770s when wine imports from the Continent came to a sudden halt and perry was adopted as an alternative.

But as the world sped up in the twentieth century, perry, with its slow and demanding fruit, was left behind. Cider making could be scaled up more easily, but perry pears just weren't suited to factory-sized production. As the First and then Second World Wars arrived and farm workers went away to fight, labour-intensive perry making became an impossible luxury. By the 1970s, most of the old perry orchards were gone, along with most of the people who knew how to turn the fruit into a drink. Around this time, Oliver, like many of his generation, upped and left the family farm. His grandfather had grown perry pears and cider apples but growing fruit now didn't look like much of a future. Instead, he moved to London and a career in the music business. Making drinks (and drinking) became a hobby. This changed when he met another amateur drink maker, a Cambridge don called Roger French. French was an eccentric 'ciderist' and perry producer who lived in an old cider maker's cottage. Beneath his kitchen he had dug out a cellar to store his concoctions. 'It was chaos,' recalls Oliver. 'Roger had to wear wellies in his cellar because it was usually under a foot of water.' He would rise up from his subterranean store-house clutching mouldy-looking bottles with rusting tops and no labels. When French took the tops off, there would be a ssshhhhhh spritz of fizz. 'Those drinks changed my life,' says Oliver. As he sipped, he thought to himself, 'This is what I want to make.' It was like finding the Holy Grail, he said. 'I'm still searching for those flavours today.' In the 1990s, Oliver began planting a new perry orchard and exploring Herefordshire in search of forgotten perry trees.

To make perry, first the pears are milled into a porridge and the milled fruit is left to macerate for twenty-four hours to help temper the harshest tannins. This is pressed to extract as much juice as possible which is then stored inside barrels. The first wave of fermentation in the autumn is explosive, but this almost grinds to a halt during winter when the temperature falls. Then in spring, microbial life reawakens and another wave of fermentation begins, as sharp, tangy malolactic acid is converted into softer-tasting lactic acid. Throughout the process, Oliver (just like Belgian lambic brewers) hands control to nature, relying only on the work of wild yeasts and spontaneous fermentation. 'Good perry making is about striking a deal with yeast and then standing back and allowing nature to do its thing,' he says. 'It's such a simple process, which is what makes it so terrifying. When it goes right, it's unassailable. When it goes wrong, it's unsellable, a complete disaster.'

Some of the yeasts that drive the process come from the fruit itself, the rest from the air blowing through the farm or spores resting on the stone of the buildings, the wood of the rafters and on the surface of the barrels. It is only when the yeasts have exhausted most of the sugars in the juice that Oliver takes control and begins his work as a blender. This involves what he describes as 'a conversation' with the barrels. Fermentation will have given each barrel its own personality and this reveals itself to Oliver as he tastes each one. 'One perry might say to me, "I am not going to taste better than this, you'll want to bottle me just like I am." And I'll reply, "You're dead right, you're perfect, you're gorgeous."' These perries he leaves as they are. But another perry might reproach him, telling him he should have paid more attention in the orchard or in the pressing room, 'and they're saying, "Sort me out, will you?" Whereas others say, "I'm boring and ordinary just like the rest of the world, pep me up, give me some purpose, let me have a chance to sing."' Oliver brings perries such as these together in a blend, creating something exceptional. When he is living his other life, working with musicians and sound, he adjusts the bass, middle and treble frequencies, to create layers and harmony. 'It's the same with perry,' he says. 'Barrels full of perry are like a mixing desk.' The sign of a successful perry for Oliver is less a taste and more a sensation. 'When it comes out of the barrel, and I take a sip I want it to make me want to chew,' he says. 'Good perry is chewy.'

I helped to crush and press the Coppy pears we had collected in the morning along with sacks of other varieties that grew on Oliver's farm. By the end of the afternoon, we had filled two barrels. When I returned a year later, we sat down to drink a little of what we had made. 'Lovely slab of pear in the middle,' Oliver said as we sipped, 'like soft velvety wine.' And at the end of the glass he smiled and said, smacking his lips, 'That's it. Chewy.'

May Hill

It wasn't so long ago that most of us could have almost literally drunk in our surroundings. Wherever we were in the world, there would have been a brewer, distiller, winemaker or an orchardist who bottled the biodiversity of the landscape. In Pajottenland, in Imereti and in the Three Counties of England, that connection still exists (just), but for most of us it has been lost. Charles Martell has made saving that link between place and product his life's work.

Martell lives over the border from Tom Oliver, in the Gloucester-shire village of Dymock. In the early 1970s he was filmed for a BBC television series about endangered foods, called *A Taste of Britain*. In it, Martell can be seen attempting to produce the first real farmhouse Double Gloucester cheese since the war. 'I was young, with a head full of dreams,' he said as we watched the archive footage together. 'They came to film me because the cheese was dying, but I was saying, "No, this can't be an epitaph. I can't let that happen."' In fact, making the cheese was just a means to an end. The real motivation was to save a cow, the Old Gloucester. At the time there were only nine bulls and seventy cows left. Wherever Martell travelled in the country, he kept seeing the same black-and-white cows, Holstein-Friesians. 'Over centuries, so many places had developed their own breeds, but these were disappearing.' Gloucestershire was his county, and he believed it should have its own breed. 'I wasn't going to sit back and let it disappear.' He made cheese and by doing so saved the breed. In the process, he became one of the most important farmhouse producers of his generation.

Then, in 2000, in a part of the farm he calls Perry Croft, Martell planted an orchard. I visited one autumn when the trees were covered in mahogany, gold and auburn leaves and the branches were heavy with small, red, round perry pears. Over the fence was his herd of Old Gloucester cows and miles in the distance was a knot of trees. This was May Hill, the centre of the universe for anyone who grows perry pears. Legend has it that perry trees will only prosper within sight of that hill. And here was Martell in the centre of it all. He had his sense of place in the world, the feeling of belonging to a landscape. But that hadn't come easily.

Back in the early 1970s, when his own farm was struggling, Martell worked as a lorry driver to make ends meet, picking up animals to take to market. He went from farm to farm, most within sight of May Hill, and usually saw enormous, magnificent perry trees. The farmers he visited explained which varieties they were. But as the years passed, on his rounds, he noticed trees had been chopped down or left abandoned and overgrown. By then, perry was just a memory and perry trees weren't thought to be worth keeping.

Martell is now planting trees for the future and trying to reverse the decline. From the ground, he picks up a perry pear, a pyramid-shaped fruit flecked with crimson and about the size of a golf ball. It was Dymock Red, named after the village nearby. People thought it had gone extinct and Martell, depressed at this thought, had taken action. He told his wife he was going out and wouldn't be back until he had found the pear. He drove to the farm where the last known sighting had been back in the 1950s and then travelled in an ever increasing circle, looking in every farm and garden that had pear trees. It took him two weeks (during which time, he admits, he did go home) and he did eventually rediscover the Dymock Red. Nine trees of this pear variety are now growing in Martell's garden. 'I suspect that's now all that's left in the world.' Martell says his perry orchard is a 300-year plan. 'Why three hundred years?' I ask. 'Because it's appropriate,' he says. In a hundred years' time, it'll be time for the cider apple trees to be cut down as they reach the end of their lives and the perry trees will begin to fill the space over the next two centuries. 'They make such big trees, and perry is such a fine drink, with such a strong connection with this place. They belong here.'

In a barn nearby were hundreds of heavy bottles, corked but unlabelled, perry that was made twenty years ago waiting to be used to wash one of the cheeses Martell makes, Stinking Bishop. Next to the barn was a distillery, home to a beautiful, tall, pear-shaped copper still. Here, Martell was turning some of his perry into a spirit, an eau de vie. From a wooden beam above the still was a small bell tied by a piece of rope, itself held in place with wax. In the old days, if a worker fell asleep and the still overheated, the wax would melt, free the rope and the bell would make a noise, waking up the distiller just in time to stop the still exploding. 'Like so much of what they did years ago, it was simple, but it worked,' said Martell. We sipped some of the strong, saffron-coloured liquid that had been aged in barrels. 'A fitting tribute to perry pears,' Martell said as we drank, the spirit taking effect. We looked out towards Perry Croft. 'When you walk amongst those big trees it's like being inside a cathedral. You feel the sense of something bigger than yourself.'

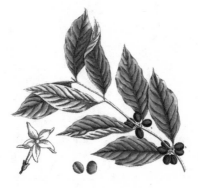

Part Nine
Stimulants

They have a very good drink … almost as black as ink,
and very good in illness … this they drink in the morning
early in open places before everybody, without any fear
or regard, out of China cups … as hot as they can; they
put it often to their lips but drink but little at a time.

Leonhard Rauwolf, Aleppo, 1573

When people talk about Proust's madeleine moment – when, biting into a cake, a lost memory is instantaneously unlocked – they usually forget to mention that the sweet sponge had first been dipped in a 'warm liquid' before the 'extraordinary thing' happened. The over-looked liquid was an infusion of blossom from the lime tree (a species of *Tilia*), linden-flower tea. Perhaps it receives less attention because hot drinks are so omnipresent in our lives. From the time humans had the means to heat water, they have created infusions, some purely for medicinal reasons, others for their calming effects (including Proust's linden-flower tea), but most for their ability to stimulate the senses.

Take cassina, for example. For one thousand years, in parts of the southern United States, the toasted leaves and bark of the yaupon tree were used by Catawba and Timucua indigenous people to make this concoction also known as 'black drink'. Spanish conquistadors described watching people make the brew and drink it only to vomit (the plant's scientific name is *Ilex vomitoria*). But cassina wasn't just a means of purifying the body; its main appeal was its high levels of caffeine. The genuine kick the drink provided led it to featuring in all of the important events in Catawba and Timucua life, from religious ceremonies to war.

Cassina is one of thousands of examples of infusions past and present drunk around the world. Wherever you find humans you will find a stimulating drink, even in places where barely any plants grow: in Iceland, a brew was made using Arctic alpine flowers (*Dryas octo-petala*), while the nomadic Sami in northern Sweden made an infusion with a fungus, *Piptoporus betulinus*. In drinks, humans have found many things: enhanced physical prowess, improved mental agility, appetite suppression, pain relief, reduced fatigue and an increase in euphoria.

But out of all the contenders, just two plants came to stimulate humans in every habitable continent on Earth: *Camellia sinensis* (tea) and *Coffea arabica* (coffee). Early converts to these drinks conferred sacred status on both: Buddhists in China drank tea to improve meditation, while Sufi monks in the Arabian Peninsula used coffee to lead them to higher states of concentration and more intense prayer. Coffee and tea share a bitter alkaloid, the psychoactive drug caffeine, one of nature's most potent defence mechanisms. Concentrated in the leaves of both plants, it acts as a natural pesticide capable of repelling insects and putting off hungry herbivores. When leaves of tea or coffee plants fall to the ground, caffeine can even leach into the soil where it acts as a herbicide and keeps other plant competitors in check. Enjoying a caffeine fix isn't an exclusively human trait either. Nectar infused with caffeine will encourage pollinating insects to make return visits to plants, so in exchange for spreading pollen some bees receive a caffeinated buzz.

In the places where wild tea and wild coffee began (south-western China for tea, East Africa for coffee), hunter-gatherers, aware that these plants were stimulants, first chewed the leaves and (in the case of coffee) seeds. Fermentation and other processing techniques came later, a means of not only preserving plant material but also unlocking more of the plants' powers. Pottery started to be made around 20,000 years ago, and sometime after that (we don't know when exactly) dried and fermented leaves and seeds were being brewed into drinks. From their centres of origin, tea and coffee radiated out around the world, and wherever they arrived, people fell in love with them – or more likely became addicted. In 1610, the Dutch East India Company transported the first shipment of tea into Europe, and in 1615 coffee followed suit, this time care of Venetian traders. Caffeine was on its way to becoming the world's favourite drug. Within fifteen minutes of drinking a cup of coffee, the effects of caffeine race through our central nervous systems, making our hearts beat faster, activating neurons and triggering the release of dopamine. For most of us, one cup is never enough. We rely on both these drinks, they're part of our lives, an unrivalled ingredient in countless daily rituals. The two plants, *Camellia sinensis* and *Coffea arabica*, have transformed entire economies (coffee generates nearly $5 billion a year for Brazil in exports alone, and in India, the tea industry employs 1.2 million people). So why, when they are so widely drunk, do tea and coffee belong in a book about endangered food and drink?

The answer to that question lies in the origins of the two drinks. In this part the focus is on a wild tea and a wild coffee, both from tropical forests, both victims of some of the most urgent problems we now face: climate change, deforestation and the loss of biodiversity. Tea and coffee can provide a lens for seeing what's happening to our planet.

30

Ancient Forest Pu-Erh Tea

Xishuangbanna, China

In the summer of 2019, a Hong Kong auction house sold one of the rarest collections of teas ever assembled. Included among the lots, wrapped in yellowing, fraying bamboo leaves and bound together by twine, was a stack of circular cakes of compressed tea. On the surface of these, just barely visible, were small paper tickets with a series of symbols. This provided evidence that the tea had been made in the 1920s by a company called Tong Xing Hao based in Yunnan, the south-western province of China and the birthplace of tea. The bidding for this vintage batch of dried leaves closed at $1.08 million. How this hundred-year-old block of tea came to be so sought-after and valuable was the result of thousands of years of ingenuity and just a few decades of economic change in China.

The solid cakes were a type of tea called pu-erh (pronounced *poo-err* or *poo-ahr* and also spelled pu'er). Long before people worked out how to make loose-leaf tea (during the fourteenth-century Ming dynasty), wild tea leaves were always withered, sun-dried and turned into solid bricks or cakes. Thanks to yeasts and bacteria these cakes of tea had lives of their own as they fermented over years (in some cases decades), their flavours, like a maturing wine, continuously shifting and changing. Most of the world's tea is now picked ('plucked' is a more accurate word) from modern cultivars of waist-high bushes grown as monocultures in huge plantations. This is the model that now exists across most of China and in the world's sixty or more tea-growing countries. But as with wild Arabica in the highlands of south-western Ethiopia, there are mountains in China filled with forests of wild tea. This is in southern Yunnan, where China meets Myanmar, Laos and Vietnam; northern Thailand is also within reach.

Here, left to its own devices, the tea plant *Camellia sinensis* grows into sprawling, tall, spindly trees, big enough to climb, some as high as fifteen metres and with broad leaves. Occupied by indigenous groups such as the Dai, the Blang, the Yao and the Lahu, this region was – and still is – like no other part of China. In their isolated mountain villages surrounded by thick forest, it's likely the ancestors of these people were the world's very first tea drinkers.

While in most of the world's vast plantations leaves are skilfully manipulated, oven-dried and blended to create particular flavours, the rarest pu-erh (what is referred to as raw or unripened pu-erh) is more like natural wine; a minimalist approach is taken when processing it, the idea being that (for good or bad) by drinking this tea you can travel without travelling. One cup, in other words, will transport you to other places, the villages and forests in Yunnan's three main pu-erh regions. The northernmost region is Lincang, closest to the border with Myanmar. East of Lincang is the Pu-Erh region (and the city of Pu'er itself); the third is Xishuangbanna (or Banna), on the border with Laos. Banna is one of the world's richest biodiversity hotspots. It covers just 0.2 per cent of China's land area but harbours a quarter of all mammals found in the country, a third of all its birds and nearly a fifth of all its plants.

This biodiversity helps to explain why people obsess over pu-erh made from the leaves of the oldest trees. Each cake contains the very essence of a specific part of a forest, from the soil and the nutrients drawn up by the tree, the plantlife that surrounds it, to everything that tree has experienced over centuries (in some cases, millennia). This is what scientists call 'plant apparency', in that every trauma suffered by a tree (drought, disease and attacks by pests) affects the plant's chemistry (as a defence mechanism it can produce protective compounds called 'secondary metabolites', including terpenes and phenolic acid). In an ancient tea tree, this is believed to create unique flavours. Or as indigenous people in Xishuangbanna put it, the trees develop a deeper character in the same way a human who has endured greater hardships does. The different ways the mountain villagers pick, process and store the leaves also adds a cultural dimension to pu-erh's uniqueness. Pu-erh expert Don Mei describes the drink as a 'celebration of impermanence'. On one level it is just a beverage, a psychoactive stimulant, 'but when you brew your way through leaves of pu-erh and drink, the experience is ephemeral. You can never taste the same tea twice.'

To make a cake of pu-erh, after the leaves are plucked, they are sun-dried on long wooden racks to wither and darken (this helps develop flavour). Next, they are cooked in woks over hot fires to stop oxidation. The leaves are then rolled and kneaded (which drives out more moisture, breaks down the membrane of the leaf and activates chemical compounds that add yet more flavour). Once they are pressed into cakes, fermentation over years intensifies the complexity of the tea. One pu-erh might have woody, leathery notes; another a subtle tang of dried fruit; another still, an earthy, mushroom-like taste.

Pu-erh tea cakes are beautiful to look at. Round ones are usually smaller than a dinner plate but bigger than a saucer, and a couple of centimetres thick. Others are square or rectangular, the size of a paperback. The texture might be a solid mass of dark autumnal leaves and broken twigs, or like pressed potpourri, a tangle of brown, yellow and orange plant material. As if leaving an artist's signature, some pu-erh makers embed a small piece of card within their cakes, while others press them in moulds that leave behind a raised or indented symbol. These messages tell where the tea came from. The cakes are then wrapped in paper.

If you want to drink some pu-erh, you crumble a small piece of the cake to make a brew. A few pu-erh cakes, however (including the record-breaking pu-erh made in 1920s Yunnan), are so valuable they will probably never be drunk. Instead, they are collected like works of art. People are not only drawn to their flavours but to their stories too. The most valuable vintage teas were made by now renowned factories such as Menghai, Xiaguan, Fu Yuan Chang and Tong Xing Hao, which all orginate in the pre-revolutionary era. These are the Krug, Taittinger or Pol Roger of the tea world. Today, investors as well as a number of extremely wealthy tea obsessives drive the global trade in cakes, both old and new. And therein lies one of the problems facing pu-erh tea. An ancient indigenous tradition has been turned into one of the most lucrative food businesses on the planet.

As the 2019 Hong Kong auction illustrated, demand for pu-erh is booming. Most of this demand is coming from within China. In the 1990s, as the country got richer, pu-erh went from being a relatively obscure tea drunk by indigenous people and agricultural workers to becoming a status symbol. Today pu-erh cakes made from regions such as Xishuangbanna can sell for tens of thousands of dollars per kilo. The trade is inevitably having an impact, both positive and negative, on the mountain villages. While the indigenous people have retained their veneration for the forests, the ancient trees and pu-erh making, outsiders have moved in and have started to turn the tea into a mass-produced commodity. Villages are being amalgamated to manufacture pu-erh on a larger scale and distinctive natural flavours are being lost as a result. 'More consistent teas are being made,' says Don Mei, 'and we're losing the highs and lows that come with the wilder, smaller batches.' Pu-erh's individuality is at risk of disappearing.

The villages themselves have also been transformed including Lao Banzhang, one of the most prestigious of all pu-erh making locations. At the beginning of this century, it was so isolated and mountainous it could take days to reach it. In the rainy season, getting here was near impossible, the journey considered far too dangerous, although obsessive tea hunters were prepared to risk their lives in search of its particular pu-erh. The altitude of the village (almost 2,000 metres) and the age of the trees can give the pu-erh a drunken effect, an almost overpowering sensation created by all the psychoactive chemicals in the tea. Since the pu-erh boom, new roads have been built into Lao Banzhang and it has become a tourist destination. This is the positive impact, an example of rural development; it means indigenous people are at last being rewarded for their work. The downside is that checkpoints have been introduced around some of the prefecture's most celebrated villages, including Lao Banzhang, because their fame has resulted in other teas being brought in and then labelled as locally produced pu-erh. Meanwhile, in Nannuo Shan, another pu-erh region in Xishuangbanna, villagers built a barrier around the trunk of an 1,800-year-old tree. 'The idea was to protect it from the growing numbers of tourists,' says Don Mei, 'but the concrete they used in its defence ended up killing the tree.' These are just a small number of tragic stories, but they illustrate a trend: a culture and ecosystem under pressure. All of this feels a very long way from the origins of pu-erh.

The first definitive reference to tea making and tea drinking appeared just over 2,000 years ago. The document, titled 'Tong yue', 'Contract with a Servant', was written by Wang Bao in southern China during the Western Han dynasty in 59 BCE (the contract stated that Wang Bao expected a daily fix of tea, almost like a dose of medicine). At this time, tea picked and processed into cakes in the mountains of Xishuangbanna was making it as far north as Chang'an, China's ancient capital (home of the terracotta warriors). Here it was given as 'tribute tea' to Han royalty. Evidence of this comes from the second-century BCE Yang Ling mausoleum, the tomb of a queen that was excavated in the 1990s, where fragments of pu-erh cake were found. This tea would have travelled along trade routes that radiated out from the tea-growing mountains of Yunnan. Less well known than the Silk Road, the Tea Horse Road turned the city of Pu'er into a trading hub (which resulted in the tea being named pu'er or pu-erh). Its tentacles went in all directions; the Guan Ma route took tea north (including to Chang'an) and west, where it joined the Silk Road; to the south was Meng La, which transported cakes of tea to Laos and then further into what is today called Vietnam and Cambodia. But for centuries, the most important path on the Tea Horse Road was the Guan Zang, the one that reached into Tibet.

In the extreme conditions of this mountain kingdom, everyone from kings to bandits depended on solid cakes of tea. The ancient trade route, one of the harshest trails in all of Asia, stretched nearly 1,500 miles from Pu'er city to Tibet's capital Lhasa, a climb of 12,000 feet (making it among the highest cities in the world). This epic journey involved taking the cakes through the subtropical valleys of Yunnan, along the wind-blown and snow-packed Tibetan Plateau, across the freezing Yangtze, Mekong and Salween Rivers, through the 400-mile-long Nyainqêntanglha Mountains, climbing a three-mile pass and finally dropping down into the holy Tibetan city. Along the way, the superhuman tea porters had to survive snowstorms, torrential rain, collapsing cliffside ledges and robbers. Each porter transported around 90kg of tea (the more they carried, the more they were paid) which they took along passages where snow could be waist-high and six-feet long icicles hung from rocks above their heads. These journeys lasted months and are probably the most arduous ever undertaken by any merchants or travellers in history; an illustration of the power and prestige of tea.

Once in Tibet, cakes of (by now) fermented leaves were turned into hot, stimulating brews that aided survival (before, the only other drinks on offer here had been snowmelt, yak milk or a fermented barley gruel). As little vegetation grew around the kingdom, tea was an important source of vitamins and minerals and helped ward off scurvy. Salt and cereals were also traded along the tea route to Tibet – and these became the ingredients for butter tea, a fatty, salty, sharp-tasting brew heated and drunk from morning to night, bowl after bowl, up to sixty a day. In the 1890s, the English adventurer and painter Arnold Henry Savage Landor shared bowls of butter tea and *tsampa* (a thick porridge made with roasted barley) with a gang of bandits. 'With their dirty fingers,' he wrote, 'they stirred the mixture in the bowl until a paste was formed, which they rolled into a ball and ate.'

By the eighth century, a drink closer to the look and taste of modern pu-erh was being made in Xishuangbanna. By then, tea making and tea drinking had become more sophisticated, enough for Lu Yu (considered to be the 'sage of tea') to write *Cha-jing* (*The Classic of Tea*), a text that took readers from the myths and legends surrounding the drink to instructions on how to perform a tea ceremony. Lu described how different regions had their own approach to making tea. South-east of the Yangtze River they tied cakes together with bamboo strips, whereas upstream, they used cord made from the bark of mulberry trees.

One thousand years later, making pu-erh cakes had gone from being an indigenous craft to a factory process. In the 1700s, small family-owned factories in Xishuangbanna and in Pu-er city had developed unique house styles with reputations that spread across China. These included Tong Xing Hao (the maker of the million-dollar pu-erh cakes). Supplying these factories with wild tea leaves were the indigenous tribes who lived in the wild tea forests. This 'antique age' of pu-erh came to an end in the middle of the twentieth century when not only the culture of pu-erh became endangered, but also the ancient wild trees themselves. The Communist Revolution in 1949 closed many of the tea factories, a fact which today adds cachet to the pre-revolutionary cakes. Under Mao, pu-erh returned to obscurity and became more of a rural tradition. Large tea plantations producing loose-leaf tea dominated. During the Great Leap Forward in the 1950s, villagers in Yunnan were told to build steel furnaces and help industrialise the countryside. In the process, wild tea trees were cut down and used as firewood. By the 1980s, pu-erh producers were paid pennies for a kilogram of their tea. As one pu-erh trader, American-born Paul Murray, puts it, 'It had become tea for "your average Joe" someone who might be shearing yaks high up on the Tibetan plains, a functional tea, one that could be brewed all day and just got the job done.' Murray has pu-erh cakes from this period with bits of glass and rock inside them, a reflection of how production standards had fallen along with prices. More threats to the wild tea forests came in the 1990s. As China got richer, people swapped bicycles for cars, creating a surge in demand for rubber. Historically, rubber was grown in regions around the equator such as Indonesia, but farmers there were switching over to growing palm trees to supply the food industry's demand for palm oil. Between 2001 and 2010, global rubber prices tripled, so in a push for self-sufficiency, the Chinese government handed out subsidies to farmers to abandon traditional crops and grow rubber instead. The project was so relentlessly pursued in Xishuangbanna that nearly a quarter of its forests were turned into monocultures of rubber trees. At its peak, the rubber price went so high, even tea growers in high-altitude, frost-prone villages (unsuited to growing rubber) cleared out ancient tea trees to switch to the new crop. But rubber didn't bring the change in fortunes that tea farmers were hoping – and some of them were left with failed rubber plantations where before they had had tea trees.

The recent pu-erh boom should have brought unqualified good news for the tree forests of Xishuangbanna but this hasn't proved to be the case. In the early 2000s, some villages cleared out slow-growing ancient trees and replaced them with monocultures of high-yielding bushes so more tea labelled as being from Xishuangbanna could be turned into cakes. Meanwhile, the indigenous people who have tended the tree forests for centuries are unlikely to get to sip pu-erh from the oldest trees left in Xishuangbanna. These leaves don't even make it onto the market – they are auctioned off each year to the highest bidder. One such tree grows in a village called Bangdong on the western tip of Yunnan, a survivor amid so much destruction. It is more than four hundred years old, the height of a three-storey building, so tall that scaffolding has to be used to pluck the leaves from the highest branches. According to local pu-erh traders, the tea from this tree is likely to be drunk by government officials or business leaders in Beijing. Just like the cakes found inside the Yang Ling mausoleum, pu-erh made from the most ancient trees has once again become a tribute tea, a privilege for a twenty-first-century elite.

31

Wild Forest Coffee

Harenna, Ethiopia

I met my first coffee tree in a shaded forest north of La Paz in Bolivia, far from the birthplace of coffee. The small community of Chu-chuca, made up of a handful of houses and farms, was the setting for the encounter. It was late afternoon, hot and humid, and a wall of sound was building, created by the succession of birds that were joining in the dusk chorus. Parrots, toucans and hummingbirds were busy settling in for the night. I was with Don Fernando Hilaquita, a coffee farmer in his sixties. Wearing a broad straw hat, he led me on a trail beneath tall cedars and towering laurels. Dry leaves crunched beneath our feet as Hilaquita pointed out wild edible mushrooms and birds' nests lodged inside the holes of tree trunks. Within this semi-managed wilderness and growing under the canopy, we found the coffee trees; young and spindly-looking. Against their tough, leathery, green leaves, bright red berries, the size of marbles, stood out. I reached up and picked a handful of these coffee cherries. Popping one in my mouth, I bit into sweet and sticky flesh until my teeth hit seed, more accurately a pair of seeds, oval halves that nestled together within the fruit. Their shape and the groove running along their centre made the seeds recognisable, but instead of roasted brown they were a grey-green colour. Nothing about their taste gave any clue this could be the ingredient in a pitch-black, nerve-jangling espresso.

To me, the forest looked beautiful and full of life, but all was not well in this part of the coffee world. A disease the farmers had named *la roya* ('the rust') had caused serious damage in the region, and coffee trees and people's livelihoods had been ruined. The disease wasn't new, but the scale of the damage was. Since the middle of the nineteenth century, coffee growers have had to contend with this fungus (*Hemileia vastatrix*) which one Victorian botanist described as 'the vampire of the vegetable world'. But in the twenty-first century, with the world more globalised and the climate warmer and wetter, the capacity of *la roya* to wreak devastation has been amplified. *La roya* also loves coffee trees planted closely together, with branches and leaves low to the ground, as they are in the modern coffee industry. The fungus causes tiny blotches to appear on the leaves; each blotch contains around two hundred spores which eventually burst out and infect the plant's neighbours.

First, an orange powdery surface covers the underside of the host leaves, which then turn yellow. The fungus then covers the entire leaf, making photosynthesis impossible. After struggling to feed itself, the plant starves to death. Even if a tree survives and produces seed, it will have been rendered unsellable. So far, no cure has been found for *la roya*. In 2012, following a succession of mild and moist winters, outbreaks of *la roya* erupted across Central and South America. It left coffee harvests in Colombia reduced by 30 per cent and in El Salvador by more than 50 per cent. By 2017, the cost of damaged crops and lost profits reached $3 billion and almost two million farmers left the land. Theirs was already a precarious existence; coffee is an agricultural commodity, traded in the world's financial centres, so a bumper crop in Brazil one year can send global prices crashing downwards. Add in a devastating disease and the human cost is enormous. Migrant caravans travelling north through Latin America into Mexico and towards the US border exist for many reasons, but when reporters have asked people why they have left their homes, some of them have provided a two-word answer: 'La roya.'

The disease also affected the life of Don Fernando Hilaquita, the farmer who introduced me to my first coffee tree. In 2014 *la roya* wiped out most of his trees. 'We replanted, because we didn't want to give up,' he told me. But for most of the other growers it had proved too much and they had left to find work elsewhere. Hilaquita was one of the few farmers left, but even he was worried there were more problems to come. 'If the climate keeps changing or the disease comes back, more trees will die, and we might as well die with them.'

Coffee's past may be able to guide us to a solution, but it's also part of the problem. Coffee grows in an imaginary belt that wraps around the world between the tropic of Cancer and the tropic of Capricorn, taking in Costa Rica and Nicaragua in Central America,

Bolivia and Brazil further south, sub-Saharan Africa (between Came-
roon in the west and Somalia in the east), South Asia (southern India),
South East Asia (Vietnam, Indonesia and Papua New Guinea), and
Jamaica and the Dominican Republic in the Caribbean. This belt was
only completed in the nineteenth century with the founding of plantations across parts of South East Asia and other tropical regions, but
all of the coffee grown in it can be traced back to the wild forests in
the highlands of southern Ethiopia. How coffee made its way out of
East Africa and ended up creating that 'belt' is crucial in understanding
why coffee is under threat, and not just from *la roya*. This is because
almost all of the coffee grown around the world today comes from
the descendants of a handful of plants that spread around the world
in the eighteenth century.

In the cool, upland forests of south-western Ethiopia, as far back as
one million years ago, a rare biological event took place. Two different
coffee plants, *Coffea canephora* and *Coffea eugenioides*, hybridised to create
a new species. That cross was successful and, luckily for us, stabilised.
This is how Arabica (*Coffea arabica*) came into existence, the source of
most of the world's coffee. The other species grown around the coffee
belt is one of Arabica's parents, *Coffea canephora*, more commonly
known as robusta. Arabica is the more refined of the two and the one
that has filled most of the world's coffee-drinking history. Robusta,
mostly used in instant coffee, was only known to science at the end
of the nineteenth century, and only became an important commodity
coffee in the twentieth. But long before coffee was a drink, it was a
food.

In Ethiopia, the biological centre of coffee, hunter-gatherers first
interacted with wild Arabica plants by eating the flesh of its sweet
berries. In some cases the seeds were spat out, in others the raw beans
were chewed. Today, the Oromo people of southern Ethiopia carry
on a tradition of taking ripe coffee berries from wild trees, grinding
them using stone mortars and then blending the mashed seeds with
butter to make small balls that can be carried as an energy snack on
long journeys. At some point, we don't know when, people started
sun-drying and roasting coffee seeds and then brewing them.

The wild coffee trees in Ethiopia's highland forests and in a small
area of neighbouring South Sudan are the main storehouse of genetic

diversity for Arabica (just as the wild trees around the Tian Shan in
Kazakhstan are the gene pool for the apple). At its simplest, these
forests are split into two main regions, east and west of the Great Rift
Valley. In the west are the Wellega, Illubabor, Tepi, Bench Maji, Kaffa
and Jimma-Limu coffee areas, and in the east, across the Rift, are
Sidamo, Bale and Harar. In each of these areas, and in each of the
forests, are genetically distinct populations of Arabica. Each area has
a unique flavour profile, or even range of profiles. Coffee has an
'origin', in the same way the term 'terroir' is used for wine, to identify
the difference between one vineyard and another. Each of the distinct
populations of wild coffee trees has evolved and adapted to its own
environment over hundreds of thousands of years. This diversity
explains why, in the west in the Agaro region, in the Jimma-Limu
zone, coffee may be sweet and subtle, with notes of citrus, tropical
flowers and stone fruit (such as peach), whereas coffee from the Bale
Mountains is usually fruity and floral but with added notes of vanilla
and spice. Each of these coffee areas is also home to different
communities.

One of the lesser-known wild coffee forests (and one of the hardest
to reach) is Harenna, 250 miles south-east of Addis Ababa, set within
the Bale Mountains which has some of the highest peaks in East
Africa. This is a biodiversity hotspot; thousands of plant species can
be found here, along with endangered punk-haired Bale monkeys,
lions and the rare Ethiopian wolf. Much of the mountain forest here
has been so inaccessible that this biodiversity remained largely
undocumented until the end of the twentieth century. Harenna is
dwarfed by the Bale Mountain massif, which has peaks of over 4,000
metres, and even in the dense forest where the coffee grows (at 1,500
to 1,800 metres) there's often a cloud of mist above the high canopy.
Harenna might appear to be completely given over to nature but
within the coffee forest are villages, hamlets and single smallholdings.
The forest is currently home to around 3,000 people, and for most of
them coffee is their life. Their livelihoods depend on gathering beans
from trees that can be completely wild or semi-wild (tending them
makes harvesting easier). The wildest coffee grows on wiry branches
of tall, spindly trees; the red, cherry-like fruits are picked and tossed
into long, cylindrical straw baskets draped over shoulders. Some of
the wild coffee is sold on to traders, but much of it stays in the forest.

Every social occasion, including births, deaths and marriages, features coffee. Even the processing and brewing of the beans is a ritual. The sundried beans are roasted until they darken and become shiny and brown. The little moisture left inside the bean builds up until each one is forced open with a crack and the heavy aroma of roast coffee fills the air. Once cooled, the seeds are ground in a wooden pestle until they are fine enough to be gently simmered in water inside a terracotta pot, called a *jebena*. Guests look on as this is happening, sharing food, talking and breathing in the scent of the roasting beans.

We don't know how far back these traditions go, but the Scottish travel writer James Bruce who visited Ethiopia in the 1760s (in search of the source of the Nile) described forests of wild coffee, the drink and the rituals surrounding it. In Europe where people had been drinking coffee for more than a century, Bruce's story was dismissed. There were good reasons for people to doubt his claim. At the time, Europeans regarded Yemen, on the Arabian Peninsula, as the birthplace of coffee. This is where it had been seen growing, where modern coffee drinking started, and where it was traded from. When Carl Linnaeus, the Swedish botanist and father of taxonomy, was shown a handful of coffee seeds in the 1730s, he named the plant *Coffea arabica*, coffee 'from Arabia'. It wasn't until the nineteenth century, after similar accounts to Bruce's from other travellers, the connection between coffee and Ethiopia was established. Coffee plants and seeds had been transported centuries before from Ethiopia, across the short but dangerous stretch of water in the Red Sea, the Bab-el-Mandeb (the 'Gate of Tears'), to the west coast of Yemen. One theory is coffee crossed the Red Sea with pilgrims travelling in their thousands through Ethiopia to reach Mecca. More likely coffee was transported by Arab traders moving through East Africa, via Harar. (Because of the presence of the volcanic glass obsidian in Ethiopia, we know trade routes existed during the Neolithic.)

In Yemen, the potency of the drink gave it sacred status. It became known as *qahwa*, a word which originally referred to the stimulating *khat* potions used by Sufi mystics to stay alert for night-time prayers or to transport them into trance-like states. In the fifteenth century, coffee became the new *qahwa* and the religious drink of choice. Some accounts credit the Sufi scholar Gemaleddin Abou Muhammad Bensaid with the shift. He was said to have sanctioned coffee drinking among dervishes, 'so that these devout Muslims, might spend the night in prayers or other religious exercises with more attention and presence of mind'. Other accounts mention Muhammad al-Dhabani, a Sufi mufti who realised coffee's powers after the drink helped him recover from illness. What is clear is that by the beginning of the sixteenth century, coffee plantations had spread along the western edge of Yemen and beans were being exported across the Islamic world from the port of Mocha.

By the end of the sixteenth century, there were coffee shops in Cairo, Aleppo and Damascus and in the Grand Bazaar of Constantinople. Coffee arrived in Venice in 1615 and in 1650 England's first coffee shop opened (by the end of the century, there were six hundred). New Yorkers had their first taste of coffee in 1696. Consider the timing. It's likely this new drink, a stimulant, helped inspire the ideas and innovations that shaped the modern world, not alcohol, the older drink of choice (a depressant). The Age of Enlightenment was fuelled by caffeine.

For centuries Yemen maintained its monopoly on coffee cultivation; no viable seeds or coffee plants were allowed to leave the Arabian Peninsula, being so valuable they were carefully guarded. This changed in the 1690s when an infinitesimally small number of coffee plants left the country and went on to provide the genetic base for most of the coffee grown in the coffee belt that now wraps around the world. As we know from the stories of wheat and bananas, lack of diversity is never good in the long term. These plants were sent out from Yemen and across the globe on two major separate trajectories. The first batch was taken by the Dutch East India Company thousands of miles to the Indonesian island of Java (a Dutch-controlled territory at the time). Then, in 1706, one coffee plant was transported from Java to Holland and planted in the Amsterdam Botanical Garden. Six years later, as a gift to the Sun King, Louis XIV, a coffee tree from the botanical garden was sent to France, where it was eventually planted in the Jardin du Roi in Paris, inside France's first ever greenhouse. A decade later, a French naval officer called Gabriel Mathieu de Clieu took some coffee plants from the Jardin du Roi on a boat bound for the Caribbean. All of the plants except one died on the voyage, and even that one had a lucky escape. When a fellow passenger saw de Clieu tending to it with their limited water rations he tried to destroy the plant. But de Clieu kept it alive, and it was eventually planted on the Caribbean island of Martinique in 1720. It wasn't until 1727 that a descendant of de Clieu's plant made a further and perhaps more important journey, smuggled into Brazil by a Portuguese diplomat, Francisco de Melo Palheta. This plant, so the story goes, was hidden inside a bouquet of flowers, a gift from de Melo Palheta's lover.

The second trajectory involved French traders. In 1718 they took coffee plants from Yemen to Réunion Island, east of Madagascar. From here coffee plants were dispatched first to colonies in East Africa to create large-scale plantations in Kenya and Tanzania, and then west to Brazil. So, most of the world's coffee came from two sets of plants, one that passed through a French botanic garden and another through an island in the Indian Ocean. The two did have different character-istics. The ancestors of de Clieu's plants were given the name *typica*, and the other type, a more delicate, sweeter- and brighter-tasting coffee, was called *bourbon*. What made this narrow genetic selection more of a problem for the future was the biology of Arabica; it is self-pollinating, meaning it doesn't have to mix its genes with those of another plant for fruits to be produced. Because of its history and its narrow genetic base, a cultivated Arabica plant today has a fraction of the gene vari-ation (the alleles) of those found in the wild. In the face of climate change, water shortages and increasing disease, the concern is that Arabica might not have a big enough genetic toolkit to adapt fast enough, or even at all.

There have been attempts to add greater diversity to the global crop. A century ago, when the coffee industry was dealing with earlier waves of *la roya*, the response was to create diversity through plant breeding. As with any crop, farmers spotted mutations and adaptions in their coffee plantations and these were picked up and used by plant breeders. One example was cultivar 'Maragogype', a mutation of typica found in Brazil in 1870 which had fruit twice the size of other coffee and large seeds. Then there was 'Villa Sarchi', a mutant of *bourbon* found in Costa Rica, attractive to farmers because it produced shorter trees, making harvesting easier. Other mutations were taken up by breeders to create crosses such as 'Sarchimor' (a hybrid coffee of Villa Sarchi and a plant known as the Timor hybrid). On the plus side, the newer cultivars showed more resistance to *la roya*, but on the downside most were descendants of the plants that came via Paris and Java; all originated from the same narrow gene pool.

Another response to the threat of disease was to introduce new, and potentially resistant, Arabica plants from forests in Ethiopia. The most celebrated of these is Geisha. Originally from a remote forest near the village of Gesha, in south-eastern Ethiopia, near the South Sudan border, it was planted by coffee growers in Kenya and then taken to Central America where it ended up in a botanic collection in Costa Rica. A farm in Panama (Hacienda Esmeralda) took an interest and started to grow it, but for many years it was overlooked until one of the sons roasted a batch of Geisha beans and was amazed by what he tasted. Word of Geisha spread and, in 2004, it became the most expensive coffee ever sold at auction, fetching $130 per pound, around one hundred times more than a commodity-grade Arabica. Because of that record price, farmers across Central and South America began to grow Geisha at an astonishing rate and it is now spreading around the world's coffee belt. The variety illustrates the benefits of saving wild coffee diversity for its amazing flavour and its genetics, which are essential for the future of coffee plant breeding. But just as we're realising the value of the coffee genetics in the Ethiopian highlands, the wild coffee trees are under threat.

To produce fruit and good-quality beans Arabica coffee needs specific conditions: warm (but not hot) days followed by cool nights. This is why it's most often grown at higher altitudes. If temperature and rainfall deviate too much between optimal conditions, the quality of the fruit quickly deteriorates, productivity starts to fall, and the plant may become weaker and more vulnerable to disease. Scientists at the Royal Botanic Gardens in Kew have calculated that during the twenty-first century, because of climate change, more than 65 per cent of the places where Arabica grows today in Ethiopia could become unsuitable for this crop by the end of the century. Other research shows a similar pattern for the rest of the world. It will simply be too warm, and in many cases too dry. One option for coffee farmers is to start planting trees at higher altitudes where temperatures are cooler, especially in Ethiopia. But at the Harenna forest, around the high Bale Mountains, the potential to move to higher elevations is limited. They are already approaching the limit of where coffee grows.

The worst-case projection made by the scientists at Kew is that up to 80 per cent of Ethiopia's wild coffee population could be wiped out, before the end of the century, from climate change alone. This is a scary prospect for the 125 million farm workers around the world who depend on coffee, and for everyone who drinks it; if the forecast proves true, we will have lost much of Arabica's wild gene pool. Climate change is not the only problem. This wild coffee ecosystem is also under pressure from deforestation, in some cases to create new pasture for Ethiopia's expanding cattle herd. All of this is happening before the full diversity of wild coffee has been understood. Scientists are now in a race against time to map the surviving coffee diversity before more of it disappears.

If Arabica's future is precarious, perhaps we could drink more robusta, which already makes up around 45 per cent of the global coffee trade. First identified in 1897 by botanists exploring the forests of the Belgian Congo (today's Democratic Republic of Congo), it started to be grown on a large scale in the 1920s. This was because of *la roya*. While Arabica was vulnerable to the disease, robusta wasn't and being more robust gave it its name (it also grows at lower altitudes than Arabica and in warmer, wetter climates). Its proportion of the global crop grew considerably during the 1970s and 80s when production expanded in Asia, particularly in Vietnam. But although robusta has a higher caffeine content than Arabica, its taste is inferior. If the best Arabica is sweet, delicate, bright, floral and fruity, robusta is coffee's sledgehammer blow, a full-on caffeine kick with notes of woodiness, hints of tobacco and even rubber. If you've ever stood at a marble-top counter in a French or Italian coffee bar and drunk a one-euro espresso, it is likely you've experienced robusta, as it is often blended with Arabica to add body and improve *crema*. If you drink instant coffee, again, that is most likely robusta. It's no substitute for Arabica.

In Bolivia, Don Fernando Hilaquita showed me his own approach to saving Arabica. The Chu-chuca community's recovery from *la roya* has involved not changing coffee varieties but changing the farming system. Hilaquita rejected the old plantation model, monocultures of densely planted trees in which all other life had been eradicated. Instead, he has revived the forest around the village and started growing coffee with Arabica trees planted under the shade of the wild canopy and among other plants. As we walked further into his coffee forest it was growing dark and the birds started to fall silent. The warm, sun-beaten day had become starlit and cool. This, he told me, handing me more cherries, was a wilder way of farming. 'La roya might still find its way in,' he said, 'but at least I'm not fighting nature to grow coffee. Maybe she'll be kind.'

Stenophylla

Unlike cereal crops, coffee can't be preserved inside the vault in Svalbard or in any of the world's seedbanks. Coffee species have to be maintained as living plants, in botanic gardens, research stations, or in laboratory conditions. Once their habitat is gone, there is little chance of bringing an endangered coffee back. In 2019, Aaron Davis, a botanist at Kew and an expert on coffee diversity, published a paper with colleagues listing the conservation status of 124 coffee species (of which Arabica and robusta are just two), and found that at least 60 per cent are threatened with extinction.

With time against us, Davis is taking a radical approach to ensuring the future of coffee diversity – by tracking down and tasting some of the at-risk species, especially the ones we know little about. He is hoping to find types of coffee worth considering for cultivation in a changing world. These have been found around the world from Upper West Africa to the northernmost tip of Australia. About thirty new species have been named by Davis himself. He and his colleagues have roasted as many of them as possible, to find out if they produce a drinkable coffee. 'All very fascinating, but most of them are just about acceptable and some of them taste disgusting,' he says. A few have little or no caffeine and the coffee they make can be unbearably acidic.

But Davis is convinced there is more special coffee waiting to be discovered, or rediscovered, ideally something as robust as robusta but as drinkable as Arabica. One candidate is the endangered species called *Coffea stenophylla*. Once known as Highland Coffee it is now usually referred to just as stenophylla. Native to Sierra Leone, Guinea and Ivory Coast its slender trees can grow to a height of thirty feet and the fruits it produces are purple-black. Davis knew from dried plant specimens held at the herbarium at Kew that the tree had last been recorded in Sierra Leone in 1954; people suspected it had been wiped out in the country's so-called 'development decade' when huge areas of forest were cleared to make way for cash crops. From Kew's archives and library, Davis also knew that this species had a reputation of being superior in terms of its flavour. To the very few people who remembered tasting it in Sierra Leone, stenophylla was a much finer cup than robusta and perhaps even superior to Arabica. But it disappeared from cultivation, despite being farmed and exported from Sierra Leone up to the early twentieth century. By the beginning of the twenty-first century it was thought to be extinct. In 2018, Davis and fellow coffee scientist Jeremy Haggar from the University of Greenwich were invited by the government of Sierra Leone to have one last attempt at finding the lost species. On their journey they took copies of some of the archives from Kew's herbarium and library and their colleagues put up 'Wanted' posters of the missing coffee.

Their quest began with a visit to the last known location of a stenophylla tree, which they then travelled around in concentric circles (just as Charles Martell had done when he went in search of a lost pear tree). After several false leads and substantial amounts of trekking, they found a single tree. Although this was a great achievement, it was about as useful as finding a lone panda because, unlike Arabica, stenophylla needs to be pollinated by another tree if it is to produce seeds. They travelled even further afield and after hacking through dense forest, close to the Liberian border, they reached the top of a hill and found a cluster of stenophylla trees. They had just made it in time, the surrounding area had been heavily deforested. In the summer of 2020, a small batch of stenophylla (just nine grams) was roasted by a team of coffee experts in London, accompanied by Davis. It was the first time in nearly a century that anyone had tasted it. 'It was fragrant, fruity and sweet,' said Davis. 'A coffee with real potential.' It can also tolerate higher temperatures than Arabica and has greater resistance to la roya. Other species may not be found and saved in time.

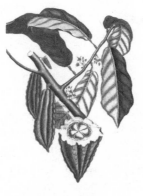

Part Ten
Sweet

If the enemy is taking his ease ... harass him;
if well supplied with food ... starve him out.

Sun Tzu, *The Art of War*, fifth century BCE

Like all good menus, we end with sweet things, foods traditionally associated with moments of pleasure, conviviality and celebration. Yet what also unites the three foods in this part is the reason for their being endangered: conflict. Whereas most of the other ingredients in this book have been pushed towards extinction by agricultural change, habitat loss, disease or economic forces these foods are victims of strife.

A story linked to the sacking of Carthage by the Romans in 146 BCE tells us that after the destruction of that prosperous city, located in present-day Tunisia, the Roman general Scipio Aemilianus passed a plough over the site, sowing salt in the furrows to ruin the soil, literally salting the earth so Carthage would be destroyed for good, its fertile lands rendered barren like a desert. This was how it was retold by nineteenth-century historians, but it was pure myth. It has been calculated that it would have taken a fleet of 10,000 Roman ships, all fully loaded with salt, to have made the soil of Carthage infertile.

But the myth does brilliantly encapsulate the way in which food (or lack of it) can be used as a weapon of war. In September 1864, to bring a speedier end to the American Civil War, the Union Army Generals Sherman and Sheridan ordered their men to make non-combatants in the South feel the 'hard hand of war'. They did this by destroying crops, attacking food stores and killing livestock, leaving people with little to eat as winter approached.

During the First World War, naval blockades by the British in the Atlantic resulted in German citizens living through the 'turnip winter' of 1916–17 when food supplies declined. Less than three decades later, during the Second World War, Herbert Backe, Nazi Germany's Minister of Food and Agriculture, devised *der Hungerplan*. If this had been implemented it would have resulted in 30 million citizens in Eastern Europe dying of starvation so that food supplies could be diverted to Germany and its soldiers on the front lines of Europe. Resistance by the Red Army meant this never came to pass but Backe's *Hungerplan* shows how hunger has the potential to be a lethal weapon in any conflict.

In the twenty-first century, food and farming continue to be among the first casualties of war, and conflict is also the fastest way in which a food can go extinct. The stories that follow are testimony to that fact. We'll see how a food culture, which evolved over thousands of years, can be all but eradicated in no time at all by conflict. We will also see how food (and memories of food) can be a source of hope during troubled times. Ingredients and recipes help give us a sense of our place in the world. For people who have lost everything, a food tradition or taste from home can take on new meaning.

32

Halawet el Jibn

Homs, Syria

Located within the Fertile Crescent, Syria is among the world's oldest agricultural sites and its place on the Silk Road meant that it developed one of the most sophisticated and diverse cuisines. The recent war, however, has devastated land, displaced farmers, wiped out unique crops and placed traditional ingredients and food knowledge at risk of extinction. In a cruel twist, food was one of the causes of the war. Between 2007 and 2010, the country experienced one of the worst droughts in recorded history. Aquifers, lakes and rivers were running dry because of overambitious government targets for wheat production. The knock-on effects hit rural communities hard and pushed one million Syrians off the land and into cities where they were impoverished and marginalised. Tensions climaxed in street demonstrations in the spring of 2011, which were met by a brutal crackdown from the government of Bashar al-Assad. Civil war followed.

A decade on, the United Nations estimates that 700,000 people have been killed; 5 million people have fled the country as refugees to live in Turkey, Jordan, Lebanon and Egypt; 6 million more Syrians are internally displaced; 90 per cent of survivors inside Syria are categorised as food insecure, a predicament not helped by the spiralling cost of food (between 2019 and 2020 prices inside the country doubled).

In 2015, the world looked on in horror as Syrian (and world) heritage sites came under attack. ISIS militants stormed the ancient oasis city of Palmyra in the Syrian Desert. They blew up the 2,000-year-old Temple of Bel and destroyed what had been some of the world's best-preserved Roman monuments. Less visible, however, was the destruction of the nation's food system, which will have long-term consequences for Syrians once the war ends. Many of the battle front lines were in or around agricultural areas, which meant an enormous

number of casualties in farming communities and confiscation of land
by warring parties. It is estimated that before the conflict, agriculture
provided employment for 50 per cent of the population. Syria had
been one of the leading food exporters in the region, producing cereals,
fruit and vegetables for its neighbours and the Gulf states. Early on
in the war, farmers' fields were deliberately targeted, trees in orchards
set on fire, and markets in towns and cities bombed. Various armed
factions levied taxes on food aid as it moved from one besieged area
to another and supply chains were choked off. Unable to find their
own food, and close to starvation, millions of Syrians became entirely
dependent on these rations.

As this was all unfolding, a small team of scientists based near
Aleppo was working behind the scenes, desperately trying to save a
food resource valuable not just for Syria but for the world. Twenty-
five miles west of Aleppo in the town of Tel Hadya was one of the
world's most important seed collections, part of a network of twelve
sites strategically placed around the globe, each responsible for a
different type of food. The seed bank in Tel Hadya was run by the
International Centre for Agricultural Research in the Dry Areas
(ICARDA) and held the widest range of wheat, barley, lentil and
chickpea in the world, in effect 12,000 years of farming history. This
genetic resource was important for the future of all our food as it
contained seeds with drought- and disease-resistant traits. It was now
in a war zone and at risk.

In 2012, a militia group attacked the research station, stealing
vehicles; and later, as the conflict escalated, kidnapping staff. Yet the
remaining workers stayed with the collection, somehow finding
enough diesel to run the generators and keep the temperature inside
low enough to preserve the seeds. Just as Nikolai Vavilov's colleagues
had risked their lives to protect seeds during the siege of Leningrad,
so the ICARDA team set about ensuring the 150,000 samples stored
in Tel Hadya were safe.

At one point the scientists were forced to strike a deal with the
rebels: the fighters agreed to protect the seed bank and keep the
generator running if, in return, the scientists provided them with food
grown in the centre's experimental gardens. The deal lasted until the
spring of 2016, when the Assad regime bombarded Aleppo and nearby
towns, including Tel Hadya. The scientists knew they had no choice

but to move the seeds to safety. Those who were left loaded up a truck with as many boxes of seeds as it could hold and headed south, escaping across the border into Lebanon.

Luckily, years earlier, they had backed up most of the collection by sending duplicate seeds to Svalbard, the vault built into the ice of the Arctic. ICARDA built a new seed bank in Lebanon, and those backup seeds were used to replace what was lost in Syria. With Lebanon reeling from its own economic and political crises, these seeds again find themselves in an unstable location. What makes this even more tragic is that seeds salvaged from Iraq's national seed bank in Abu Ghraib, which was destroyed in the second Gulf War, had been added to the collection in Syria. Back then, it had been seen as the safest place in the region to store them.

The Tel Hadya collection represented more than plant genetics; it contained landrace seeds important to Syrians. Over millennia, the country had absorbed ideas and ingredients from many of its diverse neighbours and inhabitants, including Assyrians, Turks, Alawis, Druze and Yazidi, influences that have played out in thousands of traditional Syrian recipes. One seed that was part of this cultural history was Hourani, a durum wheat collected from farmers around Homs. Because of its unique properties, Hourani wheat was ideal for making exquisite semolina pastries, including one called *halawet el jibn*. Bakers made this by creating a dough to which they added sugar syrup and majdouli (a salty, stringy cheese which gives the dough its elasticity). Thin strips of this dough are then filled with a cream called *qoshta* (or *ashta*), rolled, cut into bite-size pieces, covered in rose-petal syrup and sprinkled with ground-up pistachios.

Halawet el jibn belongs to a larger family of sweet delicacies found across the Levant including, most famously, baklava, also made with semolina flour. The origins of these foods can be traced back to the Roman Empire via the influence of Byzantine cooking and the later spread of baking techniques through the Ottoman Empire. In Syria, these foods, and others like them, became part of the social glue; sweet pastries were either made in the home or bought from bakeries (much loved and famous institutions, feted for their creations) and exchanged with friends and family. The war brought a violent end to much of this tradition.

Why worry about the fate of a cake during a war? Well, when you start to deconstruct *halawet el jibn* down to its individual ingredients, you begin to see the scale of the damage that has been wreaked on Syria's food system. Consider Hourani wheat, which like Kavilca in eastern Turkey had adapted to Syria's soil over millennia, now lost because so many farmers have fled the country. And consider the Tel Hadya collection where its seeds had been saved, now gone from Aleppo. Meanwhile, thousands of acres of pistachio fields have been destroyed, the trees targeted by fighters, the farms bombed, mined and set on fire, all with the aim of causing as much damage as possible to rural communities.

These attacks also go to the heart of Syrian identity. In the first century, the pistachio was such a quintessential feature of Syrian agriculture and cuisine that Pliny considered Syria to be the place where the nut originated. Pistachios had in fact come from further east in Iran and Afghanistan, but to the Romans it was clear the nut's culinary use had been perfected in the kitchens of Aleppo, Damascus and Homs. Syria went on to become the largest source of pistachio for the Middle East and Europe. 'The pistachio tree is the lung that allows our villages to breathe,' said one of the farmers who was driven off his land by the war. 'I will only be fine as long as my orchard is fine.' Before the war, in the farmland around the town of Morek, just north of Homs, 40,000 tonnes of pistachios a year were harvested, about half of all the pistachio nuts Syria produced. But after 2011 and the start of the war, farming them became too dangerous. In desperation, thousands of trees were cut down and used for fuel and firewood.

Further north of Morek, on the border with Turkey, is Kobani, a Kurdish area and another pistachio-growing region. For nearly a year, Kobani came under siege after ISIS took control of the city and the outlying villages. Hundreds of people were killed or kidnapped, and thousands more fled to refugee camps across the border in Turkey. When the US-led coalition launched airstrikes, backed by Kurdish soldiers on the ground, ISIS fighters set fire to field after field of pistachio trees as they retreated. 'All that was left was their blackened remains,' says Leyla Asmen, an aid worker who is helping with the work to rebuild Kobani. 'When ISIS retreated, they used explosives to blow up ancient wells and irrigation channels.' Even after the locals returned to their farms, they couldn't harvest pistachios from the surviving trees because landmines had been buried in the soil.

A food can easily become endangered if the source of its ingredients, say a farm, is destroyed. But if the place where food is prepared and processed is attacked, along with the people who possess the skills to make it, then that food will be at risk of extinction. In Syria, bakeries were targeted even as people were outside queuing for bread and cakes. One bakery that had to close because of the conflict was Salloura in Aleppo. For 150 years, the family-run store had been renowned for its range of pastries, including *halawet el jibn*, the cheese and pistachio pastry. Two years into the conflict, as the fighting intensified and sugar, flour and pistachio fell into short supply, the family shut up shop and fled across the border into Turkey and on to Istanbul, joining the half a million other Syrian refugees already in the country. In the city's Aksaray neighbourhood, now referred to as 'Little Syria', the Salloura family recreated the shop they had left behind in Aleppo and started making traditional pastries, including *halawet el jibn*. On a WhatsApp group called 'Syrians in exile', refugees in different parts of the world share pictures of the desserts on offer at the Salloura bakery and they post comments too. 'You are bringing me back to my home,' wrote one Syrian now living in North America. 'Like a fire, it burns me and hurts me to look at it.'

In the summer of 2020, Syria's pistachio farmers started to return to their orchards with pruning scissors in hand. Many fields hadn't been touched for eight years; some trees had dried out, their branches withered. There were the landmines to contend with, too. The other features of Syrian culture that made *halawet el jibn* celebrated, however, are still scattered around the world; the seed bank with the 'just right' variety of wheat remains in Lebanon; the bakers, the Salloura family, are still in their temporary home in Istanbul; and the customers they served, like millions of Syrians, are refugees overseas. Living on in the hearts and minds of Syrians around the world, Syrian food culture will endure until peace descends and people can return home.

33

Qizha Cake

Nablus, West Bank

'Nablus has the best bakers, the best cakes and definitely the best tahini,' Vivien Sansour told me as she was giving me a rundown of the various Palestinian seeds and flavours that she is trying to save. Raised in Beit Jala, near Bethlehem, she grew up, she says, 'with soil beneath my fingernails', growing food with her grandmother and learning to cook with her mother, aunts and grandparents. A child of the West Bank in the 1980s, all Sansour had known was conflict; she had lived through occupation, witnessed the arrival of illegal settlers and seen the Second Intifada (the uprising) unfold across the Palestinian territories. This had resulted in loss of land and traditional crops: fruits, vegetables and cereals, landrace varieties farmers had grown for generations. 'How can people farm under these pressures?' Sansour asked herself. 'How is it possible to grow food?'

She left the West Bank to study in the US and took to anthropology. A research project led her to Mexico, where she met seed-saving farmers growing heritage maize and squash. When she heard their message of *sin maíz no hay país* it made her think of home, and what was being lost, and she decided to return. She had her own farming heritage to save. Back in the West Bank, she launched the Palestine Heirloom Seed Library, a one-woman mission to track down and conserve the crop varieties that had vanished during the conflict.

She started with the courgettes, tomatoes and beans she had loved as a child. After posting pictures of jars filled with seeds on Facebook, she was inundated with messages. People wanted to know if she could find the vegetables their grandparents used to grow and their mothers had cooked. 'I touched a raw nerve, they understood something was missing, and they were almost begging me for help.' She started to travel around the West Bank, from Hebron in the south to Jenin in the north – places where agriculture went back almost 12,000 years.

Every community she visited and every farmer she met had stories of seeds they wanted to share. They showed her pictures of farms long gone, described dishes made with vegetables since disappeared and sang songs that had traditionally been sung during the harvest time. Her project wasn't just about saving the biodiversity of the West Bank, it was also, she says, about saving Palestinian culture. This part of her mission became clear in Jenin. The older people kept mentioning a fruit they had once loved which was now thought to be extinct, the *jadu'i* watermelon. The fields around Jenin were once filled with these big, green fruits. People told her that, until the 1960s, many Palestinian farmers had made their living growing this watermelon, which was popular across the Levant, from Beirut to Damascus. Women described how, during the harvest, they had given birth in the *jadu'i* fields. But when Sansour asked if she could taste this cherished watermelon, the answer was always the same. 'The watermelon is extinct, you may as well look for a dinosaur.' On her travels across the West Bank, she kept asking farmers if they had any *jadu'i*. The answer was always 'no' until one day she met Abu Ghattas, a farmer turned shopkeeper. Ghattas led her to a drawer at the back of the shop. 'It was full of screws and nails,' Sansour says, but at the back was a packet of watermelon seeds. '*Jadu'i*,' he told her. He thought that people no longer remembered the fruit, let alone cared, but he had saved the seeds just in case. 'All that time he couldn't bring himself to throw them away,' Sansour says. By growing the watermelon and saving its seeds, she has helped to bring the *jadu'i* back.

Further success came with wheat. In Shawawra, south-east of Bethlehem, farmers had saved their traditional seeds, including an endangered emmer variety called *Abu Samra* ('the handsome one'). The wheat's awns (its whiskers) are almost black in colour, its grains have a distinctive flavour and, most important of all, it needs little irrigation. 'It takes what it can from the rain,' Sansour says. For farmers in the West Bank, this trait is now more essential than ever, because since the occupation many have lost seeds, land and a reliable water supply.

*

The Arab-Israeli conflict is about land, but an equally crucial factor in the dispute is water. Water was one of the triggers of the Six Day War in 1967 (there had been moves to divert the River Jordan, Israel's main source of drinking water). With its victory in that war Israel more than tripled in size and embarked on a plan of agricultural expansion (including growing oranges, bananas, wheat and cotton). The control of water became an even bigger source of conflict. It has remained so ever since. Israel and Israeli settlements (the latter considered to be illegal under international law) remain in control of most of the West Bank's water. Palestinian farmers say this has stifled their agricultural economy. In 2014, the World Bank highlighted concerns that some weren't even able to draw their agreed allocation.

Among the crops that have been in decline in the West Bank are landrace varieties of sesame. Farmers used to grow this seed across much of the West Bank, particularly on the fertile plains around Nablus. So embedded is sesame in Palestinian culture that folk songs make reference to the seed, including 'Ya Zarain El Semsem'. Sung at weddings, it includes a pledge by the groom to always grow sesame for his bride and her family. Some traditional dances even feature the hand motions made by farmers in the fields as they harvest the sesame. Like *Abu Samra* wheat, it is a rain-fed crop capable of thriving in an arid climate. Dark-coloured landrace varieties of sesame were once used by Palestinian bakers as an ingredient in a paste and a cake; both are called qizha and both are pitch-black in colour.

In the city's small factories, sesame seeds are ground into a thick paste with the main ingredient of qizha, nigella seeds. This creates a shiny, inky black mixture that looks like treacle and has an earthy taste with hints of mint (the oil from the sesame gives it a smoother texture). Bakers blend this dark paste with semolina flour, sugar and nuts to make a sweet, moist and pitch-black qizha cake. The best versions of these cakes are still made in Nablus, but sesame imported from Ethiopia and Sudan has now replaced the Palestinian varieties.

For a young farmer from west of Ramallah, Muhab Alami, bringing traditional sesame back into production in the West Bank to sell to bakers is a long-term ambition, but it's proving tough. 'The water is controlled, and the land is controlled,' he says. 'There is a permanent feeling of uncertainty. It's stressful to be a farmer here. As a result,

our food heritage is disappearing before our eyes.' Even after crops
have been harvested, trying to sell them presents a whole new set of
challenges. 'The military impose restrictions; new settlements are an
obstacle and checkpoints are sometimes impossible to pass.'

The majority of the West Bank (and most of its agricultural land)
is found in the territory referred to as 'Area C'. Since the early 1990s,
this has been under Israeli military control and Palestinian access to
land and markets became more restricted, says Alami. Growing sesame
was already challenging: the crop needs large amounts of land on
which to grow and the seeds are labour-intensive to harvest. The
added pressures of conflict made it increasingly uneconomic to
produce. Many farmers couldn't compete against cheaper imported
sesame and switched to what they saw as more lucrative crops,
including tobacco.

But Alami wants to help preserve the old endangered varieties even
if only by finding and saving their seeds. 'They are part of my identity,
a crop grown on this land for thousands of years,' he explained. Three
years before I met him, he had worked on IT systems for a bank. 'I
felt as though I was working with air,' he said, moving his hands as
if trying to feel something that wasn't there. 'And now I am a farmer
and I am producing something real.' For him, being a farmer and
working to bring back a lost Palestinian crop is a peaceful act of
resistance. 'I have less money, but now I feel richer.'

Sansour is a cheerleader for farmers such as Alami and for traditional Palestinian food. On her travels around the West Bank, she
takes a mobile kitchen made of two wooden cabinets on wheels,
each a couple of metres long and a metre wide. On this, she chops
ingredients, prepares recipes and cooks. 'People can be moved to
tears when they taste something from their childhood that has become
hard to find,' she says. 'It reminds them of a time when life was not
so hard.' She also helps people grow their own food in community
gardens. 'You can even see violence in the soil,' she says. 'When we
dig a new garden, we often find pieces of shattered glass and empty
tear-gas canisters.' One day, she says, she will bring back other lost
varieties of sesame to the West Bank. 'To tell me that our seeds are
not worth saving and planting is like telling me that we as people
have no worth and no future,' she says.

There is an old Palestinian saying that Sansour shared with me before we said goodbye. 'He who does not eat from his own adze [a farming tool] cannot think with his own mind.' This is why a watermelon, a grain of wheat or a tiny sesame seed is such a powerful thing. Each one can be a small taste of freedom.

34

Criollo Cacao

Cumanacoa, Venezuela

When Europeans first started falling in love with chocolate around three hundred years ago, one type of cacao was famous for making the finest chocolate of all. This was criollo, the indigenous cacao of Central America. It comes from a rare and, compared with other varieties, fragile plant. Centuries of cross-breeding and efforts to create new hybrids made pure lines of criollo even rarer (today it makes up less than 5 per cent of the world's cacao supply). But there was one part of Central America in particular where the variety flourished and from where it was exported to the Old World: Venezuela. The trade in this fine cacao became so important that for many years it was Venezuela's main export. During the twentieth century, however, the country's politicians sidelined cacao growing, setting their sights on another natural resource, the country's oil reserves, among the biggest in the world. For a while, cacao's decline in Venezuela didn't seem to matter; oil made it the wealthiest and most developed country in Latin America. But when oil prices collapsed and corrupt governments entered the frame, Venezuela's economy took a nosedive, with disastrous consequences for millions of its people. It was just as this was unfolding that I arrived in Venezuela, in search of its cacao.

It was the spring of 2017 and I had travelled to the capital Caracas on a near-empty plane (most other people were attempting to make the journey in the opposite direction). There were protests on the streets, little food in the supermarkets and the city was being described as one of the world's murder hotspots. Kidnapping for ransom was the new boom industry. The economic crisis had pushed the country to near collapse. This resulted in a quarter of the 30 million population becoming in dire need of food and basic supplies and another 5 million fleeing the country. This was all happening under the presidency of Nicolás Maduro, a hero to his socialist party members but to many Venezuelans little more than a dictator and whom many governments in the Americas and elsewhere no longer recognised as a legitimate leader.

Because of its scarcity, food had become a source of conflict. Fights break out in food queues. One Venezuelan monitoring the situation told me that some people had even been prepared to commit murder over packets of rice. The shortages had kicked in around 2014, and people's anxiety over where their next meal was coming from just kept increasing. First, they waited days for basic ingredients to arrive in supermarkets, then weeks and now months. People weren't even able to buy maize to make *arepa*, Venezuela's daily bread. A black-market food economy was flourishing, with a new profession invented, the *bachaqueros:* people who because of their connections had privileged access to ingredients which they then resold at massively inflated prices. Venezuelans began losing so much weight many fell on dark humour to describe the situation. They called it the Maduro diet.

I'd travelled to Caracas to meet a woman with an idea for how some Venezuelans could find their way out of the crisis. Maria Fernanda Di Giacobbe had been a restaurant owner and a chef, but during the economic collapse she had been reborn as an activist. There was an answer to the crisis, she told fellow Venezuelans, an opportunity of work which could also help the country regain its pride. Di Giacobbe's solution was chocolate, more specifically Venezuela's rare and prized cacao, criollo. After a week in her company, I was convinced she was right.

We met inside a theatre in Caracas; hundreds of people, most of them women, had gathered to hear Di Giacobbe – supported by farmers and chocolate makers – describe her vision, learn about Venezuela's chocolate history and find out why it could be an important part of their future. Many had spent days travelling to Caracas by bus from villages further south. Some told me they had come in search of hope. Their towns were now violent places, their homes had been burgled, some had been mugged at gunpoint and all of them had experienced food shortages. This last feature of Venezuelan life I had seen for myself inside a supermarket close to the cinema. Aisle after aisle had been filled with identical bottles of whatever product was available to give an impression of abundance. There were thousands of bottles of ketchup and shampoo, but when I asked a sales assistant if there was any bread, flour or sugar, the answer was, 'No, no, no.' Away from the city, the situation was worse; there had been outbreaks of diphtheria. In a street market, I saw makeshift stalls where traders had decanted tiny portions of baby formula into medicine bottles. Venezuela's food system was broken and people were making use of what little they could find.

Di Giacobbe, who is in her fifties and has short silver hair, piercing eyes, a sculpted face and a beaming smile, took to the stage inside the theatre. She led her audience through centuries of chocolate history, a story in which Venezuela had played a lead role. Before oil (and the discovery in 1914 of reserves filled with 'black gold'), chocolate had powered Venezuela's economy. Di Giacobbe told her audience that cacao could do this again—it could help create a better future. They might live in one of the most troubled countries in the world but, as Venezuelans, they possessed the cacao seeds which made the finest and most coveted chocolate on the planet, criollo.

The oil boom had resulted in many Venezuelan farms being neglected or abandoned as people left the land. For those who had kept their criollo trees alive, the crisis had turned farming into a risky business. Robbers were prepared to seize crops from farmers' haciendas, stripping cacao pods from trees. Some farmers were employing security guards to prevent this happening. Others, in an attempt to sidestep the thieves and reduce the risk of losing a crop, were picking their cacao earlier and earlier – before it was at its peak. 'They end up being paid less because the quality is not so good,' explained Di Giacobbe.

The stress of the situation had led more farmers to leave the land. Cacao production had halved in less than a decade. Worse still, some farmers had been kidnapped, and many were too traumatised to return to their farms, even those whose families had been growing cacao for centuries. One cacao grower and chocolate maker in her seventies described to me how robbers had targeted her farm five times. 'The last time, they took everything,' she said, pausing as she started to cry, remembering the attack. They took away her cacao as well as her processing equipment. 'But we must keep going,' she said. 'Our culture and our livelihoods revolved around cacao. Venezuela *is* cacao and so we are cacao.'

Even when farmers do manage to harvest their cacao, the ongoing crisis has meant it is no longer guaranteed to reach its destination. 'A truck can be stopped thirty to forty times on the journey to Caracas,' another farmer told me, 'and drivers are forced to pay bribes.' Sometimes trucks are held at checkpoints for days, sometimes they never make it back to the depot. Seizures, the government told one news agency, were used to settle unpaid taxes. To the farmers, it felt like expropriation, plain and simple.

Now, with the country's oil exports unsteady, Di Giacobbe said it was time to remember how important cacao had been – and could be – in their country. She had grown up in a family of cooks and trained as a chef, but when the economic crisis hit, she had been forced to close her restaurants. This was when she started to make chocolate. For all of its cacao history, Venezuela exported the best cacao beans in the world for others – mostly Europeans – to turn into bars and confectionery and so reap most of the economic benefits. Di Giacobbe began experimenting, designing a DIY chocolate operation with borrowed equipment and the fridge from her home. In search of the best cacao, she took to the road and travelled thousands of miles, seeking out the few farmers left growing the highest-quality native criollo, learning how they fermented and dried their seeds to achieve the best flavours.

She sold the bars she made in small quantities, mostly in Caracas, but she managed to smuggle some out of the country wrapped inside clothes in suitcases. This way the world started to learn about her work and the rare chocolate she was making. But instead of just focusing on her own business, Di Giacobbe started to encourage other Venezuelans to join in her mission. Her little factory became a training centre where women from across the country could learn how to make chocolate: roast beans, winnow them into broken 'nibs', grind them down, 'conch' them into a smooth paste and temper them into shiny bars of chocolate. Plenty were interested; many had lost jobs and, too often, so had their husbands. Revitalised by their new skills, the women fanned out to other communities, teaching more women what they'd learned.

Word spread, and by the time I met Di Giacobbe in 2017, 8,000 chocolate makers, most working from home, had joined the network. That year she was given the prestigious Basque Culinary World Prize, awarded to chefs making a wider social impact through food. 'She is affecting every aspect of cacao and chocolate in Venezuela,' said one of the judges, the food writer Harold McGee. 'By helping farmers tend their trees, improve the way they process the beans, Di Giacobbe has given communities a chance to benefit from the chocolate.' The movement was a radical one, not only because it was launched during a crisis, but also because the transformation of cacao into chocolate has usually rested in the hands of large corporations. Di Giacobbe's work has continued through the worst of the economic crisis and the years of food shortages. When finding sugar, a basic ingredient for the bars, became a challenge (with even Coca-Cola's factories in Venezuela struggling to get enough of it) Di Giacobbe's network of chocolate makers created an alternative supply chain, sharing what they had.

Sitting inside the theatre in Caracas, a new band of recruits were listening to this story, absorbing every detail of how they too could start making chocolate in their communities, setting up their own businesses, taking criollo cacao from bean to bar. This was a rare chance to regain some independence and help bring more of Venezuela's cacao farms back into production. Making a chocolate bar might not at first seem like a life-changing act, but hearing Di Giacobbe describe it, it definitely is. 'Cacao gives us a chance to make a new country with a new economy, and to win back some dignity,' she said.

I spoke to one of the hundreds of Venezuelan women who had already followed Di Giacobbe's vision and was making chocolate. 'We can forget our problems for a little while and work,' she told me. 'Cacao is something real, we can touch, taste and smell it. This was not the case with oil.' If Di Giacobbe does succeed in helping to change her country for the better through chocolate, it will be a case of history repeating itself. Venezuelan cacao has been a revolutionary food before.

When the Spaniards arrived in present-day Venezuela, it's estimated the country was inhabited by half a million indigenous people. Some escaped the colonists by fleeing into isolation; many others were killed, mostly wiped out by diseases introduced by the Europeans. In need of a workforce, the Spaniards transported 100,000 enslaved African men, women and children to Venezuela, with the first slave ships arriving in the 1520s. Most were sent to the northern coast, to work on the newly established haciendas, where cacao had started to be grown on a commercial scale. These plantations changed Venezuela's landscape, and with the arrival of thousands of enslaved people, its population.

By the 1580s, some of the cacao was being shipped to Seville, where it was processed into drinking chocolate and by the 1620s, cacao was Venezuela's main export. As demand for cacao increased, enslaved Africans were used to create hundreds more plantations. By the middle of the century, the country had overtaken Mexico as the world's leading producer of cacao.

The popularity of chocolate spread through Italy, France and England, sweetened as it was with sugar from plantations in the Caribbean and Brazil, grown and processed by millions more enslaved Africans. At the beginning of the eighteenth century, Venezuela was supplying 90 per cent of all the cacao arriving in Europe. 'The chocolate sipped by Europeans from Pepys in London to Cosimo III in Florence,' said the chocolate historians Sophie and Michael Coe, 'came largely from the cacao groves of Caracas that had been worked by slaves.'

As the trade continued to flourish, Venezuela's cacao growers became increasingly resentful of European rule. The Spanish Crown thwarted all efforts by farmers to sell cacao independently and ran a monopoly over the colony's cacao trade through an enterprise called the Compañía Guipuzcoana. This gained a reputation for brutality against any dissenting farmers and triggered a rebellion led by a cacao farmer called Juan Francisco de León. But it was another revolutionary leader, one who had also grown up in the cacao plantations, Simón Bolívar, who liberated Venezuela from the Spanish and its cacao monopoly in 1823. Venezuela as an independent nation state was founded on chocolate.

Di Giacobbe came to realise that although Venezuela's cacao trade had fallen into steep decline, surviving in many of the historic haciendas and on parcels of land was the best cacao in the world. If this precious resource was lost to Venezuela, it would be lost to all, but if it could be restored, thousands of businesses could be created.

Criollo was the type of cacao treasured by the Mayans and the Aztecs; criollo was the cacao that had brought chocolate to the attention of the world. Unlike other types of cacao (forastero and trinitario), criollo has hardly any bitterness, and because it contains more caffeine, it's also more stimulating. Across Venezuela, as haciendas were planted in different regions, unique varieties of criollo evolved, some taking the names of the place in which they grew, such as the isolated village of Chuao (possibly the most prized of Venezuela's cacao). Others were named after their appearance, such as porcelana (when you peel back the skin of the bean it's glistening and pure white).

When Venezuelan cacao production fell into decline after the oil boom, so did the amount of criollo being grown, and chocolate's centre of influence shifted to Africa and other types of cacao. Cacao was already being grown in Spanish colonies in Equatorial Guinea at the end of the nineteenth century and from here it spread to Ghana and the Ivory Coast (these two countries now account for nearly three-quarters of all the cacao grown in the world). By the 1960s, cacao breeders had developed new F1 hybrids, including a variety called CCN51. It didn't have criollo's delicate flavours, but it was higher-yielding and profitable and so farmers in Central America planted it in place of the indigenous varieties. Venezuela, distracted by oil, didn't get to fully embrace this process of modernisation and so the most endangered cacao in the world, criollo, survived here.

Di Giacobbe wants to save every one of the surviving criollo trees. She travels thousands of miles throughout Venezuela to spread her ideas in towns and villages and to offer her support to farmers. I joined her on one of these expeditions, to a cacao farm near a town called Cumanacoa, a twelve-hour drive from Caracas. In the eighteenth century, a Spanish settler had realised how incredibly fertile the soil in the area was: 'the fruits have a flavour and a taste which they possess in few other places', he said. More colonists arrived in the 1790s, including a sailor turned farmer from the Catalan region who, with twenty enslaved Africans, established a hacienda. Over the next two centuries, the cacao they planted helped make this small Venezuelan town famous among the world's chocolate makers.

On our journey we passed through one military roadblock after another, during which time I learned to brace myself for intimidating inspections by groups of heavily armed soldiers. At blockades they peered through the car windows with cool, hard stares. By the fifth check point, I realised the best approach was to avoid all eye contact and to look straight ahead. In every town we passed, another kind of watchful gaze fell upon us. These came from the eyes of the deceased leader Hugo Chávez which seemed to be everywhere care of painted murals on walls and billboards; a reminder to the masses to stay loyal, the state was watching.

At our destination, we stepped in among the cacao trees. It was more like being in a jungle than on a farm, a beautiful wilderness bursting with life, filled with birdsong and the hum of insects. The air was warm and damp and under our feet was a thick carpet of dark, decomposing leaves. Above us were the broad, leathery leaves of banana trees creating a canopy. Beneath this, just visible in the half-light, were cacao trees. They looked unworldly and magical. The ugly-beautiful pods (the fruits), coloured purple, red and yellow, were the shape of mini-rugby balls. They were growing not from the branches but directly out of the tree trunks, and each was small enough to be held within two cupped hands, with grooves running up and down it. These pods also had a tip that curled around at the end, a sign that they were criollo.

Knowing when they are ready to be picked is an art, possibly even a musical skill. 'You can do it by sound,' Di Giacobbe told me as she tapped her fingers on a pod, making a percussive *tuk tuk tuk*. The seeds and pulp had become detached from their shell, the hollow beat a sign that they were now ripe. She nodded to one of the farmers standing nearby who took a machete and sliced through the barely visible stem. Inside were rows of seeds, each one the size of a tip of a thumb, about thirty cacao beans packed together in a moist, white, milky pulp which tasted sharp and refreshing, as if someone had taken a lychee and mashed it up with citrus and honey. I bit into a seed. It was bland, with a touch of bitterness. There wasn't the tiniest hint of chocolate.

We followed the harvest through to a nearby farm building where fermentation was used to unlock the flavours in cacao. This involves placing the seeds inside a wooden box which, over several days, becomes a cauldron of bubbling microbes. Yeasts and lactic acid bacteria present on the seeds start feeding on the sugars, creating alcohol and acetic acid. So much energy is generated by this process that temperatures within the box can reach 50°C. Acids penetrate the hard shell of the seed and kill it, causing it to break down and start to develop flavours and aromas more characteristic of chocolate. The next stages of the process, drying and roasting, serve to intensify and fix these flavours. The timing and control of each of these different steps is crucial to the final taste of the chocolate, and Di Giacobbe was teaching hundreds of small-scale farmers how to process their crop to help make the very best chocolate.

Back in Caracas, I met a couple of the farmers working with Di Giacobbe. They were two brothers who had fought for years to get their hacienda back from the government after it had been seized illegally. They had been engineers but lost their jobs during the crisis. 'We are learning to become farmers again,' they told me. 'Venezuela has something that the world wants, cacao is the only opportunity we have left.'

I tasted one of the bars Di Giacobbe had made in her 'chocolate lab' in Caracas, produced with criollo she had helped to grow on the farm near Cumanacoa. It tasted of ripe fruit and was full of bright notes that sang as the long flavour melted in my mouth. 'Chocolate represents happiness and pleasure,' she said as we broke off another piece. 'It is also a food that is full of hope.'

Cold War and Coca-Colonisation

For business watchers, an important shift took place in the year 2013; the company Apple became the world's number one brand, displacing Coca-Cola. The drinks brand had been in the number one slot since 2000 when the list was first compiled. By 2020, it had dropped to fifth place (behind Amazon, Microsoft, Apple and Google), confirming tech giants as the new drivers of our planet's shared experiences.

We know that homogenisation of the world's food and global diet goes far beyond Coca-Colonisation (a term first used in France in the 1950s). It's the wheat in our bread, the soy which feeds the chickens we eat and the genetics that underpin the global seed industry. And yet, Coca-Cola's ubiquity remains a useful shorthand for how uniformity is brought to the world. It is not just our diets that have been homogenised, but also our palates.

Take Russian kvass. A fermented, thirst-quenching, fizzy but very sour drink, it used to be made in countless homes across Russia by leaving stale bread and water to ferment together for a few days. This naturally carbonated the water as well as making it tangy and acidic (*kvass* in Slavic languages means 'sour'). When money allowed, honey, raisins or berries might have been added to elevate the flavour and speed up fermentation, which is why different versions of kvass existed across Russia as well as in Poland, Latvia, Lithuania and Ukraine. For centuries, this was a drink of the people. 'We have bread, and we have kvass, and it's all we need,' is one Russian saying. Sourness was also a sign that harmful microbes had been banished, so kvass served as a valuable alternative to water, just as beer did in Western Europe. As another saying advised, 'Bad kvass is better than good water.'

In a busy street scene in *War and Peace*, Tolstoy describes crowds around which hawkers are selling kvass (along with gingerbread and poppyseed sweets). He writes of Russian soldiers in their barracks bolstering their strength and readying themselves for action by drinking cups of kvass. Russia's own version of Mrs Beeton, the writer Elena Molokhovets, was a devotee of kvass. She collected a thousand or so recipes for it, including 'Moscow kvass from apples', made in wooden barrels in the summer and stored in cellars in the winter, a drink that would last for a year; and 'kvass from raspberries and strawberries', which was left to ferment in kegs buried in ice. Her recipes read like a celebration of sourness and national pride. Drinking kvass, she noted, is 'a culture-laden act that helped to define one's Russianness'.

Coca-Cola first arrived in Russia during the Cold War, but it wasn't until the collapse of the Soviet Union that the first hoarding advertised it, in Pushkin Square. By 1995, Coca-Cola had opened a bottling plant in St Petersburg (not far from the Vavilov Institute). Yet the drink's popularity in Russia wasn't as easily won as in other countries, or at least at first. Patriotic ad campaigns for factory-made kvass ran on Russian television with the punchline, 'Say no to Cola-nisation. Drink kvass to the health of the nation!' A dark-coloured kvass was even bottled to resemble a litre of cola; it was called Ni-Kola (pronounced in Russian, this sounds like: 'NOT cola'). But all the while, in an attempt to see off the sugary Western competition, factory kvass was made to taste sweeter and sweeter. Russian palates were being won over by sugar as Coke and other Western brands set up shop.

As the national appetite turned from sour to sweet, some types of kvass went all but extinct, including white kvass or *kislie shchi* (which translates roughly as 'sour soup'), a honey-coloured, more elegant version of black kvass. Rather than being made from stale bread, *kislie shchi* was made from fermented malted wheat and rye grains. Within a matter of days, it would have become a sparkly, white drink and it was used not just as a thirst quencher but as a type of fizzy stock that could bring a hint of sourness to chicken broth. The starters used for white kvass were treasured, shared among families and friends and passed down through generations. But people stopped making their home-made kvass, and white kvass in particular became a memory.

In 2013, a Russian drinks maker set about bringing back kvass culture (in both senses of that word). Svetlana Golubeva's idea was to make a white kvass to an old family recipe that she could bottle for sale in

Moscow. All she had to do was find the right recipe. So she set off on a 1,500-mile round trip to remote villages in southern Russia, to Tambov, Ryazan and Voronezh, knocking on the doors of the oldest residents she could find.

She came across white kvass being made in just one village and was given a starter for making it. All she needed now were some instructions. How long should the white kvass ferment for? she asked. Until it's ready, came the reply.

Will Golubeva be able to make *kislie shchi* popular again? It's unlikely, but at least while the river of sweet homogeneity gushes through the world and into Russia, Golubeva has dared to go against the flow.

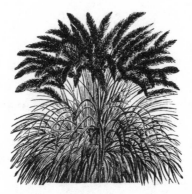

Epilogue:
Think Like a Hadza

Are we being good ancestors?

Jonas Salk

Memories of Hadza-land return to me. The images and sounds that keep replaying are ones from after the porcupine hunt. Sigwazi, the Hadza hunter, had removed the animal's sharp spines, cooked the offal on the fire and shared out the meat. After eating, we walked out of the dense bush and into a clearing where, all of a sudden, Sigwazi stopped, and with a bow hung from one shoulder, the porcupine carcass on the other, his body began to tilt and sway. During this slow-motion dance, almost hypnotised, he sang. I did not understand the words, but I could tell this wasn't a song of triumph; to me it sounded like a tribute being sent through the trees and across the hunting grounds. I remember experiencing a feeling of envy. It wasn't that I wanted to live Sigwazi's life, but I envied his connection with his surroundings.

By the time a Hadza child is five they can recognise the sounds made by animals around them and know something of each species' life cycle, even their mating habits. They are experts in biodiversity because they have to be. In an age in which not just food but the entire human experience is converging into a mass of homogeneity, the Hadza remind us that there are many ways to live and be in the world.

I've gone back to the origins and history of food in this book to help us see the speed at which we're transforming the world. That process of rapid change is the story of our times, and we all need to be active participants in deciding where that story goes next. Our ancient ancestors 12,000 years ago were ingenious in domesticating the first crops, so too were the scientists, plant breeders and food industrialists of the twentieth century who found a system to feed the world. But we now know there can't be one way for all. We cannot afford to carry on growing crops and producing food in ways that are so violently in conflict with nature; we can't continue to beat the planet into submission, to control, dominate and all too often destroy ecosystems. It isn't working. How can anyone claim it is when so many humans are left either hungry or obese and when the Earth is suffering?

The Hadza have an impact on their environment, but they know when lines are being crossed and too much is being taken; if this happens, it will always mean less food somewhere down the line. Maybe that was why Sigwazi was singing out towards the trees with the carcass on his shoulder – perhaps he was acknowledging to his part of the world that he knew he'd received a special bounty that day. When I returned home, there seemed to be little I could take from Hadza-land and apply to my life. There are no baobab trees or honeyguide birds where I live.

Help with this came from a friend, Miles Irving, who is evangelical about making connections between nature and the food we eat. His work as a professional forager has led him to study hunter-gatherer societies around the world, including the Hadza. For Irving, also, eating wild food is a way of life. In his early fifties, long-haired and lean, he scours woods, roadsides and beaches in search of birch sap, wild garlic, sorrel, seaweeds and mushrooms. He believes we should all bring wild ingredients back into our lives and into our kitchens, even if on the smallest scale. 'Eat a dandelion growing on your garden lawn,' he once told me, 'it's a revolutionary act.'

We met up one autumn morning at a beach close to his home in Kent. The tide was on its way out and a layer of chalk jutted up along the shore. Around the white rock were greens, purples and chocolatey browns. 'Seaweed,' said Irving. 'Most people wouldn't know it – but every single piece of it is edible.' We were looking at piles and piles of food. We headed further out, to the sand and rocks newly exposed by the retreating sea, and walked across a carpet of seaweed. In rock pools there was sea lettuce, like thick sheets of green polythene – 'Great in salads.' And then dulse (one of his favourites), flat ribbons of red and brown. 'Have a munch on that … ' It tasted sweet and savoury as I chewed, and then the flavour of fresh crab came through. We tried toothed rack, rubbery apart from the delicate tips, 'but you can toast them and make crisps'. We finished with Irish moss, also known as carrageen, plucked from rocks but leaving their bases intact so they could grow back again. In the palm of my hand, it looked like the silhouette of a tree in winter, its tiny, purple, delicate branches radiating from its stem. Its long mellow taste reminded me of digestive biscuits. Irving explained that these, and the five hundred other seaweed species possible to eat, were among the best food nature could provide, packed with nutrients that had long become extinct from most modern diets, and with levels of amino acids and iodine most of us never get to eat. This was food for our bodies and our brains. 'It is a gift. It's like the beach is saying to us "Here you are, you need this".' Foraging was how Irving changed his relationship with nature. 'I feel like I'm more tuned in. It reminds me to have a sense of trust and gratitude for the world.'

As the tide came further in, he looked back at the sea. 'I'm not saying we should return to being hunter-gatherers, but all of us can benefit from getting back something of that relationship with nature.' He had recently set himself the challenge of eating twenty different wild plants in a day. 'I managed eighteen. I'm working on it,' he said, excusing his shortfall, 'this is a lifelong project.' Something caught his eye. Bending down to take some dulse, he realised he had forgotten his penknife and so he smashed a piece of flint against a rock to make an improvised blade. 'When you go in search of wild food, do you sometimes feel like a Hadza?' I asked him. 'Without the roots those guys have, that unbroken culture going back thousands and thousands of years, definitely not,' he said. 'But I know I wouldn't be an impostor living in that world, because I belong there. So do you ... and so does everyone else.'

In our own way, we all need to become experts in biodiversity and to become more sensitive to the natural boundaries we are pushing against when we make decisions about what we are going to eat. Nothing could be more important. The lives of future generations depend on it. We need to learn to recognise the diversity that exists; we can only help to save it if we know it's there. Endangered foods are like the dwindling number of Atlantic salmon in rivers and the ocean, indicator species sounding a warning call that something is wrong in our world.

If we want to save endangered foods, those in this book and many others, two things need to happen. The first, which seems easier because it's in our control, is to shift our own thinking and actions around food. By thinking more like a Hadza, we can make the connection between the food we eat and the ecosystems we exist in. The second, which might appear almost impossible, is to rethink the global food system. Aside from the fact that we have to, that we have no choice, it *is* possible, because it has been done before. If Norman Borlaug's work and the Green Revolution show us anything, it is that through human efforts and ingenuity, food systems can be transformed. As we have seen, that transformation was only ever designed to be short-lived; it was a clever fix for feeding the world at a particular point in time. Borlaug himself believed it could only be sustained for twenty-five to thirty years, but the world became locked into that way of feeding itself. The system is now long past its sell-by date; ailing and propped up by unsustainable amounts of fossil fuels. We can – and we must – redesign it.

We get the food system we pay for. Every minute of every day, a million dollars is spent on agricultural subsidies around the world, whether that's for planting yet more soy in the Cerrado, more monocultures of maize in North America, fields of homogeneous wheat in Europe, or sending out more boats to already overfished West African waters. This is public money, our money, and it is supporting a system that isn't resilient, healthy or sustainable. These subsidies, between $700 billion and $1 trillion a year, can too easily distort decisions on what the world grows and how it eats. For the endangered foods in this book, this has made a level playing field impossible. The odds are stacked heavily against them – as well as the communities which produce them. The system (whether we are aware of it or not) shapes how you and I eat. It is dictating behaviours around food – behaviours that humans have only recently acquired.

I am not proposing the endangered foods and drinks featured here (and thousands of others out there) could provide the menu for our future. Most of them will (and should) only ever feed the communities that produce or harvest them. But I do believe that the food system we need – and which the planet needs – is one in which these foods can have a place and are no longer at risk of extinction. Our food system needs to embrace all forms of diversity: biological, cultural, dietary and economic.

Yes, we need to build on the very latest technology but we also need to draw on the methods that have taken our species this far, not only in the last century but also over millennia. Our future food is going to depend on multiple systems of agriculture. Some will be highly industrialised and mechanised, others smaller in scale and richer in their variety of crops and animals. Diversity can help each of these systems become as successful and resilient as they can possibly be. As we've seen, efforts are already under way to make this happen, from the reappearance of landrace fields of wheat to the work banana breeders are doing, using wild genetics and rethinking the monoculture model. Saving diversity gives us options.

From governments to individuals, everyone has a part to play. Innovative ideas within countries and within cities can promote diversity and save endangered foods. Brazil, for example, introduced a national policy in which at least 30 per cent of food for school meals had to come from local farms. In Copenhagen, businesses supplying apples to schools were given contracts based not just on volume but on the number of different apple varieties they could supply, which led to a revival of local orchards. New technology can help make the milling of crops such as Kavilca less arduous, while digital networks can create markets for people like Sun Wenxiang selling his red mouth glutinous rice over WeChat. And more of us can become like Esiah Levy, making a difference by planting seeds and sharing them. Like Charles Martell (and the Hadza), we also need to explore the environment around us, finding foods closer to home. We can be the saviours of the endangered foods in our own regions.

My main source of optimism comes from the people we have met in this book and the many others like them, guardians of the world's food diversity: the seed savers, the innovators, the big-picture scientists and the radical cooks. In the unlikely setting of the old Fiat factory, now a sprawling exhibition centre in the heart of Italy's industrial north, a biannual gathering called Terra Madre brings thousands of people together from nearly 150 countries. They are part of the global Slow Food network, and they come to share seeds and stories and to display their food. Piled precariously inside the exhibition hall there might be fifty different squashes in an assortment of sizes, shapes and colours, next to pyramids of different citrus varieties, a rainbow display of various types of beans, and wheels of cheeses from remote mountain villages. A kaleidoscope of rice, cobs of corn, edible insects, dried fish, fruit and vegetables make this, if not the biggest food market ever created, the most diverse.

The people who bring their foods here include farmers, fishers, bakers, cheesemakers, shepherds, brewers, millers, fermenters, smokers and cooks. Many arrive in their traditional costumes, from Georgian winemakers dressed in *chokha*, the high-necked, woollen warrior dress, to the red-and-gold silk shawls of Khasi people who have travelled from Meghalaya in northern India. They are the keepers of tradition, 'the preservers of fire'. Here at Terra Madre I first got to taste wild Ethiopian coffee from the Harenna forest and a rare piece of qizha cake; it was also where I met Matthew Raiford, the farmer from the American South who grows the Geechee red pea, one of the stories that first inspired me to write this book.

The symbol of the Slow Food movement is a snail, an obvious emblem for a slower, more contemplative approach to food. But there is another explanation for the symbol. When a snail constructs its shell, it starts to build in one direction, upward into a spiral; then, when the structure it has built has become too weak and vulnerable, it reverses the process and builds in the opposite direction, adding strength and stability to its home. We have made our home, our planet, far too weak and too vulnerable. Like the snail, we need to build more resilience. We can't retreat into the past; but rather than squander what went before we can use our inheritance as a source of strength, as a resource to rebuild with. The endangered foods in this book helped make us who we are; they could be foods that show us what we can become.

Further Reading

INTRODUCTION and FOOD: A VERY BRIEF HISTORY

Jennifer Clapp, *Food* (Polity Press, 2016)

Ruth DeFries, *The Big Ratchet: How Humanity Thrives in the Face of Natural Crisis* (Basic Books, 2014)

Jared Diamond, *Guns, Germs and Steel* (Vintage, 1998)

Anya Fernald, Serena Milano and Piero Sardo, *A World of Presidia* (Slow Food Editore, 2004)

Cary Fowler and Pat Moony, *Shattering* (University of Arizona Press, 1990)

Jack R. Harlan, *Crops and Man* (American Society of Agronomy, 1992)

Philip H. Howard, *Concentration and Power in the Food System* (Bloomsbury, 2017)

John Spicer, *Biodiversity* (Oneworld, 2006)

Bee Wilson, *The Way We Eat Now* (Fourth Estate, 2019)

E.O. Wilson, *The Diversity of Life* (Penguin, 2001)

Richard Wrangham, *Catching Fire* (Profile Books, 2009)

PART ONE: WILD

Hugh Brody, *The Other Side of Eden* (Faber & Faber, 2001)

Eva Crane, *The World History of Bee Keeping and Honey Hunting* (Routledge, 1999)

Jared Diamond, *The World Until Yesterday* (Allen Lane, 2012)

Yuval Noah Harari, *Sapiens: A Brief History of Humankind* (Vintage, 2015)

Robert Hughes, *The Fatal Shore* (Vintage, 2003)

E. Barrie Kavasch, *Native Harvests* (Dover Publications, 2005)

Frank Marlowe, *The Hadza: Hunter-Gatherers of Tanzania* (University of California Press, 2010)

Bruce Pascoe, *Dark Emu* (Scribe US, 2019)

Michael Pollan, *In Defence of Food* (Penguin, 2009)

Jules Pretty, *The Edge of Extinction* (Cornell University Press, 2014)

Tiziana Ulian et al., *Wild Plants for a Sustainable Future: 110 Multipurpose Species* (Kew Publishing, 2019)

PART TWO: CEREAL

Liz Ashworth, *The Book of Bere: Orkney's Ancient Grain* (Birlinn Ltd, 2017)

Michael Blake, *Maize for the Gods* (University of California Press, 2015)

Betty Fussell, *The Story of Corn* (North Point, 1992)

Jack R. Harlan, *The Living Fields* (Cambridge University Press, 1995)

Noel Kingsbury, *Hybrid: The History and Science of Plant Breeding* (University of Chicago Press, 2011)

Harold McGee, *McGee on Food and Cooking: An Encyclopaedia of Kitchen Science* (Hodder & Stoughton, 2004)

Neil MacGregor, *A History of the World in 100 Objects* (Allen Lane, 2010)

Charles C. Mann, *The Wizard and the Prophet: Science and the Future of our Planet* (Picador, 2019)

Charles C. Mann, *1491: The Americas Before Columbus* (Granta, 2006)

Francisco Migoya and Nathan Myhrvold, *Modernist Bread* (The Cooking Lab, 2017)

Magnus Nilsson, *The Nordic Baking Book* (Phaidon Press, 2018)

Michael Pollan, *The Omnivore's Dilemma* (Bloomsbury, 2011)

Catherine Zabinsky, *Amber Waves* (University of Chicago Press, 2020)

PART THREE: VEGETABLE

Dan Barber, *The Third Plate* (Penguin Press, 2014)

Christine M. Du Bois, *The Story of Soy* (Reaktion Books, 2018)

John Reader, *Propitious Esculent* (William Heinemann, 2008)

Mark Schapiro, *Seeds of Resistance: The Fight to Save Our Food Supply* (Hot Books, 2018)

David Shields, *Southern Provisions: The Creation and Revival of a Cuisine* (University of Chicago Press, 2016)

Geoff Tansey and Tamsin Rajotte (eds), *The Future Control of Food* (Earthscan, 2008)

Michael W. Twitty, *The Cooking Gene: A Journey Through African American Culinary History in the Old South* (Amistad Press, 2013)

PART FOUR: MEAT

Mark Essig, *Lesser Beasts: A Snout-to-Tail History of the Humble Pig* (Basic Books, 2015)

Dan Flores, *American Serengeti: The Last Big Animals of the Great Plains* (University Press of Kansas, 2017)

Bob Kennard, *Much Ado About Mutton* (Merlin Unwin Books, 2014)

Andrew Lawler, *Why Did the Chicken Cross the World?* (Atria Books, 2014)

Robert Malcolmson and Stephanos Mastoris, *The English Pig: A History* (Hambledon Continuum, 1998)

Maryn McKenna, *Plucked, The Truth About Chicken*, (Little Brown, 2018)

Harriet Ritvo, *The Animal Estate: The English and Other Creatures in the Victorian Age* (Harvard University Press, 1989)

Upton Sinclair, *The Jungle* (Penguin, 2002)

Joshua Specht, *Red Meat Republic* (Princeton University Press, 2019)

PART FIVE: FROM THE SEA

Rachel Carson, *The Sea Around Us* (Oxford University Press, 2018)

Paul Greenberg, *Four Fish: The Future of the Last Wild Food* (Penguin Group, 2011)

Naomichi Ishige, *History of Japanese Food* (Routledge, 2011)

Mark Kurlansky, *Salmon: A Fish, the Earth, and a History of a Common Fate* (Oneworld, 2020)

Daniel Pauly, *Vanishing Fish, Shifting Baselines and the Future of Global Fisheries* (Greystone Books, 2019)

Fred Pearce, *When the Rivers Run Dry* (Granta, 2018)

Callum Roberts, *The Unnatural History of the Sea* (Gaia, 2007)

Drew Smith, *Oyster: A Gastronomic History (with Recipes)* (Abrams, 2015)

PART SIX: FRUIT

Helena Attlee, *The Land Where the Lemons Grow* (Penguin, 2015)

Rachel Carson, *Silent Spring* (Penguin Classics, 2000)

Barrie Juniper and David Mabberley, *The Story of the Apple* (Timber Press, 2006)

Dan Koeppel, *Banana: The Fate of the Fruit That Changed the World* (Plume Books, 2009)

John McPhee, *Oranges* (Daunt Books, 2016)

Joan Morgan, *The New Book of Apples* (Ebury Press, 2010)

Joan Morgan, *The Book of Pears* (Ebury Press, 2015)

Gary Paul Nabhan, *Where Our Food Comes From* (Island Press, 2011)

Michael Pollan, *The Botany of Desire* (Bloomsbury, 2002)

Christopher Stocks, *Forgotten Fruits* (Random House, 2009)

Daniel Stone, *The Food Explorer* (Dutton, 2018)

Mary Taylor Simeti, *Pomp and Sustenance* (Alfred A. Knopf, 1989)

PART SEVEN: CHEESE

Peter Atkins, *Liquid Materialities* (Routledge, 2016)
Trevor Hickman, *Stilton Cheese: A History* (Amberley Publishing, 2012)
Sandor Ellix Katz, *The Art of Fermentation* (Chelsea Green Publishing, 2012)
Mateo Kehler (ed.), *The Oxford Companion to Cheese* (OUP, 2016)
Mark Kurlansky, *Milk! A 10,000-Year Food Fracas* (Bloomsbury, 2019)
Harold McGee, *Nose Dive: A Field Guide to the World's Smells* (John Murray, 2020)
Bronwen Percival and Francis Percival, *Reinventing the Wheel: Milk, Microbes and the Fight for Real Cheese* (Bloomsbury Sigma, 2019)
Michael Pollan, *Cooked* (Allen Lane, 2013)
Patrick Rance, *The Great British Cheese Book* (Pan Macmillan, 1988)
Michael Tunick, *The Science of Cheese* (OUP, 2014)

PART EIGHT: ALCOHOL

Carla Capalbo, *Tasting Georgia* (Pallas Athene, 2017)
James Crowden, *Ciderland* (Birlinn, 2008)
Alice Feiring, *For the Love of Wine* (Potomac Books, 2016)
Lisa Granik, *The Wines of Georgia* (Infinite Ideas, 2019)
Garrett Oliver (ed.), *The Oxford Companion to Beer* (OUP, 2011)
Jancis Robinson (ed.), *The Oxford Companion to Wine* (OUP, 2015)
Jancis Robinson, Julia Harding and José Vouillamoz, *Wine Grapes* (Allen Lane, 2012)
Tim Webb and Stephen Beaumont, *World Atlas of Beer* (Mitchell Beazley, 2012)
Tim Webb and Joe Strange, *CAMRA's Good Beer Guide Belgium* (CAMRA Books, 2018)
Simon J. Woolf, *Amber Revolution* (Interlink Books, 2018)

PART NINE: STIMULANTS

Will Battle, *The World Tea Encyclopaedia* (Matador, 2017)
Aaron Davis et al., *Coffee Atlas of Ethiopia* (Kew Publishing, 2018)
James Hoffman, *The World Atlas of Coffee* (Mitchell Beazley, 2018)
Jeff Koehler, *Where the Wild Coffee Grows* (Bloomsbury USA, 2018)
Stuart McCook, *Coffee Is Not Forever* (Ohio University Press, 2019)
Jonathan Morris, *Coffee: A Global History* (Reaktion Books, 2018)

PART TEN: SWEET

Sophie D. Coe and Michael D. Coe, *The True History of Chocolate* (Thames & Hudson, 2013)

Chloé Doutre-Roussel, *The Chocolate Connoisseur* (Tarcherperigree, 2006)

Louis E. Grivetti and Howard-Yana Shapiro (eds), *Chocolate: History, Culture and Heritage* (Wiley-Interscience, 2009)

Marcos Patchett, *The Secret Life of Chocolate* (Aeon Books, 2020)

Simran Sethi, *Bread, Wine, Chocolate: The Slow Loss of Foods We Love* (HarperOne, 2016)

EPILOGUE: THINK LIKE A HADZA

Miles Irving, *The Forager Handbook* (Ebury Press, 2009)

Notes

INTRODUCTION

2 'more and more the same': Colin K. Khoury et al., 'Increasing homogeneity in global food supplies', *Proceedings of the National Academy of Sciences*, III (II), March 2014, 4001–6, DOI: 10.1073/pnas.1313490111.

2 'just four corporations': See Philip H. Howard, *Concentration and Power in the Food System* (Bloomsbury, 2017). Also see Howard's website https://philhoward.net/ for a visual guide to concentration of power in the food system.

2 'one million years (around 40,000 generations)': This is an argument set out by Denis Burkitt, an Irish-born surgeon who worked in hospitals in East Africa in the 1960s. On his return to the UK, he realised the high levels of obesity, heart disease, cancer and stroke there were all absent in his African patients who consumed more traditional, less processed food. These so-called 'Western diseases', he concluded, were diet-related (and due to lack of fibre in particular). See also Michael Pollan, *In Defence of Food* (Penguin, 2009).

3 'reported on food stories': The programme is BBC Radio 4's *The Food Programme*, founded in 1979 by a former foreign correspondent, Derek Cooper, and presented since 2000 by Sheila Dillon.

4 'Wheat, rice and maize': I use the word maize instead of corn. The former is indigenous in origin whereas the latter is European.

4 'the Arab Spring': Most Arab countries buy 50 per cent of their food from abroad. Between 2007 and 2010, imports of cereals including wheat to the region increased by nearly 15 per cent. This was also a time of rapid food price inflation, and so in 2007–8 some staple crops doubled in price. In Egypt, food prices increased by more than a third between 2008 and 2010. See 'Food and the Arab spring, Let them eat baklava', *The Economist*, 17 March 2012.

4 '10 billion by 2050': Food and Agriculture Organisation (FAO), 'How to Feed the World in 2050', October 2009, http://www.fao.org/fileadmin/templates/wsfs/docs/expert_paper/How_to_Feed_the_World_in_2050.pdf.

4 'We've been killing life': Launch of OP2B, a coalition for biodiversity, United Nations General Assembly, New York, 23 September 2019, https://www.youtube.com/watch?v=HPlzGVAqEZo&t=1s.

4 'It's over-simplistic now': Corinne Gretler and Emily Chasan, 'Big Food Rethinks Farming To Fight a Lack of Crop Diversity', Bloomberg, 23 September 2019.

5 '213,000 different samples': Exact numbers of varieties (and cultivated varieties, cultivars) are extremely problematic: many are yet to be recorded whereas others might have been catalogued by a seed bank under two different names. Most of the figures I use come from the Crop Diversity Trust (which oversees the collection inside the Svalbard Seed Vault).

7 'The disease it causes (Fusarium head blight)': A.J. Hilton et al., 'Relationship between cultivar height and severity of Fusarium ear blight in wheat', *Plant Pathology*, 48 (2), 1999, 202–8, and see Chapter 6, for a more detailed description of how the disease attacks wheat. See also Stuart McCook and John Vandermeer, 'The Big Rust and the Red Queen: Long-Term Perspectives on Coffee Rust Research', *Phytopathology Review*, May 2015, on how in our race against crop diseases, just like Alice's Red Queen, we are having to run faster and faster, just to stand still.

7 'The physicist': Albert-László Barabási, *Linked: The New Science of Networks* (Plume Books, 2003). Barabási's ideas in *Linked* are referred to by Henry Dimbleby in the UK's *National Food Strategy* published in July 2020, https://www.nationalfoodstrategy.org/partone/. Barabási has also investigated the interaction between the biochemistry of what we eat and our health (the so called 'dark matter of nutrition'). In this he continues to highlight how much more complexity there is for us to understand about food. See Albert-László Barabási, 'The unmapped chemical complexity of our diet', *Nature Food*, 1, 33–37, 9 December, 2019.

8 'more refined grains, vegetable oils': Scientist Colin Khoury used fifty years' worth of data sourced from the FAO to measure the increasing homogenisation of diets. In an interview with the author, he summed up the process as follows: 'The Vietnamese diet is becoming more like a European diet, an African diet more like a North American one. Nutritious traditional foods are becoming marginalised, day by day, bite by bite.'

9 'porridge made with barley': Karin Sanders, *Bodies in the Bog and the Archaeological Imagination* (University of Chicago Press, 2009).

10 'quarter of the land': IPBES, 'Nature's Dangerous Decline "Unprecedented"; Species Extinction Rates "Accelerating"', 6 May 2019, https://www.un.org/sustainabledevelopment/blog/2019/05/nature-decline-unprecedented-report/.

10 'transgenics and gene editing': One example is the Gates Foundation support for genetically modified fruit in Uganda (see Chapter 22). The

desirable genetic traits being added to future 'super-bananas' are often sourced from crop wild relatives. See Bill Gates, 'Building Better Bananas', GatesNotes, https://www.gatesnotes.com/development/building-better -bananas.

10 'the Red List': The list was started in 1964 by the International Union for Conservation of Nature and has evolved to become the world's most comprehensive information source on the global extinction risk status of animal, fungus and plant species, https://www.iucnredlist.org/. This list is a critical indicator of the health of the world's biodiversity.

11 'the tediousness of fast-food': Quoted from the Slow Food Manifesto, November 1989.

FOOD: A VERY BRIEF HISTORY

14 'One billion years later': Michael Marshall, 'Timeline: The Evolution of Life', *New Scientist*, 14 July 2009.

15 'Earth's rocky surface': For a good summary of how soil was formed and how earth went from the Big Bang to the first crops, see Catherine Zabinsky, *Amber Waves* (University of Chicago Press, 2020).

16 'Between 800,000 and 300,000 years': In his book *Catching Fire*, anthropologist Richard Wrangham argues the use of fire by early humans began much earlier, possibly 1.7 million years ago. See also Rachel N. Carmody et al., 'Cooking shapes the structure and function of the gut microbiome', *Nature Microbiology*, 4, 2019, 2052–63.

16 'hunter-gatherers reached Australia': S. Anna Florin et al., 'The first Australian plant foods at Madjedbebe, 65,000–53,000 years ago', *Nature Communications*, 11, 2020, 924.

16 'In the Black desert': Helen Briggs, 'Prehistoric bake-off: Scientists discover oldest evidence of bread', BBC News, 17 July 2018, https://www.bbc.co.uk /news/science-environment-44846874.

16 'our saliva and our gut microbiomes': Jens Walter et al., 'The Human Gut Microbiome: Ecology and Recent Evolutionary Changes', *Annual Review of Microbiology*, 65 (1), June 2011, 411–29, DOI: 10.1146/annurev-micro-090110 -102830.

17 'Why go to the trouble': Professor Dorian Fuller, Inaugural Lecture, 'Growing Societies: the Archaeobotany of Food Production and Globalization of Agriculture', UCL, 2014, available on Soundcloud: https://soundcloud .com/ucl-arts-social-science/growing-societies-professor-dorian-fuller.

17 'Globalisation in the ancient world': There are important exceptions, including *Coffea arabica* (coffee) and *Camellia sinensis* (tea). Both were (and still are) harvested from wild forests. Tea cultivation began around 3,000

years ago, for Arabica coffee it was probably less than 1,000 years ago. See Muditha Meegahakumbura et al., 'Domestication Origin and Breeding History of the Tea Plant (Camellia sinensis) in China and India', *Frontiers in Plant Science*, 8, 2270, January 2018, DOI: 10.3389/fpls.2017.02270.

17 'ate the storms': E.O. Wilson, *The Diversity of Life* (Penguin, 2001).

18 'toxic tuber cassava': Andri Frediansyah, 'Microbial Fermentation as Means of Improving Cassava Production in Indonesia', in *Cassava*, Viduranga Waisundara (ed.), Intech Open, 20 December 2017, DOI: 10.5772 /intechopen.71966.

PART ONE: WILD

20 'life in the industrialised world': The colonial (and Hobbesian view) of pre-agricultural societies as being nasty, brutish and short continued well into the twentieth century. Helping to change mainstream thinking was a late-1960s landmark conference and book (Richard B. Lee and Irven DeVore, *Symposium on Man the Hunter*, Aldine Pub. Co., 1966), which demonstrated how hunter-gatherer societies were knowledgeable, sophisticated and, above all, different from one another.

20 'just a few thousand people continue': Nutritional anthropologists and human ecologists who work with hunting and gathering communities argue there are no populations left who source 100 per cent of their diet from wild, hunted or gathered foods, all year long. One reason is that most populations are in some way integrated into the global economy. Also, when GIS remote sensing has been used to track isolated populations in the Amazon, the imagery often shows the existence of garden plots, so these groups are subsistence farmers who forage wild foods.

20 'three hundred different species': For a good overview of the different roles of wild food in traditional societies, see Zareen Bharucha and Jules Pretty, 'The roles and values of wild foods in agricultural systems', *Philosophical Transactions of the Royal Society*, 2010, B3652913–26, DOI: 10.1098 /rstb.2010.0123.

21 'Across India, 1,400 wild plant species': A. Ray et al., 'How Many Wild Edible Plants Do We Eat – Their Diversity, Use, and Implications for Sustainable Food System: An Exploratory Analysis in India', *Frontiers in Sustainable Food Systems*, 4 (56), 2020, DOI: 10.3389/fsufs.2020.00056.

21 'wild bush meat': The growing trade in wild meat (legal and illegal) and the increasing consumption of this meat in Asia has been linked to the Covid-19 outbreak of late 2019/early 2020. For more on this, see 'Spillover' in Part Four.

21 'Deforestation to make way for monocultures': For causes of habitat loss and the loss of food, see FAO Commission on Genetic Resources for Food

and Agriculture, 'Wild Foods: The State of the World's Biodiversity for Food and Agriculture', 2019, p. 160, section 4.4, 'Wild Foods', http://www.fao .org/3/CA3129EN/CA3129EN.pdf.

21 'indigenous people who make up': According to the World Bank there are approximately 476 million indigenous peoples worldwide, in over ninety countries. World Bank, 'Understanding Poverty: Indigenous Peoples' (updated 1 October 2020), https://www.worldbank.org/en/topic/indigenous peoples.

22 'stewards of the natural world': John Fa, a professor of biodiversity and human development, calculates more than one-third of the world's remaining pristine forests are within land that's either managed or owned by indigenous peoples. John E. Fa et al., 'Importance of Indigenous Peoples' lands for the conservation of Intact Forest Landscapes', *Frontiers in Ecology and the Environment*, 18 (3), 2020, 135–40, DOI: 10.1002/fee.2148. See also the World Bank, 'The Role of Indigenous Peoples in Biodiversity Conservation: The Natural but Often Forgotten Partners', 2008, https://siteresources.worldbank .org/INTBIODIVERSITY/Resources/RoleofIndigenousPeoplesinBiodiversity Conservation.pdf.

22 'higher proportion of nutrients': Mongabay interview with Chris Kettle of Biodiversity International: 'Making room for wild foods in forest conservation', 22 July 2019, https://news.mongabay.com/2019/07/making-room -for-wild-foods-in-forest-conservation/. See also D. Rowland et al., 'Forest foods and healthy diets: Quantifying the contributions', *Environmental Conservation*, 44 (2), 2017, 102–14, DOI: 10.1017/S0376892916000151.

22 'hard to find': Herman Pontzer et al., 'Hunter-gatherers as models in public health', *Obesity Reviews*, 19: 24–35, 2018, DOI: 10.1111/obr.12785.

24 'fraction of that time': On the value of the honeyguide in finding concealed bees' nests, see Brian Wood et al., 'Mutualism and manipulation in Hadza–Honeyguide interaction', *Evolution and Human Behavior*, 35, 2014, DOI: 10.1016/j.evolhumbehav.2014.07.007.

25 'shared among the rest of the group': The Hadza are an egalitarian society. If a hunter has a run of bad luck and has weeks without a kill, others will share their meat with him. Attempts to preserve and store meat away for private consumption are regarded as immoral, and all members of the group consider it their right to have a piece of an animal once it's butchered. See Frank Marlowe, *Why the Hadza are Still Hunter-Gatherers, Ethnicity, Hunter-Gatherers in Africa* (Smithsonian Institution Press, 2002), pp. 247–75.

25 'the Hadza's favourite food': When a team of anthropologists surveyed a large number of the Hadza and asked them to list their most preferred foods, honey came out on top. Honey ranked well above meat, berries and

tubers for both men and women (meat came second for men, for women it was berries). See J. Berbesque and F.W. Marlowe, 'Sex Differences in Food Preferences of Hadza Hunter-Gatherers', *Evolutionary Psychology* 7 (4), 2009, 601–16, DOI: 10.1177/147470490900700409.

25 'made the human brain larger': Alyssa N. Crittenden, 'The Importance of Honey Consumption in Human Evolution', *Food and Foodways*, 19 (4), 2011, 257–73, DOI: 10.1080/07409710.2011.630618.

27 'waiting for its share': Some researchers have described the Hadza burying or hiding honeycomb, to keep them 'hungry and thus more eager to guide them'. This is not what I witnessed.

29 'One-third of the Earth's land': United Nations report, 'Nature's Dangerous Decline "Unprecedented"; Species Extinction Rates "Accelerating"', 6 May 2019, https://www.un.org/sustainabledevelopment/blog/2019/05/nature-decline-unprecedented-report/. See also, Global Forest Watch, 'We Lost a Football Pitch of Primary Rainforest Every 6 Seconds in 2019', 2 June 2020, https://blog.globalforestwatch.org/data-and-research/global-tree-cover-loss-data-2019/.

29 'tens of thousands of hectares': Carbon Tanzania, a forest conservation scheme which runs projects in Hadza country, says as much as 160,000 hectares a year were being deforested in the part of Tanzania occupied by the Hadza. Author interview with Marc Baker, December 2018.

29 'cattle closer to the Hadza's camps': Ann Gibbons, 'Farmers, tourists, and cattle threaten to wipe out some of the world's last hunter-gatherers', *Science*, May 2018 https://www.sciencemag.org/news/2018/05/farmers-tourists-and-cattle-threaten-wipe-out-some-world-s-last-hunter-gatherers.

29 'risk of becoming degraded': ELD Initiative & UNEP, 'The Economics of Land Degradation in Africa: Benefits of Action Outweigh the Costs', 2015, www.eld-initiative.org.

30 'interaction with humans becomes rarer': The work of evolutionary biologist Claire Spottiswoode is important here. Spottiswoode recorded the sounds of the honeyguide and their human callers in Zambia and Mozambique and reported on the decline in the interaction in 'Natural Histories: Honeyguide', BBC radio documentary, 2016. See also Claire Spottiswoode et al., 'Reciprocal communication in human-honeyguide mutualism', *Science*, 353, 2016, 387–9.

31 'One was a cemetery': Author interview with Bruce Pascoe, October 2018.

32 'roamed the Western Desert': Michael Symons, *One Continuous Picnic* (Melbourne University Press, 2007), Introduction.

33 'meat of the country': Most of the historical references to murnong cited here are from Beth Gott's groundbreaking paper, 'Ecology of Root Use by

the Aborigines of Southern Australia', *Archaeology in Oceania*, 17, No. 1, 1982, 59–67. See also Bruce Pascoe, *Dark Emu* (Scribe US, 2019), which also draws on the diaries and journals of settlers to argue that Aboriginal people were agriculturalists. A blog on the subject of murnong by Australian botanist John Morgan is also worth reading, 'Where have all the Yamfields gone?', Morgan, Plant Ecology, April 2016, http://morganvegdynamics.blogspot.com/2016/04/where-have-all-yamfields-gone.html.

35 'Myall Creek in 1838': Robert Hughes, *The Fatal Shore* (Vintage, 2003), Chapter 8.

36 'Prior to first contact': ABC News, 'Watershed moments in Indigenous Australia's struggle to be heard', 3 July 2018. Also author interview with Bruce Pascoe, October 2018, and Dave Wandin, Wurundjeri elder, July 2020.

36 'symptoms of their diabetes reversed': Kerin O'Dea, 'Marked improvement in carbohydrate and lipid metabolism in diabetic Australian aborigines after temporary reversion to traditional lifestyle', *Diabetes*, 33(6), June 1984, DOI: 10.2337/diab.33.6.596. See also, Michael Pollan, *In Defence of Food* (Penguin, 2009), Part II.

36 'Murnong is making a slow return': Author interview with Dave Wandin, Wurundjeri elder, July 2020.

38 'I watched a meal': The author's field trip was in September 2018.

38 'Apache, Navajo and Pueblo': According to the Department of the Interior Bureau of Indian Affairs, in 2018 there were 573 federally recognised Native American tribes. See United States Department of the Interior, 'Indian Entities Recognized and Eligible To Receive Services from the United States Bureau of Indian Affairs', https://www.govinfo.gov/content/pkg/FR-2018-07-23/pdf/2018-15679.pdf.

42 'impossible to cultivate': Karlos Baca told me he remembers his grandfather having some success growing bear root outside his porch at home.

42 'multi-billion dollar herbal medicine trade': There's a long history of traditional medicines becoming global drugs. Salicylic acid is one of the most famous examples. Found in dried willow and myrtle leaves it was used by ancient Egyptians and Native Americans, and then later by nineteenth-century European chemists who synthesised the compound into the drug we know today as aspirin.

43 'highest rates of type 2 diabetes in America': Centres for Disease Control and Prevention, 'Native Americans with Diabetes', January 2017, https://www.cdc.gov/vitalsigns/aian-diabetes/index.html.

44 'each one a sovereign nation': Author interview with Elizabeth Hoover, July 2018.

44 'a taste of the lakes': Author interview with Winona La Duke, January 2021

47 'one billion citrus trees': Pierre Laszlo, *Citrus: A History* (University of Chicago Press, 2007).

48 'true ancient ancestor of all of the world's citrus': Author interview with Albert Wu, September 2018, and see G.A. Wu et al., 'Genomics of the origin and evolution of Citrus', *Nature*, 554, 2018, 311–16, DOI: 10.1038/nature25447.

48 '8-million-year-old citrus leaves': In 1931 Nikolai Vavilov identified the origins of citrus in 'Eastern Asia ... the upper course and the valleys of the great rivers of China, Hun-ho and Yangtze-Kian'. More recent research into the genetics of citrus placed the birthplace closer to the south-east foothills of the Himalayas, the eastern area of Assam, northern Myanmar and western Yunnan.

49 'fruit of ghosts': Author interview with Kalkame Momin, an ethno-botanist who has researched traditional uses of citrus in the Garo Hills, and see Kalkame Momin et al., 'An ethno-botanical study of wild plants in Garo Hills region of Meghalaya and their usage', *International Journal of Minor Fruits, Medicinal and Aromatic Plants*, 2 (1), 2016, 47–53. See also Anamika Upadhaya et al., 'Utilization of wild Citrus by Khasi and Garo tribes of Meghalaya', *Indian Journal of Traditional Knowledge*, 15 (1), January 2016, 121–7.

49 'keep bugs away from the bodies of the deceased': My thanks to Professor Monique Simmonds, Deputy Director of Science, Royal Botanic Gardens, Kew, for her insights into the possible uses of citrus in traditional medicine.

50 'Illegal logging, road building and agriculture': In the most recent surveys, plant geneticists were still able to find more than twenty different citrus species in the region and sixty-eight different varieties, confirming the area's status still as a 'treasure house of citrus'. A Biosphere Reserve as well as a Citrus Gene Sanctuary have been founded to protect biodiversity. However, India's National Bureau of Plant Genetic Resources found populations of species have been reduced by illegal logging and deforestation to make way for other food crops.

51 'The genome of *Citrus indica*': Author interview with Fred Gmitter, Professor Horticultural Sciences, University of Florida, November 2018, and also author interview with Tracy Kahn, curator of the Citrus Variety Collection, California Riverside University, October 2018.

52 'centres of diversity': It should be noted that archaeologists have revised (and continue to revise) Vavilov's 'centres of origin' (because of more recent excavations and new analytical techniques). However, Vavilov's maps remain an important guide to genetic diversity historically, i.e. what was growing wild and cultivated in different parts of the world in the first half of the twentieth century.

53 'little to protect the seed bank': An important exploration of Vavilov's work and legacy is Gary Paul Nabhan, *Where Our Food Comes From* (Island Press, 2011).

54 'students of Vavilov': Author interview with Cary Fowler, January 2021.

PART TWO: CEREAL

58 'University College London': The thousands of seeds I was surrounded by (both ancient and modern) make up the archaeobotany reference collection at University College London. This record of thousands of years of wild food, domestication and farming was established by Gordon Hillman, a pivotal figure in the development of archaeobotany.

58 'like a swimmer doing breaststroke': 'Wild wheat shows its muscles', Phys.org, 10 May 2007, https://phys.org/news/2007-05-wild-wheat-muscles .html.

59 'true fairy tale of genetics': Jacob Bronowski, *The Ascent of Man* (BBC Books, 1973).

60 'landrace': The term is used in different ways by different people. The approach I am taking is to regard a landrace as a local population of a particular crop that has been selected over many years for its particular ability to thrive in that particular place. They have a narrower gene base than the species as a whole (because they have been 'selected') but are still genetically diverse. Varieties are bred more formally: selected not only for their ability to survive but also for special characteristics, such as high protein, colour and flavour. These are also referred to as 'cultivars', and are usually at some point crossed with other varieties to gain new features.

62 'shingle on a beach': A more ancient technique (used in Turkey and Egypt) was to moisten the spikelets (the packets of grain) and then pound these by hand in a mortar as explained by Mark Nesbitt, Senior Research Leader at the Royal Botanic Gardens, Kew, who, like me, had travelled in the Kars region in search of emmer wheat.

63 'fat dripped down and cooked the grains': Compared with the modern bread wheats that followed emmer in wheat's evolution, Kavilca has low levels of gluten, so it is a grain for making flatbreads rather than fluffy loaves but most often it is cooked into a pilaf or added to soups or stews.

64 'I'm getting the same chill': Author interview with John Letts at his farm near Oxford, August 2018.

64 'Hard basalt rock': Even older evidence of humans eating grain in the Fertile Crescent came from a cave in northern Iraq, south of the Karacadag Mountains, thought to have been the resting place of a Neanderthal man. Tartar found on his 45,000-year-old teeth showed his diet had included a

porridge made from cooked grains. How this was done before the invention of pottery remains a mystery. See Amanda Henry et al., 'Microfossils in calculus demonstrate consumption of plants and cooked foods in Neanderthal diets', *PNAS*, January 2011.

64 'charred remains of ancient flatbreads': Amaia Arranz-Otaegui et al., 'Archaeobotanical evidence reveals the origins of bread 14,400 years ago in northeastern Jordan', *PNAS*, 115 (31), July 2018, 7925–30, DOI: 10.1073/pnas.1801071115.

64 'he became a hunter-gatherer': Jack R. Harlan, *The Living Fields* (Cambridge University Press, 2010).

65 'double the number of grains': Emmer also had twice the number of chromosomes as einkorn, which gave it far more genetic diversity, i.e. a bigger genetic 'toolkit' to adapt to a wider range of environmental conditions.

65 'This is how things stayed': Emmer also evolved into *Triticum turgidum*, what we now call durum (pasta wheat), and after a hybridisation with a goat grass (*Aegilops tauschii*) it also developed into spelt wheat.

66 'bread wheat eventually displaced emmer': The persistence of emmer in ancient Egypt, long after the spread of bread wheat (and the development of sophisticated grain stores), puzzled archaeobotanists for generations. The reason might be as simple as they loved the grain, and had a cultural preference for the way it made their food (and beer) taste.

66 'was also chemically different': Bread wheat also had an extra set of chromosomes. As with emmer's advantage over einkorn, this increased wheat's abilities to adapt.

66 '560,000 different samples of wheat': These are the number of accessions recorded by the Genesys database of Plant Genetic Resources. See https://www.genesys-pgr.org/c/wheat

67 'most widely grown crop': Wheat is grown on 215 million hectares of the Earth's surface – an area the size of Greenland and distributed from Scandinavia to South America and across Asia. See the CGIAR Research Programme on Wheat, https://wheat.org/.

67 'an incomprehensibly vast cloud of dreams': Charles C. Mann, *The Wizard and the Prophet: Science and the Future of our Planet* (Picador, 2019), which also provides the best (and most balanced) account of the Green Revolution.

67 'crossing it with traditional Mexican varieties': At the time Mexico was coming out of years of revolution and civil war. The Roosevelt administration and the Rockefeller Foundation, a wealthy philanthropic organisation with White House connections, offered to help. They funded research to improve the crops in the hope this would in turn improve the lives of rural peasant farmers. Because of the Green Revolution's dependence on fertilisers and irrigation, it's argued the main beneficiaries were instead large landowners.

68 'across the wheat-growing world': Thomas Lumpkin, 'How a Gene from Japan Revolutionized the World of Wheat', *Advances in Wheat Genetics*, 2015.

68 'Nearly half of all the crops': Charles C. Mann, *The Wizard and the Prophet: Science and the Future of our Planet* (Picador, 2019).

69 'bred for yield and homogeneity': Endashaw Girma, 'Genetic Erosion of Wheat (Triticum spp.)', *Journal of Natural Sciences*, 7 (23), 2017.

70 'causes the plant to commit suicide': I was lucky to have numerous discussions about FHB with Claire Kanja of Rothamsted Research who helped me to better understand the sneaky ways of the fungus. Also recommended (not least for its clever title): K. Kazan et al., 'On the trail of a cereal killer: recent advances in Fusarium graminearum pathogenomics and host resistance', *Molecular Plant Pathology*, 13 (4), 2012, 399–413.

70 'billions of dollars': Research points to crops facing bigger risks in the future, mostly because of climate change. For each 1°C increase in global temperature, yields of wheat are forecast to fall by 6 per cent, just as the world's population is growing. See 'Climate change will cut crop yields: study', Phys.org, 15 August 2017, https://phys.org/news/2017-08-climate-crop-yields.html.

70 'the most promising solution': Einkorn has been found to have the greatest resistance to FHB, but types of wild emmer also have resistance. See Tomasz Goral, 'Fusarium head blight resistance and mycotoxin profiles of four Triticum species genotypes', *Phytopathologia Mediterranea*, 56, 1, 2017, 175–86, DOI: 10.14601/Phytopathol_Mediterr-20288.

71 'botanist named Arthur Watkins': R.J. Gutteridge et al., 'Assessment of the A.E. Watkins wheat collection in 2008 for resistance to foliar, stem base and root diseases', Department for Environment, Food and Rural Affairs (DEFRA), 2008, https://repository.rothamsted.ac.uk/download/c01d7f443 f9fd97538d1ca48f79bbda3e6d06122e186c67f1ccc9eeoc3ad387e/3931418/WGIN StakeholderNewsletterOctober2008.pdf.

72 'botanist named Mirza Gökgöl': Nusret Zencirci et al., 'Mirza (Hacızade) Gökgöl (1897–1981): the great explorer of wheat genetic resources in Turkey', *Genetic Resources and Crop Evolution*, 65, 2018, 693–711, DOI: 10.1007/s10722 -018-0606-9.

73 'to be 1 per cent': United Nations FAO, 'Traditional wheat varieties of Tajikistan, Turkey, Uzbekistan are subject of research', Regional Office for Europe and Central Asia, 28 January 2016, http://www.fao.org/europe /news/detail-news/en/c/381431/.

74 'levels of minerals such as zinc and iron': Peter R. Shewry et al., 'Do "ancient" wheat species differ from modern bread wheat in their contents of bioactive components?', *Journal of Cereal Science*, 65, 2015, 236–43, DOI: 10.1016/j.jcs.2015.07.014.

75 'Bere (Anglo Saxon for barley)': for a good overview of the grain, its history and recipes, see Liz Ashworth, *The Book of Bere: Orkney's Ancient Grain* (Birlinn Ltd, 2017).

75 'From flag leaf ': In the wild, barley grows in pairs of grains, one either side of the ear, a 'two-row barley'. Another mutation created barley with six rows. It was the six-row variety, which is also a more resilient crop, that arrived on Orkney, and gives the island its bere. Brewers prefer two-row barley because it is easier to work with, and so when beer culture spread across Europe from the fourteenth century, six-row barley fell out of favour but not on Orkney.

77 'flatbreads and *knäckebröd*': Author interview with Magnus Nilsson, April 2019. See also *The Nordic Baking Book* (Phaidon Press, 2018).

77 'barley flour and tea': Dry-roasted barley grains are also a common snack in Ethiopia, eaten when having a drink particularly in the southern highlands (Gamo-Baroda region).

78 'disappearing landrace varieties': 'Bere Barley (*Hordeum vulgare L*)', Scottish Landrace Protection Scheme, https://www.sasa.gov.uk/variety-testing /scottish-landraces/scottish-landrace-protection-scheme-slps/bere-barley.

78 'all important in the human diet': H.E. Theobald et al., 'The nutritional properties of flours derived from Orkney grown bere barley', *Nutrition Bulletin*, 31(1), 2006, 8–14, DOI: 10.1111/j.1467-3010.2006.00528.x.

81 'more than 1,300 varieties': Liu Xu, 'China moves to protect its crop biodiversity', *China Dialogue*, 18 June 2019.

81 'mostly red to mostly white': A second trait in the domestication syndrome is loss of seed dormancy. A wild plant all of whose seeds sprouted at the first shower or warm spell would risk disaster, so most wild species hedge their bets and stagger the germination of seeds. But in the more controlled agricultural environment, where the seeds are sown all at once and reaped all at once, there is strong selection against seeds with this trait.

81 'primary food of three billion people': 20 per cent of the world's calories also come from rice, and across South Asia it provides more than half of all protein consumed. See Bienvenido O. Juliano (ed.), *Rice in human nutrition* (International Rice Research Institute and FAO, 1993), Chapter 2. The contribution of rice to protein in traditional diets is 70 per cent in South Asia and 51 per cent in South East Asia. These percentages are higher than the contribution of any other cereal protein in any region of the world.

82 'they engineered wetlands': The birth of the paddy system (based on current archaeological evidence) took place around modern Hunan and Zhejiang, when the foragers began managing the wetlands to cultivate rice. In Hunan this happened mostly around river tributaries both to the north and south of the main Yangtze. In Zhejiang it happened in the smaller upland valleys south of Hangzhou.

82 'how the paddy system was born': Author interview with Susan McCouch, November 2018. See also M. Sweeney and S. McCouch, 'The complex history of the domestication of rice', *Annals of Botany*, 100 (5), 2007, 951–7, DOI: 10.1093/aob/mcm128.

83 'The paddy system is so productive': While only 50 per cent of rice farming today happens in paddies, they produce 70 per cent of all the world's rice.

84 'largest collection of rice': International Rice Research Institute (IRRI), International Rice Genebank, https://www.irri.org/international-rice-gene bank.

84 'huge amounts of fertilisers': China's farmers pour more fertiliser onto every hectare of land than farmers anywhere else; twice as much as their European counterparts and more than fifty times the amount being applied in China in the early 1960s. This adds up to about 30 per cent of all global fertiliser use and, because of inefficient practices, vast amounts of that fertiliser never reach crops but wash into drains, rivers and ultimately the ocean.

85 'IR8 wasn't the tastiest rice': Author interview with Ruaraidh Sackville Hamilton, December 2018, former head of the seed bank at IRRI, who explained that it was perhaps the poor eating quality of IR8 that led so many farmers to keep growing their old varieties on tiny parcels of land. At their local markets, they made money by selling the new, approved varieties they cultivated, but at home they preferred to eat their traditional rice. They also knew from experience that if something went wrong and the modern crop failed, the traditional varieties provided a reassuring safety net.

85 'A later iteration, IR64,': Gurdev Khush, 'Green Revolution: The Way Forward', *Nature Review Genetics*, 2, 815–822 (2001), DOI: 10.1038/35093585

85 'Genetics of Disaster': Jack Harlan, 'Genetics of Disaster', *Journal of Environmental Quality*, 1(3), 1972

87 'regarded as a maverick': King was convinced soil was a living organism crucial to the productivity of farming. This was at odds with a prevailing view within USDA at the time that nutrients in soil would last indefinitely without the need for them to be replenished. He is now considered to be one of the pioneering thinkers of what would become the organic movement. See John Paull, 'The making of an agricultural classic: Farmers of Forty Centuries or Permanent Agriculture in China, Korea and Japan, 1911–2011', *Agricultural Sciences*, 2, 2011, 175–80, DOI: 10.4236/as.2011.23024.

88 'zero growth in fertiliser': The target date set was 2020 (the Ministry of Agriculture and Rural Affairs reported this had been achieved in 2018). See OECD Agricultural Policy Monitoring and Evalution, Section 8, China,

https://www.oecd-ilibrary.org/sites/049d4bd3-en/index.html?itemId=/content/component/049d4bd3-en.

89 'an American plant scientist': Allen Van Deynze et al., 'Nitrogen fixation in a landrace of maize is supported by a mucilage-associated diazotrophic microbiota', PLoS Biology, 16(8) 2018.

89 'fierce and well-armed': Hernán Cortés, Letters from Mexico, trans. Anthony Pagden (Yale University Press, 1986), p. 318.

90 'enormous economic value': Eric Triplett, 'Diazotrophic endophytes: progress and prospects for nitrogen fixation in monocots', Plant Soil, 186, 29–38 (1996), DOI: 10.1007/BF00035052.

90 'Chew on it and you'd break teeth': Author interview with Logan Kistler, December 2019, curator of archaeobotany and archaeogenomics at the Smithsonian National Museum of Natural History. See also Logan Kistler, 'Multiproxy evidence highlights a complex evolutionary legacy of maize in South America', Science, 14 December 2018, 1309–13, https://science.sciencemag.org/content/362/6420/1309.

90 'lived in small groups': We have no hard evidence of the exact size of the groups the early maize-eating hunter-gatherers lived in, but based on our understanding of how these societies operate, small groups of around fifty seems likely.

91 'dependent on the grain': There are parts of the Americas in which maize stayed as a minor crop or part of a highly diversified crop system, for example in the eastern Amazon from about 4,000 years ago onward.

92 'You have selected wisely': Author interview with Paul Ermigiotti, Crow Canyon Archeological Centre, Colorado.

92 'bound the heads of their newborns': This has been suggested by Meso-American expert Karl Taube, see Neil MacGregor, A History of the World in 100 Objects (Allen Lane, 2010).

92 'popcorn in other words': As was found in Paredones, an archaeological site on Peru's northern coast dated 2500 BCE. This was a pre-ceramic age, so the maize would have been popped using clay-lined baskets placed in the embers of fires.

92 '1,078 landraces': Botanist Flaviane Malaquias Costa discovered this huge diversity after visiting 2,049 farms in seventy rural communities in far western Santa Catarina, southern Brazil. Santa Catarina, she concluded, was a 'microcenter of diversity of Zea mays L'. See F.M. Costa et al., 'Maize diversity in southern Brazil: indication of a microcenter of Zea mays L', Genetic Resources and Crop Evolution, 64, 2017, 681–700, DOI: 10.1007/s10722-016-0391-2.

92 '24,000 samples of maize': H. Perales et al., 'Mapping the Diversity of Maize Races in Mexico', PLoS ONE 9 (12), 2014, e114657, DOI: 10.1371/journal.pone.0114657.

93 'successful human inventions ever created': Charles C. Mann, *1491: The Americas Before Columbus* (Granta, 2006).

93 'deficiency in the vitamin niacin': Pellagra was a huge problem particularly among poor US Southerners in the early twentieth century. Farmers were under pressure to grow cotton which crowded out more balanced food-production regimes and unmodified corn made up the majority of the diet.

94 'as soft as pillows': Author interview with Martha Willcox, Senior Scientist, Maize Landrace Coordinator at CIMMYT, November 2018.

94 'two different types of maize': Joanne A. Labate et al., 'Molecular and Historical Aspects of Corn Belt Dent Diversity', *Crop Science* 43, no. 1, 2003, DOI: 10.2135/cropsci2003.8000.

95 'into the "Corn Belt"': Based on the author's interview with expert in corn genetics, Dr John Doebley of the University of Wisconsin, October 2018.

96 '50 per cent of globally traded maize': Karen Braun, 'How the 19th century boosted America to the top of the world corn market: A history of US grain trade', *Reuters*, 12 June 2020.

96 'taking stones from the foundation': Betty Fussell, *The Story of Corn* (Knopf, 1992).

96 'molded into such uniformity': Arnold Ullstrup, 'The effects of the southern corn leaf blight epidemic of 1970–1971', *Annual Review of Phytopathology*, 1972, 10:37–50, DOI: 10.1146/annurev.py.10.090172.000345.

96 'birthplace of maize itself': 'Where does United States export Corn to?', Observatory of Economic Complexity, 2016, https://oec.world/en/visualize/tree_map/hs92/export/usa/show/21005/2016/.

97 'closer to 10 million': Author interview with Alyshia Galvez, October 2018. See also Alyshia Galvez, *Eating NAFTA: Trade, Food Policies, and the Destruction of Mexico* (University of California, 2018).

97 'US government subsidies': The US government paid out a record $46 billion to farmers in 2020. See Allen Rappeport, 'Trump Funnels Record Subsidies to Farmers Ahead of Election Day', *New York Times*, 12 October 2020, https://www.nytimes.com/2020/10/12/us/politics/trump-farmers-subsidies.html. The primary beneficiaries are the largest producers of commodities like maize, soybeans, wheat, cotton and rice.

98 'only one-fifth of the farmers had saved the seeds': Francis Denisse McLean-Rodríguez et al., 'The abandonment of maize landraces over the last 50 years in Morelos, Mexico', *Agriculture and Human Values*, March 2019, DOI: 10.1007/s10460-019-09932-3. See also, : George A. Dyer et al., 'Genetic erosion of maize', *PNAS*, Sep 2014, DOI: 10.1073/pnas.1407033111.

99 'That's maize we don't cook with': Author interview with Enrique Olvera, December 2019.

99 'different complex sugars ': Author interview with Alan Bennett, Professor of Plant Sciences at UC Davis, December 2019. See also, *Nitrogen Fixing and Corn*, Talking Biotech podcast (154), hosted by Dr Kevin Folta, October 6 2018, http://www.talkingbiotechpodcast.com/154-nitrogen-fixing-and-corn/. And see Allen Van Deynze et al., 'Nitrogen Fixation in a landrace of maize is supported by a mucilage-associated diazotrophic microbiota', *PLoS Biology*, 16(8), August 2018, DOI: 10.1371/journal.pbio.2006352.

100 'fifty–fifty arrangement': The Davis team has involved the Sierra Mixe community in the research project. The legal agreement ensuring that any future benefits from this research will be shared with the community has been praised by Mexico's environmental agency, as a 'win–win solution'. See also Ed Yong, 'The Wonder Plant That Could Slash Fertilizer Use', *The Atlantic*, 9 August 2018.

100 'generations of farmers in the Sierra Mixe': There is a debate in Mexico about who should benefit from any future application of the maize. For more on this see, Martha Pskowski, 'Indigenous Maize: Who Owns the Rights to Mexico's "Wonder" Plant?', *Yale Environment 360*, Yale School of Environment, 16 July 2019.

101 'American botanist Cary Fowler': Author interview with Cary Fowler, January 2021.

PART THREE: VEGETABLE

104 'agricultural and nutritional harmony': As we know from corn and pellagra, cereals provide plenty of energy but lack many micronutrients, and only some of the essential amino acid called lysine that our bodies need but can't make. Legumes contain an abundance of lysine. This is why, on every level, these two plant species complement each other.

105 'Mixed crops are the rule': Sir Albert Howard, *An Agricultural Testament* (Benediction Classics, 2010).

105 'they *bred true*': Alys Fowler, 'Prepare for Brexit with home-grown seeds', *Guardian*, 17 November 2018.

106 'seemeth not strange': Thomas Tusser, *Five Hundred Pointes of Good Husbandrie*, W. Payne and Sidney J. Herrtage (eds), (Leopold Classic Library, 2016).

106 'a tenth of that diversity had survived': There are several reasons for a decline in the diversity of the world's vegetables, including farms becoming increasingly mechanised and so uniformity becoming a higher priority. As we'll see later in the book (Part Six), refrigeration and the rise of the 'cool chain', also favoured a smaller number of varieties. But in this section I'm going to focus more on other factors.

106 'just four companies': James M. MacDonald, 'Mergers in Seeds and Agricultural Chemicals: What Happened?', United States Department of Agriculture, Economic Research Service, February 2019, https://www.ers .usda.gov/amber-waves/2019/february/mergers-in-seeds-and-agricultural -chemicals-what-happened/. BASF, is also a major player, and took over one of Bayer's seed divisions in 2017 for $7 billion. See also Geoff Tansey and Tamsin Rajotte (eds), *The Future Control of Food* (Earthscan, 2008).

106 'buying up small seed businesses': see a visual representation of this process, care of Philip H. Howard, https://philhoward.net/2018/12/31 /global-seed-industry-changes-since-2013/.

108 'Great Pyramids of Giza': Author's conversation with seed expert and trader of heirloom crops, Glenn Roberts of Anson Mills, September 2018.

108 'antique wedding ring': Author interview with David Shields, June 2018. See also, David Shields, *Southern Provisions: The Creation and Revival of a Cuisine* (University of Chicago Press, 2016).

109 'food for the slaves': John Ranby, *Observations on the evidence given before the committees of the Privy Council and House of Commons in support of the bill for abolishing the slave trade* (1791) (Gale ECCO, 2010). See also Thomas Clarkson, *The History of the Rise, Progress and Accomplishment of the Abolition of the African Slave-Trade, by the British Parliament* (1839) (Palala Press, 2016).

109 'white owners paid a premium': Michael Twitty, *The Cooking Gene: A Journey Through African American Culinary History in the Old South* (Amistad Press, 2018) p. 239, quoting historian Walter Edgar.

111 'Always in these secret gardens': Author interview with Jessica Harris.

111 'stained red rings': Author interview with Glenn Roberts.

112 'connections to Sierra Leone': In some parts of the South, Gullah is also used, and Geechee-Gullah words can be heard on some of the other Sea Islands as well as a few pockets of South Carolina and Georgia.

113 'Don't be a farmer': Author's interview with Matthew Raiford, September 2018.

113 '14 per cent of America's farmers': Emily Moon, 'African-American farmers make up less than 2 per cent of all US Farmers', *Pacific Standard*, April 2019.

115 'the Löwenmensch figure': Harald Floss, 'The Oldest Portable Art: the Aurignacian Ivory Figurines from the Swabian Jura (Southwest Germany)', *Palethnologie*, 7, 2015, DOI: 10.4000/palethnologie.888.

116 'Saskatchewan started to experiment': Wheat prices there were falling and the Canadians were looking for alternative, higher-value crops.

116 'part of a much bigger system': My thanks to Professor Dr Peter Poschlod, Chair of Ecology and Conservation Biology at the University of Regensburg for explaining the loss (and recovery) of the Alb-linse.

118 'The Franchti cave': D. Natalie et al., 'Zooarchaeological Evidence for Early Neolithic Colonization at Franchthi Cave (Peloponnese, Greece)', *Current Anthropology*, 56 (4), August 2015, 596–603.

121 'dwindling group of shamans': The Kallawaya are identified as an endangered culture by UNESCO, and because they live in one of the most ecologically diverse places on Earth and can recall the medicinal and nutritional properties of as many as nine hundred different species, they are regarded as a precious resource for the world. UNESCO, 'Intangible Cultural Heritage of Humanity, Andean cosmovision of the Kallawaya Bolivia', Nomination file No. 00048, 2008, https://ich.unesco.org/en/RL/andean-cosmovision-of -the-kallawaya-00048.

123 'attacks from harmful organisms': The toxic compounds are solanine and tomatine.

124 'Without the potato': W. McNeill, 'How the Potato Changed the World's History', *Social Research*, 66 (1), 1999, 67–83.

125 'Spaniards have enriched themselves': Clements R. Markham, *The Travels of Pedro de Cieza de Leon* (Hakluyt Society, 1864).

125 'summer by day, winter by night': All environments are diurnal by their nature, but the Andes are particularly marked at either end of the spectrum.

126 'New Zealand being one exception': It is the only other country which has managed to replicate these conditions and produce an important commercial crop of oca which is exported around the world. Elsewhere oca remains in the hands and gardens of amateur growers. See Alys Fowler, 'Ocas', *Guardian*, 14 March 2015.

128 'Among them is Eve Emshwiller': Author's interview with Eve Emshwiller, December 2018.

128 'villages are being emptied': I travelled to the Andes with the Wildlife Conservation Society which is finding ways to create economic opportunities for villagers using food.

129 'temperatures are warming': Ben Walker, 'Climate Change Is Making This Bolivian Village a Ghost Town', *Inside Climate News*, August 2017.

132 'hotter, humid weather': The earliest classification of soybeans by botanists was based on how quickly they matured (early, medium or late). For domestication, see E.J. Sedivy, F. Wu and Y. Hanzawa, 'Soybean domestication: the origin, genetic architecture and molecular bases', *New Phytologist*, 214 (2), April 2017, 539–53, DOI: 10.1111/nph.14418.

132 'farmers began domesticating the plant': Like lentils and cowpeas, this plant grows as a creeper. In the wild, it produces small pods containing tiny black seeds. Gradually, through selection, these became bigger and easier to harvest.

132 'break the bean down': The bitterness of soy in its uncooked form is why edamame – steamed soybeans, salted and eaten straight from the pod – have to be picked when they are very young and tender.

132 'condiment called *jiang*': This became *koch'ujang* in Korea with the addition of hot pepper.

132 'pressing it into blocks': In Indonesia, a different technique for making tofu was developed where the spores of a mould sourced from the hibiscus tree were added to soybeans. As the mould grows, it knits the legumes together, forming a solid, wrinkly block of food called tempeh.

132 '*shima-dofu* (island tofu)': On Okinawa as in China, the hard, dried yellow beans are soaked overnight making them elongated and plump. Fresh water is added and the beans are ground into a frothy, milky white liquid. The cold liquid is ladled through a piece of muslin placed over a sieve and the soya milk is heated at a later stage. With Japanese tofu the heating is done before the filtering happens. The approach on Okinawa is said to result in a firmer style of tofu. In both cases, after the seawater is added and the milk coagulates, it is passed through a muslin cloth and the solids left over are pressed together to make tofu.

133 'long and healthy lives': In 2005, in a *National Geographic* article, explorer and writer Dan Buettner coined the term 'Blue Zone'. This referred to five different regions around the world which had a much higher than average number of centenarians: Ogliastra in Sardinia; Ikaria in Greece; Okinawa in Japan; Loma Linda in California; and the Nicoya Peninsula in Costa Rica. See also Hiroko Sho, 'History and characteristics of Okinawan longevity food', *Asia Pacific Journal of Clinical Nutrition*, 10 (2), 2001, 159–164.

133 'Around forty were approved': Christine M. Du Bois, *The Story of Soy* (Reaktion Books, 2018). This is essential reading for the history, culture and science of soy.

134 'tinned American pork (Spam)': Sarah Crago, 'Born in the USA, eaten in Okinawa', *Japan Times*, 23 October 2015, https://www.japantimes.co.jp/life/2015/10/23/food/born-u-s-eaten-okinawa/.

134 'anchovy harvest dropping': this also contributed to one of the most infamous events in British food and farming history. The lack of fishmeal for livestock led the beef industry to look to slaughterhouse waste and the use of meat and bonemeal as a protein source, a decision that led to the appearance of BSE or 'mad cow disease' in British cattle. After the shock of this crisis abated, the industry turned instead to a protein source that was safe and plentiful: soy meal.

135 '90 per cent of all soy': Christine M. Du Bois, *The Story of Soy* (Reaktion Books, 2018).

135 'complex, globalized and financialized': Oxfam Research Reports, 'Cereal Secrets: The world's largest grain traders and global agriculture', August 2012, https://www-cdn.oxfam.org/s3fs-public/file_attachments/rr-cereal -secrets-grain-traders-agriculture-30082012-en_4.pdf.

135 'Food prices, deforestation': Cargill, along with ADM, Bunge, COFCO and Louis Dreyfus Company are all members of the Soft Commodities Forum, which has pledged to eliminate deforestation from their supply chains worldwide.

135 'the picture changed': Gustavo Bonato, 'New titans on the block: ABCDs lose top Brazil grains spot to Asian rivals', Reuters, 23 March 2016.

135 'future of the Cerrado': Kenneth Rapoza, 'In Brazil, Bolsonaro's Deforestation Might As Well Be China's', Forbes, 6 June 2019.

136 'Since the soy boom': See Our World in Data, 'Meat and Dairy Production', article by Hannah Ritchie and Max Roser first published in August 2017, last revision in November 2019, https://ourworldindata.org/meat -production.

137 'Just 20 per cent': Aline C. Soterroni et al., 'Expanding the Soy Moratorium to Brazil's Cerrado', Science Advances, Vol 5, No. 7, 03 July 2019.

139 'Everyone has a part to play': My thanks to the documentary-maker Jason Taylor who produced a film about Esiah Levy and seed collecting for The Gaia Foundation.

PART FOUR: MEAT

142 'a "big five" emerged': Jared Diamond points out that most domestic animals, including even recently domesticated trout (and presumably salmon), have smaller brains and less acute sense organs than do their wild ancestors. Powerful brains and sharp eyes are essential to survival in the wild, but on a farm or inside a barn this represents a significant waste of energy as far as humans are concerned. Gerald Crabtree, a geneticist at Stanford University, has also claimed the same applies to humans (i.e. we are all less intelligent today than our hunter-gatherer ancestors). Jared Diamond, 'Evolution, consequences and future of plant and animal domestication', Nature, 418 (6898), 8 August 2002, 700–7.

143 'bigger, faster-growing animals': It is worth considering that Robert Bakewell was running his experiments in animal genetics two hundred years before Norman Borlaug fundamentally changed wheat in the Green Revolution and a century before Darwin completed On the Origin of Species and Mendel had carried out his experiments with peas. See David L. Wykes, 'Robert Bakewell (1725–1795) of Dishley: Farmer and Livestock Improver', Agricultural History Review, 52 (1), 2004, 38–55.

143 'Before Bakewell's radical advances': In many parts of Britain and France one of the main reasons for keeping sheep was to add fertility to arable land. Pigs not only ate surplus food but also waste (which would otherwise attract vermin) and in some places, e.g. China, human faeces. The animals helped to keep the place clean. Simply put, the pig was the preferred animal of settled people, whereas ruminants (sheep and cattle) worked best for more nomadic populations.

143 'he transformed ancient breeds of cattle': Robert Bakewell's innovative ideas need to be seen in the context of wider changes in British agriculture; the conversion of arable land to pasture and enclosure both encouraged improvements in livestock breeding.

143 'least possible time': H Cecil Pawson, *Robert Bakewell, Pioneer Livestock Breeder* (London Crosby Lockwood & Son, 1957).

143 'Darwin would later cite': Selective breeding as practised by Robert Bakewell, and its demonstration of variation under domestication, was an important source of inspiration for the theory of natural selection set out by Darwin in *On the Origin of Species* (Darwin described selective breeding as artificial selection). See David L. Wykes.

144 'meat production has quadrupled': Hannah Ritchie and Max Roser, 'Meat and Dairy Production', *OurWorldInData.org.,* https://ourworldindata.org/meat-production.

145 'far more could be at risk': In 2000 the UNFAO announced that one thousand animal breeds had gone extinct in the last hundred years. 'As much as novel biotechnology may attempt to improve breeds, it is not possible to replace lost diversity,' said the organisation's head of Animal Genetic Resources. 'Extinction is forever. Biotechnology will not be able to regenerate breeds if they are lost.' See: FAO, 'One third of farm animal breeds face extinction', http://www.fao.org/News/2000/001201-e.htm. See also UN News, 'World "off track" to meet most Sustainable Development Goals on hunger, food security and nutrition', July 2019, https://news.un.org/en/story/2019/07/1042781.

147 'The winds are exceedingly uncertain and violent': Peter Ludwig Panum, *Observations Made During The Epidemic Of Measles On The Faroe Islands In The Year 1846* (Franklin Classics Trade Press, 2018).

148 'layers of intramuscular fat': In the sixteenth century, the Faroese sheep were crossed with an equally hardy sheep from the Scottish Isles, and so the 80,000 sheep on the island today are hybrids.

149 'the chef Fergus Henderson': Nose to tail eating is also referred to as the practice of eating 'everything but the squeal', i.e. the complete animal and not just the prime cuts.

149 'lambs to the slaughter': For the history of mutton, its rise and fall (and recipes), see Bob Kennard, *Much Ado About Mutton* (Merlin Unwin Books, 2014).

151 'Parmesan cheese and death': Rebecca Mead, 'Koks, The World's Most Remote Foodie Destination', *New Yorker*, June 2018.

151 'food traditions were viewed with suspicion': A Danish priest visiting the island in the 1670s set out an outsider's perspective of Faroese food: 'Other parts of the world have been blessed with great wealth, precious stones, grains or wine but God and nature have denied all of these things to the Faroese.'

153 'cooked whale blood': It is legal for islanders to catch pilot whales. Of the estimated 380,000 animals in the eastern North Atlantic, around 600 are caught and killed around the Faroes each year.

154 'one billion chickens slaughtered': Department for Environment Food and Rural Affairs, 'Latest poultry and poultry meat statistics: Monthly statistics on the activity of UK hatcheries and UK poultry slaughterhouses' (figures from November 2019), https://assets.publishing.service.gov.uk/government/uploads/system/uploads/attachment_data/file/928469/poultry statsnotice-22oct20.pdf.

155 'signal is the modern chicken': Carys E. Bennett et al., 'The broiler chicken as a signal of a human reconfigured biosphere', *Royal Society Open Science*, 5:180325, DOI: 10.1098/rsos.180325.

155 'twenty-four stone': 'A Growing Problem, Selective Breeding in the Chicken Industry: The Case for Slower Growth', ASPCA report, Nov 2015.

155 'sometime after 7500': Ming-Shan Wang et al., '863 genomes reveal the origin and domestication of chicken', *Cell Research*, 30 July 2020, 693–70, DOI: 10.1038/s41422-020-0349-y.

156 'In Hawaii, these ceremonial objects': Neil MacGregor, *A History of the World in 100 Objects* (Allen Lane, 2010).

156 'walking pharmacy': For the full story on chicken domestication and of the Chicken of Tomorrow, see Andrew Lawler, *Why Did the Chicken Cross the World?* (Atria Books, 2014).

157 'The bird is completely black': Jang-il Sohn et al., 'Whole genome and transcriptome maps of the entirely black native Korean chicken breed *Yeonsan Ogye*', *GigaScience*, 7 (7), July 2018, giy086, DOI: 10.1093/gigascience/giy086.

157 'even the bird's faeces': Author correspondence with Lee Seung Sook in Yeonsan with thanks to journalist Yolanta Siu for help with translation.

158 'Single-Comb White Leghorns': *American Poultry Journal* (online archive), Vol. 51, 1920, https://babel.hathitrust.org/cgi/pt?id=uc1.c2578787&view=1up&seq=20.

159 'by the early 1950s': H L Shrader, The Chicken of Tomorrow Program; Its Influence on "Meat-Type", Poultry Production', Poultry Science, Vol 1 (1), January 1952.

159 'restock their sheds': Maryn McKenna, *Plucked, The Truth About Chicken* (Little Brown, 2018).

160 'Tens of millions of pounds': Competition and Markets Authority, 'Decision on relevant merger situation', February 13 2018. https://assets .publishing.service.gov.uk/media/5a9592ec40f0b67aa5087b04/aviagen-hubbard -decision.pdf.

160 '2 kilos in around 35 days': Eat, Sit, Suffer, Repeat: The Life of a Typical Meat Chicken, RSPCA report, March 2020. This is not the same as the slaughter weight. For chickens in the US this is typically 42 days.

160 'increased risk of lameness': As well as the RSPCA report see also Ann Rayner et al., 'Slow-growing broilers are healthier and express more behavioural indicators of positive welfare', Scientific Reports, September 2020, DOI: 10.1038/s41598-020-72198-x.

160 'wearing diapers': The claim comes from Oxfam's 2016 report 'No Relief: Denial of Bathroom Breaks in the Poultry Industry', https://s3 .amazonaws.com/oxfam-us/www/static/media/files/No_Relief_Embargo .pdf. At the time of the report the industry denied the problem existed. See also Roberto Ferdman, '"I had to wear Pampers": The cruel reality the people who bring you cheap chicken allegedly endure', Washington Post, 11 May 2016.

162 'Bigger, faster and, for our benefit, even blind': Ahmed Ali et al., 'Early Egg Production in Genetically Blind Chickens in Comparison with Sighted Controls', Poultry Science, 64 (5), May 1985, 789–94. See also Peter Sandøe et al., 'The Blind Hens' Challenge: Does It Undermine the View That Only Welfare Matters in Our Dealings with Animals?', Environmental Values, 23, 2014, DOI: 10.3197/096327114X13947900181950.

164 'pigs couldn't be left free to roam': Essential reading on pig history and the story of how the two main lines of pig domestication crossed paths is Sam White, 'From Globalised Pig Breeds to Capitalist Pigs: A Study in Animal Cultures and Evolutionary History', Environmental History, 16 (1), January 2011, 94–120. See also Robert Malcolmson and Stephanos Mastoris, The English Pig: A History (Hambledon Continuum, 1998).

164 'captured in language': Qiu Gui Su, 'What Does the Chinese Character 家 Mean?', ThoughtCo, 04 December 2017. My thanks also to Fuchsia Dunlop for her help with Chinese characters.

164 'The Meishan, one of the oldest': Steven McOrist and Rex Walters, 'Native Pig Breeds of China', Pig Progress, 25 (3), 2009.

165 'factories on four legs': Mindi Schneider, Brian Lander and Katherine Brunson, 'How the pig became a 'pork factory' in China', China Dialogue, 23 July 2019.

166 'The small low bellied hog': Both quotes feature in Sam White, Environmental History.

169 'Pregnant sows live in gestation crates': The Humane Society of the United States, 'Scientists and Experts on Gestation Crates and Sow Welfare',

October 2012, https://www.humanesociety.org/sites/default/files/docs/hsus-expert-synopsis-gestation-crates-and-sow-welfare.pdf.

169 'antiobiotics used as growth promoters': Melinda Wenner Moyer, 'How Drug-Resistant Bacteria Travel from the Farm to Your Table', *Scientific American*, 1 December 2016.

170 'death follows within days': As with avian flu, all pigs in all systems are vulnerable. However, the scale of some intensive systems means that when swine fever hits thousands of animals can quickly become infected.

171 'the death of 5 million pigs': Detailed breakdowns of these pig mortalities don't exist, but many deaths are likely to be the result of a slaughter policy introduced by the government as an emergency measure.

171 'These pigs do fly': Kees van Dooren, 'Planes full of breeding pigs head to China', *Pig Progress*, 6 May 2020.

172 'The mass slaughter of bison': *American Serengeti: The Last Big Animals of the Great Plains* (University Press of Kansas, 2017).

172 'Thirty million bison': Hanna Rose Shell, 'Last of the Wild Buffalo', *Smithsonian Magazine*, February 2000.

172 'herds were so huge': One theory is that bison numbers had boomed at the start of the nineteenth century, because the population of indigenous hunters had been decimated by smallpox introduced by Europeans.

172 'a group of hunters': Dan Flores, 'On the History of Bison in the American West', symposium talk, 'Albert Bierstadt: Witness to a Changing West,' 16 June 2018.

173 'When I am dust and ashes': Quoted from Smithsonian Institution archives, https://siarchives.si.edu/collections/siris_sic_14832.

173 'A book published the same year': *The Extermination of the American Bison* was written in 1889 by William Temple Hornaday.

174 'agents of conquest': Joshua Specht, *Red Meat Republic* (Princeton University Press, 2019).

175 'the only other invasion', Nicholas St Fleur, 'A Start Date for the Bison Invasion of North America', *New York Times*, 13 March 2017.

175 'homesteads had been burnt out': Author interview with bison historian Jack Rhylan, October 2020.

176 'I aimed at the public's heart': Quoted in A.F. Kantor, 'Upton Sinclair and the Pure Food and Drugs Act of 1906, "I aimed at the public's heart and by accident I hit it in the stomach"', *American Journal of Public Health*, 66 (12), 1976, 1202–5, DOI: 10.2105/ajph.66.12.1202.

178 'first serious effort': The effort to save the bison became more concerted in 1905 when William Hornaday, Theodore Roosevelt and others launched the American Bison Society (ABS), a national campaign to create wild bison reserves.

179 'people started crying': Author interview with Jennifer Barfield, October 2020.

179 'the foot of the White Mountains': Elliott Coues, *The Expeditions of Zebulon Montgomery Pike* (Harper, 1810) (Palala Press, 2018).

180 'shimmering, tremulous': Theodore Roosevelt, *Ranch Life and the Hunting Trail* (Cosimo Classics, 2008).

182 'Many animals are kept alive': Someone who has studied wet markets is Professor Andrew Cunningham, an expert in zoonotic diseases (diseases that can jump from animals to humans) at the Zoological Society, London. He identified a cultural preference for fresh, so-called 'warm meat' in some parts of China. This makes it possible for humans to come into contact with blood and other bodily fluids at markets.

183 'the deaths of 105 people': L.M. Looi, 'Lessons from the Nipah virus outbreak in Malaysia', *Malaysian Journal of Pathology*, 29 (2), December 2007, 63–7, PMID: 19108397.

183 'we shake viruses loose': David Quammen, 'Why Weren't We Ready for the Coronavirus?', *New Yorker*, 11 May 2020.

PART FIVE: FROM THE SEA

185 'Some shoals were the width': Jane Grigson, *The Best of Jane Grigson: The Enjoyment of Food* (Grub Street, 2015).

187 'Since the advent of industrial fishing': Any collapse in the population of a fish species will involve numerous contributory factors, e.g. climatic conditions and water quality (both of course influenced by humans), but in the case of the Pacific bluefin tuna and sardine, and the Mediterranean swordfish, overfishing is a major contributory factor. The figures given refer to biomass and include data sourced from the International Scientific Committee for Tuna and Tuna-like Species in the North Pacific Ocean (ISC).

187 'keystone species such as the Pacific sardine': Oceana, 'The Modern Day Pacific Sardine Collapse: How to Prevent a Future Crisis', https://usa.oceana.org/responsible-fishing/modern-day-pacific-sardine-collapse-how-prevent-future-crisis. A keystone species is an organism that helps define an entire ecosystem. Without its keystone species, the ecosystem would be dramatically different or cease to exist altogether. In the case of the Pacific sardine (which for humans is high in omega-3 fatty acids), they are a critical source of food for many larger species including whales, sea lions, salmon, brown pelicans and terns.

187 'The global fishing effort': David Agnew et al., 'Estimating the Worldwide Extent of Illegal Fishing', *PLoS ONE*, 4(2): e4570, 2009, DOI: 10.1371/journal.pone.0004570.

187 'significantly altered': United Nations, 'UN Report: Nature's Dangerous Decline "Unprecedented"; Species Extinction Rates "Accelerating"', https://www.un.org/sustainabledevelopment/blog/2019/05/nature-decline-unprecedented-report/.

187 'China alone has': Ian Urbina, 'How China's Expanding Fishing Fleet Is Depleting the World's Oceans', *Yale Environment 360*, 17 August 2020, https://e360.yale.edu/features/how-chinas-expanding-fishing-fleet-is-depleting-worlds-oceans. See also Miren Gutiérrez et al., *China's Distant-Water Fishing Fleet*, Overseas Development Institute, June 2020, https://www.odi.org/sites/odi.org.uk/files/resource-documents/chinesedistantwaterfishing_web_1.pdf.

187 '3.3 billion of us': For some of the most authoritative data available on fish stocks and consumption trends, see *The State of World Fisheries and Aquaculture 2020*, UNFAO, 2020, DOI: 10.4060/ca9229en.

188 'Fishing is most likely the oldest': One school of human evolution believes we became bipedal as it helped us find food more efficiently in estuarine environments. This also explains, so the theory goes, our loss of body hair. If you look at where civilisations started (along estuaries, rivers and coasts) the theory starts to make sense. See Carsten Niemitz, 'The evolution of the upright posture and gait – a review and a new synthesis', *Die Naturwissenschaften*, 97 (3), 2010, 241–63, DOI: 10.1007/s00114-009-0637-3.

188 'fish event horizon': Gala Vince, 'Intensive fishing was an ancient practice', *New Scientist*, 24 November 2004.

188 'evil of fishers': Richard C. Hoffmann, 'Economic Development and Aquatic Ecosystems in Medieval Europe', *American Historical Review*, 101, No. 3, 1996, 631–69, DOI: 10.2307/2169418.

188 'increased carbon dioxide levels': Acidifying oceans are going to be particularly problematic for shellfish such as oysters, crabs and lobsters.

190 'It's that simple': For a much wider exploration of this idea, read Mark Kurlansky, *Salmon: A Fish, the Earth, and the History of Their Common Fate* (Oneworld Publications, 2020).

192 'Salmon Fisher to the Salmon': in Seamus Heaney, *Door into the Dark* (Faber & Faber, 1969).

192 'only 30,000 will do so': Author interview with Mark Bilsby, Atlantic Salmon Trust, November 2018.

193 'hunter-gatherers here survived on salmon': This is the Mount Sandel Neolithic campsite where, based on the bones excavated at the site, fish dominated the diet: salmon (48 per cent), trout (32 per cent), eel (7 per cent), bass and flounder, all from the nearby River Bann. The fish were probably caught using harpoons, nets or baited lines. Fish traps and wicker baskets may also have been used. At the campsite, archaeologists also found evidence of wooden racks, over which the fish would have been dried or smoked to help preserve them. 'Mount Sandel, a Mesolithic Campsite', *Irish Archaeology*, July 2013.

194 'monasteries had control': The exclusivity of salmon fishing continues to this day. To fish on a private beat (a beat is a stretch of river) on the Spey

in Scotland with a ghillie (an expert fishing guide) can cost around £400 per rod per day (which is cheap compared with some rivers in Iceland, £1,500 per day). This isn't just down to the salmon's rarity – private landownership around rivers is the biggest factor.

194 'Poor Bann!': Augustus Grimble, *Salmon Rivers of Ireland*, Vol. 1, 1903. Quoted in Anthony Netboy, *The Atlantic Salmon: A Vanishing Species?* (Faber & Faber, 1968).

195 'destroyed all vestige of fish life': Anthony Netboy, *The Atlantic Salmon: A Vanishing Species?* (Faber & Faber, 1968).

195 'made newspaper headlines': Maria Herlihy, 'Salmon make a welcome return to local stream', *Corkman*, 31 December 2016.

197 'off the coast of Norway': Mark Kurlansky, 'Factory-farmed salmon: does it make sense to grow fish in indoor tanks?', *Guardian*, 07 December 2020.

199 'animal breeders stepped in': Paul Greenberg, *Four Fish: The Future of the Last Wild Food* (Penguin, 2011).

199 *'Salmo domesticus'*: The idea that this farmed fish is a distinct species and should be called *Salmo domesticus* comes from Martin R. Gross, a Canadian evolutionary biologist.

200 'A battering from Storm Brendan': John Evans, '74,000 salmon escape Mowi Scotland farm after storm', Intrafish News, 20 January 2020.

200 '"farmed" lice can spread out': Government scientists in Scotland say the evidence showing lice from farms are damaging the wild salmon population is inconclusive, however research from Norway suggests they are having a detrimental effect. See, Thorstad, E.B. & Finstad, B, 2018. 'Impacts of salmon lice emanating from salmon farms on wild Atlantic salmon and sea trout', NINA Report 1449: 1-22. https://brage.nina.no/nina-xmlui/bitstream/handle/11250/2475746/1449.pdf?sequence=1&isAllowed=y.

201 'mixing of genes': Kevin Glover et al., 'Half a century of genetic interaction between farmed and wild Atlantic salmon: Status of knowledge and unanswered questions', *Fish and Fisheries*, 18, 2017, 890–927, DOI: 10.1111/faf.12214.

205 '€60 million a year': Neil Munshi, 'The fight for west Africa's fish', *Financial Times*, 13 March 2020. See also European Parliament, 'Fisheries in Mauritania and the European Union', Research for PECH Committee, https://www.europarl.europa.eu/RegData/etudes/STUD/2018/617458/IPOL_STU(2018)617458_EN.pdf.

205 'seafood consumed in the EU': Harry Owen and Griffin Carpenter, 'Fish Dependence 2018 Update. The Reliance of the EU on Fish From Elsewhere', New Economics Foundation, 2018.

205 'Chinese boats, subsidised by government': D. Belhabib, U.R. Sumaila et al., 'Euros vs. Yuan: Comparing European and Chinese Fishing Access

in West Africa', *PLoS ONE*, 10 (3), 2015, e0118351, DOI: 10.1371/journal.pone .0118351.

205 'China pays the biggest amount': For an overview (and history) of the role of China in global fisheries, see Roland Blomeyer, 'The role of China in World Fisheries', European Parliament, 2012, https://www.europarl .europa.eu/meetdocs/2009_2014/documents/pech/dv/chi/china.pdf.

206 'Foreign-owned processing plants': 'A Waste of Fish: Food security under threat from the fishmeal and fish oil industry in West Africa', Greenpeace International, 19 June 2019.

206 'most of the fishmeal (and fish oil)': Fish oil is also an ingredient used in the feed of penned salmon, and it's used in the pharmaceutical industry too.

206 'biologists describe as 'leaky'': Author interview with Callum Roberts, Professor of Marine Conservation in the Centre for Ecology and Conservation at the University of Exeter.

206 'In the 1990s': Fred Pearce, 'Breaking the Banc', *New Scientist*, 30 June 2001.

206 'bigger and more powerful boats': On the intensification of fishing by small-scale boats in West Africa, see Daniel Pauly, 'Size Matters: The Impact of Artisanal Fisheries in West Africa', *Sea Around Us*, 19 April 2017, http://www.seaaroundus.org/size-matters-the-impact-of-artisanal-fisheries-in-west -africa/. WWF, 5 May 2004, https://wwf.panda.org/wwf_news/?12984.

206 'lucrative and also endangered': In 2003, an agreement was reached between the park's managers and the Imraguen to end the targetting of shark and ray.

207 'continuous and significant': Banc d'Arguin National Park, *IUCN World Heritage Outlook*, Conservation Outlook Assessment 2020, https://worldher itageoutlook.iucn.org/explore-sites/wdpaid/20388.

211 'heavily tattooed ruffians': Quoted in Naomichi Ishige, *History of Japanese Food* (Routledge, 2011), an excellent account of the nineteenth-century transformation of Japanese food culture

211 'and inferior fish': Author interview with Trevor Corson, April 2019.

211 'One of the team, Akira Okazaki': This story is told in Sasha Issenberg, *Globalization and the Making of a Modern Delicacy* (Avery, 2007).

213 '*Ostrea edulis*': For detailed descriptions of the two main species of oyster in this chapter, see FAO, Fisheries Division, '*Ostrea edulis* (Linnaeus, 1758)' and '*Crassostrea gigas* (Thunberg, 1793)', www.fao.org.

213 'oyster reef habitats': The global picture isn't much better; 85 per cent of the worldwide oyster reef habitats have been destroyed over the course of the last century. See Bernadette Pogoda, 'Current Status of European Oyster Decline and Restoration in Germany', *Humanities*, January 2019, https://www.mdpi.com/394114.

214 'create a safe haven': The oyster creates a hard substrate over a soft one so other species can grow on it and that again attracts other life forms.

214 'unselfishness of an oyster': The reference appears in the short story, 'The Match-Maker' by Saki.

215 'when there's an "R" in the month': The reason is not because oysters caught in months with an R in are unsafe, it's because they mark seasons in which the animals are in their reproductive phase and less meaty.

216 'survived on oysters': Curtis Marean, a paleoanthropologist, puts forward the idea that as the world was in a glacial stage 125,000 to 195,000 years ago, much of Africa was dry to mostly desert; food was difficult to find and humans could not have survived. This is why they moved to the coast (and survived on oysters). Curtis Marean et al., 'Early human use of marine resources and pigment in South Africa during the Middle Pleistocene', *Nature*, 449, 2007, 905–8.

217 'oysters could be served': Drew Smith, *Oyster: A Gastronomic History (with Recipes)* (Abrams, 2015).

217 'oyster traders and boatmen': Henry Mayhew, *Mayhew's London* (Spring Books, 1851).

219 'overwhelm the natives': There is an ongoing debate (for some other species too) about when an invasive species becomes naturalised. The Pacific oyster is an interesting case as it fulfils the same functions as the flat oyster (which seems to be in terminal decline). Some marine biologists believe it's better to have some oysters than none. For conservation purposes, others see the invasive species as a problem.

220 'if the native oyster is eventually outcompeted': The 'enemy release hypothesis' explains why introduced species can become so successful in new environments. All plants and animals co-evolve with the pathogens and diseases in their native area, which help keep its populations in check. Introduced species run amok as they are no longer being held in check by their usual foes.

220 'including the native': Restoration projects for the native oyster are taking place across Europe, including one led by the Zoological Society of London which has created an 'oyster sanctuary' on the south coast of England to try to kick-start new populations of the species. Elsewhere, spat (oyster larvae) are being taken from the Limfjorden and placed along European coastlines in the hope they will take hold and survive.

221 'magical underwater world': Author's interview with Callum Roberts, February 2019 and November 2020.

222 'more full of fish': Callum Roberts, *The Unnatural History of the Sea* (Gaia, 2007).

223 'Cabo Pulmo on the west coast of Mexico': Models published in October 2020 by Reniel Cabral of the University of California, Santa Barbara, found

that designating a modest 5 per cent more of the world's oceans as MPAs (which would triple the area currently protected) the future global catch of the 811 species they looked at would increase by more than 20 per cent. That corresponds to an extra 10 million tonnes of food a year.

223 'more quickly than life on land': Daniel Pauly, *Vanishing Fish, Shifting Baselines and the Future of Global Fisheries* (Greystone Books, 2019).

PART SIX: FRUIT

226 'oldest depiction so far discovered': The most recent analysis of the plants and different fruits depicted on the Warka Vase was made by Naomi Miller, an archaeobotanist who works in Western and Central Asia and is based at the University of Pennsylvania. See Naomi Miller et al., 'Sign and image: representations of plants on the Warka Vase of early Mesopotamia', *Origini*, 39, 2016, 53–73, University of Pennsylvania Scholarly Commons, Philadelphia.

227 'date, olive or fig': The Sumerians had the perfect growing conditions for fruit in Uruk; gardens were shaded by tall date palms where they grew grapes, apples, melons and figs. Pears and pomegranates followed later. The date palm (which did not fruit further south in the cooler climate of Assyria) was essential to this system.

227 'the origins of nationhood': See Jules Janick, 'The Origins of Fruits, Fruit Growing, and Fruit Breeding', *Plant Breeding Review*, 2010, Department of Horticulture and Landscape Architecture, Purdue University.

227 'grafting, effectively cloning': There are several different ways of cloning fruit trees. Some species produce new roots more easily from cuttings, e.g. fig, grape, pomegranate and olive, and these were the earliest to be cloned. More difficult were apples, pears and plums, species that do not root easily from cuttings, and so the varieties couldn't be saved and reproduced until the discovery of the type of grafting I have described (the beginning of the first millennium BCE).

228 'naturally cool environments': The Italian producer Melinda stores 20,000 tonnes of fruit it harvests inside a cave system under the Dolomites. This network of abandoned mines is 275 metres below ground in the Val di Non valley in Trentino.

228 'extend the shelf life': In 1920, scientists at Cambridge University (Franklin Kidd and Cyril West) launched the first systematic studies of 'gas storage' of fruit in the world. The pair were pioneers of the new science of 'post-harvest physiology'. See 'CA storage has become staple of the fruit industry', *Fruit Growers News*, July 2011.

228 'controlled atmosphere': Using the apples stored by Melinda in the Dolomites cave system as an example, a controlled atmosphere is created as

follows: air is pumped through oxygen filters into each storage cell, creating an environment that is 99 per cent nitrogen and 1 per cent oxygen. This means the apples can still breathe, but very slowly. Within four days inside this atmosphere, the fruits' maturation slows to the point where they can be kept fresh for almost a year.

228 'the cold chain': In 1940, Frederick McKinley Jones patented a refrigeration system for trucks that would allow them to transport perishable foods for longer distances. Through his company Thermo King, Jones had a long-lasting, global impact on agriculture. His technology made international trading of fresh food possible, and changed forever the notion of 'seasonal' foods.

228 'twenty feet deep': The containers have grown in size so that today the industry standard is forty feet deep. The global fleet is equivalent to 17 million of these larger containers.

228 'ninefold increase in trade': Philip Coggan, *More, The 10,000-Year Rise of the World Economy* (The Economist Books, 2020).

228 'big metal box': Tim Harford, *Fifty Things That Made the Modern Economy* (Abacus, 2017).

229 '"marketing groups" and "clubs"': The roots of club varieties can be traced back to the first patented apple, the Honeycrisp, developed in 1960 by the University of Minnesota. The university obtained a patent on the cultivar which meant any grower who bought a Honeycrisp tree in the USA paid a $1 royalty fee for each one.

229 'To reach a global audience': Despite all the money spent on fruit breeding, some of the winners emerge by chance or were bred by amateurs. The Gala was raised by James Hatton Kidd, a Scotsman whose family emigrated to New Zealand. He took up fruit breeding (Kidd's Orange Red is one of his). He crossed Kidd's Orange Red with Golden Delicious which gave the Gala. When he died, his seedlings passed to the research station in New Zealand where Gala was selected. My thanks to Joan Morgan for making that point to me.

231 'sent these apples further afield': See Barrie E. Juniper, 'The Mysterious Origin of the Sweet Apple: On its way to a grocery counter near you, this delicious fruit traversed continents and mastered coevolution', *American Scientist*, January–February 2007.

231 'Like the bears': It is also thought dung beetles were important in spreading wild apple seeds around the forest.

231 'a man named John Chapman': Michael Pollan, *The Botany of Desire* (Bloomsbury, 2002).

232 'the Dutch and the English': more recently the creation of large-scale fruit plantations has taken place in the southern hemisphere in countries such as Peru and Chile.

232 'Stiff with cold': Nikolai Vavilov, *Five Continents* (International Plant Genetics Research Institute, 1996)..

232 'Given his genius': Quoted in Gary Paul Nabhan, *Where Our Food Comes From* (Island Press, 2011).

233 'brought me to my knees': Interview by Catherine Peix, for the film 'The Origins of the Apple', included in the book *The Wild Apple Forests of the Tian Shan*, edited by Giuseppe Barbera (International Carlo Scarpa Prize for Gardens, 2016).

233 'diluting the wild gene pool': M.Y. Omasheva et al., 'To what extent do wild apples in Kazakhstan retain their genetic integrity?', *Tree Genetics & Genomes*, 13, 2017, DOI: 10.1007/s11295-017-1134-z.

234 'every day for more than four years': In 1883, the Royal Horticulture Society held an Apple Congress at which fifty fruit experts collected and identified every known apple variety in Britain. The total number of named varieties was 1,545. It was the biggest collection of apple diversity ever assembled. See Joan Morgan, *The New Book of Apples* (Ebury Press, 2010).

234 'a nutty warm aroma': One of the many glorious descriptions of fruit featured in Edward A. Bunyard's *The Anatomy of Dessert: With a Few Notes on Wine* (Modern Library Food, paperback 2006). Bunyard (1878–1939) was a nurseryman and England's foremost pomologist.

235 'yellow plastic spheres': This appeared in the *Daily News*, New York and is cited in Joan Morgan, *The New Book of Apples* (Ebury Press, 2010).

236 'high-yielding, picked early': The ability of a single apple variety to grow in different countries around the world is an important characteristic in explaining the decline in apple diversity. A good example is the Golden Delicious. First discovered by a farmer in West Virginia, USA, it was grown by the Stark Brothers Nursery in Missouri (home of the Red Delicious), and from there the variety was also planted in the Loire Valley in France where it grew well. After the Algerian war and independence in 1962, returning colonists were given free land on the condition they grew Golden Delicious (to help boost the French fruit industry). It worked so well that in the 1970s the variety flooded British supermarkets and contributed to the downfall of hundreds of British orchards unable to compete.

236 'For the supermarkets': It should also be noted there are different types of licensing agreement. Cripps Pink, for example, is a free 'open source' variety that can be grown by anyone without paying a royalty. It's only when you want to market that variety using the 'club name' Pink Lady that you are obliged to purchase a licence.

236 'The scale of the investment': M Sharon Baker, 'Marketing Campaign for the Cosmic Crisp Heats Up as Debut of Washington's New Apple Nears', *Seattle Business*, July 2019.

238 '20 billion tonnes': Our World in Data, 'Fruit consumption by fruit type, World, 1961 to 2013', https://ourworldindata.org/grapher/fruit-consumption -by-fruit-type?stackMode=relative. Consumption figures for oranges and mandarins are slightly higher but this includes fruit processed into juice, whereas bananas are typically eaten whole.

239 'herb and not a tree': The suckers are the basal shoots of the banana, which are clones of the main plant. This form of reproduction is known as vegetative, clonal or asexual.

239 'Panama disease or Fusarium wilt': TR4 belongs to the same genus as *Fusarium graminearum* (the fungus attacks cereal crops including wheat). Agriculturally and economically speaking, it is the most significant fungal genus on the planet.

240 'most valuable plant ... a native of China': This description is given in *Paxton's Magazine of Botany, and Register of Flowering Plants*, Vol. 3 (W.S. Orr & Co., 1837, accessed online).

240 'English missionary John Williams': Douglas Marin et al., 'Dissemination of Bananas in Latin America and the Caribbean', *Plant Disease*, 82 (9), DOI: 10.1094/PDIS.1998.82.9.964.

240 'more popular than apples': Dan Koeppel, *Banana: The Fate of the Fruit That Changed The World* (Plume Books, 2009).

241 'promise of cheap labour': Stephen Schlesinger and Stephen Kinzer, *Bitter Fruit, The Story of the American Coup in Guatemala* (Harvard University, 2005).

241 'state within a state': Douglas Farah, 'A Snubbed Revolutionary Looks Back', *Washington Post*, November 13, 1995.

242 'forty different varieties': Ugandan banana diversity: F.B.M. Kilwinger et al., 'Culturally embedded practices of managing banana diversity and planting material in central Uganda', *Journal of Crop Improvement*, 33 (4), 2019, 456–77, DOI: 10.1080/15427528.2019.1610822.

243 'East African Highland bananas': Banana domestication in Africa: ProMusa website: East African Highland Banana (EAHB), https://www .promusa.org/East+African+highland+banana+subgroup.

243 'hard work and effort': Author interview with Edie Mukibi, October 2018.

244 'more disease-resistant hybrids': 'New $13.8 million project aims to boost banana production in Uganda and Tanzania', *International Society for Horticultural Science*, October 2014.

244 'one of the main testing areas': See Bill Gates, 'A Bunch of Reasons: Building better bananas', GatesNotes, 31 January 2012, https://www .gatesnotes.com/development/building-better-bananas.

244 'need this new technology': Author interview with James Dale, December 2020.

247 '300 million individual pieces of fruit': John Dickie, *Cosa Nostra* (Hodder, 2007).

248 'bit by bit everything changes': Leopoldo Franchetti, *Condizioni politiche e amministrative della Sicilia*, quoted in Alexander Stille, *Excellent Cadavers: The Mafia and the Death of the First Italian Republic* (Vintage, 1995).

248 'this is my Mafia': Michele Greco, obituary, *Daily Telegraph*, 15 February 2008.

249 'Domenico Casella': He described Sicily's citrus diversity in a book, *Varieta Di Arancio Coltevate in Sicilia* (University of Catania, 1935).

251 'an Italian diplomat': The diplomat's name was Leopoldo Zunini.

251 'bigger operators now dominate': An example of this is the purchase of Oranfrizer, Sicily's biggest fresh citrus supplier by one of the world's biggest fresh fruit companies, Unifrutti (based on the Italian mainland), backed by the American investment company, the Carlyle Group. See 'Unifrutti Group acquires Oranfrizer', *Eurofruit*, 2 November 2020, http://www.fruitnet.com /eurofruit/article/183393/unifrutti-group-acquires-oranfrizer.

251 'deserted citrus groves': Statistics covering 2000–2010 show the number of farm workers went down and the average size of holdings went up. See 'Agricultural census in Italy', Eurostat, 2012, https://ec.europa.eu/eurostat /statistics-explained/pdfscache/20078.pdf.

252 'We can't be the generation': Ryan Hagen, 'Why is a tent covering Riverside's parent navel orange tree?', *The Press-Enterprise*, 26 April 2018.

253 'Jobs in the citrus industry have declined': Citrus greening is caused by the huanglongbing bacteria, which is transmitted by the Asian citrus psyllid insect. See http://www.epi.ufl.edu/news/mapping-risk-of-citrus-greening -establishment.html.

253 'If we don't act quickly': Diane Nelson, '75 percent of Florida's oranges have been lost to disease. Can science save citrus?', University of California, Davis, 29 August 2019, https://www.universityofcalifornia.edu/news/75 -percent-floridas-oranges-have-been-lost-disease-can-science-save-citrus.

254 'our heedless and destructive acts': Eliza Griswold, 'How "Silent Spring" Ignited the Environmental Movement', *New York Times*, 21 September 2012.

255 'scientist Gayle Volk': Author interview with Gayle Volk, October 2018.

PART SEVEN: CHEESE

257 'If you don't like bacteria … ': J. Craig Venter interviewed by Karen Kaplan,'Seeing Earth's future in a petri dish', *LA Times*, 24 November 2007.

258 'one billion tonnes': According to the FAO, global milk production reached 852 million tonnes in 2019, mainly as a result of increases in India, Pakistan and Brazil. See FAO, 'Dairy Market Review – Overview of global dairy market developments in 2019', March 2020, http://www.fao.org/3 /ca8341en/CA8341EN.pdf.

258 'world milk production': figures from USDA, Dairy World Markets and Trade, https://www.fas.usda.gov/data/dairy-world-markets-and-trade.

258 'milk of other animals': By volume most of the world's milk comes from cows, sheep and goats, but in many cultures other sources are important, e.g. camels in Ethiopia, llamas in the Andes, moose in Russia, water buffalo in Vietnam, donkeys in Sardinia, horses in Mongolia, reindeer in Sweden and yaks in Tibet. For the endangered foods in this chapter, I focus on the milk of sheep and cows.

258 'mutation in the human genome': Like all mammals we drink milk as babies (the word 'mammal' comes from the scientific name *Mammalia*, coined by Carl Linnaeus in 1758, derived from the Latin for mammary glands). Beyond childhood our bodies weren't evolved to digest milk; 10,000 years ago no adult human would have been able to drink any milk at all. The enzyme lactase, which enables children to digest the milk sugar lactose, drops down to very low levels after weaning. The trait that allowed that production of the enzyme to continue (lactase persistence) evolved independently at least four times in human evolution and in different parts of the world. The mutation is thought to have given some humans such a big advantage it spread rapidly through natural selection. What that advantage was, we're not sure. It's possible that during the transition to farming, when crop failures and periods of starvation were common, the inability to drink milk might have decided whether people lived or died.

258 'an evolutionary advantage': Currently around 40 per cent of people globally have the lactase-persistent trait. They exist mainly in European populations – especially north-western Europe – and in parts of the Middle East, sub-Saharan Africa and South Asia (and in parts of the world where these populations migrated).

259 'blink of an eye': It could be that Asia's growing consumption of milk is possible (i.e. not causing too much discomfort) because of the way in which milk is being consumed. This is mostly in small portions in coffee, cakes and confectionary.

259 'longer fermentation': Acidification and fermentation also lead to some protein bonding (albeit fragile) and so even before rennet is added curds can start forming. Both forms of coagulation express whey and flush out some lactose; the ageing of cheese, helped by dehydration, also allows enzymes to 'pre-digest' milk.

259 'enzymes knit together proteins': Mateo Kehler (ed.), *The Oxford Companion to Cheese* (OUP, 2016).

259 'strange-looking clay fragments, 7,000 years old': For an insight into the fascinating work of finding prehistoric molecules of milk on clay (and working out what it all means): Mélanie Salque et al., 'Earliest evidence for cheese making in the sixth millennium BC in northern Europe', *Nature*, 493, January 2013, 522–5. See also Rosalind E. Gillis et al., 'The evolution of dual meat and milk cattle husbandry in Linearbandkeramik societies',

Proceedings of the Royal Society, Biological Sciences, 2017, DOI: 10.1098/rspb.2017 .0905.

259 'an American archaeologist': The archaeologist was Peter Bogucki. See John Sullivan, 'Clay pot fragments reveal early start to cheese-making, a marker for civilization', Princeton University, 2013, https://www.princeton.edu /news/2013/01/09/clay-pot-fragments-reveal-early-start-cheese-making-marker -civilization.

260 'earliest evidence of cheese-making': Gillis et al., *Proceedings of the Royal Society, Biological Sciences*.

260 'closer to ricotta': Ricotta (a very creamy cheese) is produced through the simple bonding that takes place through acidification. Mozzarella is a very different kind of cheese with a much firmer type of coagulation (although it is often seen suspended in milky whey). See Salque et al., *Nature*.

260 'temples dedicated to milk': Mark Kurlansky, *Milk! A 10,000-Year Food Fracas* (Bloomsbury, 2019).

260 'origins of Parmigiano Reggiano': The food anthropologist and cheese expert Harry West says the roots of Parmigiano Reggiano can be traced back to Alpine monasteries, and the monks in the Alps were likely to have learned cheese-making from Celtic barbarians; many Roman cheeses are Barbarian knock-offs, West says.

262 'only one of these traditional farmhouse cheeses ': This is Kirkham's of Lancashire which continues to be made with unpasteurised milk.

262 'twenty multinational companies now control': 'How Milk Went Global', Global-Rural Research Project, Aberystwyth University, 2018, https://www .global-rural.org/story_map/how-milk-went-global/.

262 'triggered an increase in disease': Milk produced in unsanitary 'swill barns' within cities was particularly problematic.

263 'fell by one-third': See 'How Milk Went Global', Global-Rural Research Project.

263 'dairies can house more than 9,000': Mike Opperman, 'How Consolidation Has Changed the Dairy Industry', *Farm Journal*, August 2019, accessed in *Wisconsin State Farmer*, https://eu.wisfarmer.com/story/news/2019/08/28 /how-consolidation-has-changed-dairy-industry/2127385001/.

263 'genetics of these animals was altered': Filippo Miglior et al., 'A 100-Year Review: Identification and genetic selection of economically important traits in dairy cattle', *Journal of Dairy Science*, 100 (12), December 2017, 10251–10271, DOI: 10.3168/jds.2017-12968. This has brought some serious problems for the breed including reduced immunity to disease and reduced fertility (without which milk isn't produced). Breeders have had to take the Holstein back a few steps in its recent history in order to reduce these issues. See L. Ma, T. Sonstegard et al., 'Genome changes due to artificial selection in

U.S. Holstein cattle', *BMC Genomics*, 20, 128, 2019, DOI: 10.1186/s12864-019
-5459-x.

265 'small stone cottages called *burons:*' Kehler (ed.), *The Oxford Companion to Cheese*, p. 633.

265 'an almost monastic existence': When Harry West spent time living with Salers makers in the Auvergne they told him the traditional approach to cheesemaking, with months spent in near isolaton up in the mountain, had strong associations with celibacy (the same levels of discipline and sacrifice were involved). This is a part of what makes the continuation of the tradition so difficult today as young men are no longer prepared to give up the prospect of a social and family life.

265 'down to the village by cart': Author interview with Harry West, September 2020.

265 'milk of an endangered dairy animal': The Cattle Site, 'Cattle Breeds – Salers: History', http://www.thecattlesite.com/breeds/beef/15/salers/.

266 'aromatic compounds called terpenes': Michael Tunick, *The Science of Cheese* (OUP USA, 2014). See also *The Oxford Companion to Cheese*.

267 'best possible home': For more on this idea, see Bronwen Percival and Francis Percival, *Reinventing the Wheel: Milk, Microbes and the Fight for Real Cheese* (Bloomsbury Sigma, 2019).

267 'too hostile an environment': Despite the cheese's long history, traditional Salers makers have had to meet regulations designed for cheese-making in modern, near-sterile dairies. According to Harry West, the situation is further complicated by Salers cheeses starting off with slightly higher microbial counts than pasteurised milk cheeses. These undesirable microbes then die off as the cheeses mature.

269 'the source of the recipe': The person most likely to have perfected the recipe for Stilton was a woman called Frances Pawlett who, in 1740s Leicestershire, was making a cheese fitting its description.

269 'famous for cheese': Mateo Kehler (ed.), *The Oxford Companion to Cheese* (OUP, 2016).

269 'full of mites or maggots': Trevor Hickman, *Stilton Cheese: A History* (Amberley Publishing, 2012).

270 'more trouble than babies': Lisa Anderson, 'Stilton: The Once and Future King of Cheese', *Chicago Tribune*, 23 January 1986.

270 'The last truckle of Stilton': There were several factors at play leading up to the decline in farmhouse cheese-making. Many farm workers didn't survive the war, contributing to a labour shortage. The depression of the 1930s also led to reduced demand for more expensive cheeses. In the same decade, the government set up the Milk Marketing Board which gave dairy farmers a guaranteed price for their milk and so reduced the incentive to add value to it by making cheese.

271 'the Milk and Dairies Act': Peter Atkins, 'The long genealogy of quality in the British drinking-milk sector', *Historia Agraria*, 2017, 35–58.

272 'visiting cheesemakers on their farms': Randolph Hodgson's mission to save British farmhouse cheeses followed that of an earlier campaigning cheesemonger called Patrick Rance. The cheese-making renaissance, which really took off in the late 1990s and into the 2000s, saw the number of farmhouse cheeses rise to around seven hundred.

273 'the fungus *Penicillium roqueforti*': *Penicillium roqueforti* is a type of mould that takes its name from the French sheep's milk cheese matured in a cave where the mould is naturally occurring.

275 'All else is subservient': Edith Durham, *High Albania* (Echo Library edition, 2009). According to Pier Paolo Ambrosi, 'blood vengeance' was just one feature of a code which regulated many aspects of life in the highlands of Albania. This code, called the Kanun, handed down orally, included how to welcome and respect a guest, how a theft should be compensated and murder punished. The management of justice, including 'blood vengeance', was governed by the Council of Elders as it was considered too important to be left to the initiative of individuals or families.

277 'hundreds of different wild flowers': Marash Rakaj, 'Floristic and chorological news from north Albania', *Botanica Serbica*, 2009, 33 (2), 177–83.

283 'a bacterial universe being saved': Chr. Hansen are exploring new applications for bacteria within its collection, including their potential to replace chemicals used in food preservation.

PART EIGHT: ALCOHOL

286 'drunken monkey hypothesis': R. Dudley, 'Evolutionary origins of human alcoholism in primate frugivory', *Quarterly Review of Biology*, 75 (1), March 2000, 3–15, DOI: 10.1086/393255.

288 'brewed from bananas': Paul Nugent, 'Alcohol in Africa', 15 November 2015, Centre of African Studies, Edinburgh, https://www.ascleiden.nl/content/webdossiers/alcohol-africa.

288 'mind-altering qualities': Andrew Curry, 'Our 9,000-Year Love Affair With Booze', *National Geographic*, February 2017.

288 '88 billion pints a year': 'Trouble Brewing', *The Economist*, 11 May 2019.

289 '60 per cent of all wine sales': Philip H. Howard, 'Recent Changes in the U.S. Beer Industry', Concentration and Power, State of Concentration in Global Food and Agriculture Industries (December 2017), https://philhoward.net/2019/12/30/recent-changes-in-the-u-s-beer-industry/and 'Concentration in the U.S. Wine Industry', https://philhoward.net/category/wine/. See also, *Wine Business Monthly*, February 2019.

289 'One of them, Gallo': Esther Mobley, 'What the wine world's mega-deal between Gallo and Constellation means for supermarket wine', *San Francisco Chronicle*, 7 January 2021.

289 '1,500 grape varieties': The number is growing; recent interest in increasing the diversity of wine styles and varieties has meant more are being discovered. See Jancis Robinson, *Wine Grapes* (Allen Lane, 2012).

290 'birth of winemaking': As with the 'centres of origin' of other foods and drinks, grape domestication and winemaking might have happened in several places, including Armenia and north-eastern Turkey as well as the South Caucasus.

291 'open-air museum of soils': Lisa Granik MW, *The Wines of Georgia* (Infinite Ideas, 2020).

291 'How is your vineyard': Author interview with John Wurdeman of Pheasant's Tears winery, Georgia, October 2018.

293 'stems inside the qvevri': Stems are used only when sufficiently ripened, which is why this technique is most likely to be found in eastern Georgia where the summers are hotter.

295 'wrapped in the mother's embrace': Author interview with Carla Capalbo, September 2020.

295 'big enough to hold a man': J.A. Hammerton (ed.), *Peoples of All Nations: Their life today and the story of their past by our foremost writers of travel, anthropology & history* (Educational Book Co. Limited, 1922). See also Alice Feiring, *For the Love of Wine* (Potomac Books, 2016).

296 'grape varieties facing extinction': Many were saved by one or two families keeping them going in their little plots, which is why around 470 of the original 515 varieties survived.

296 'state monopoly, Samtrest': Granik, *The Wines of Georgia*.

296 'Truth is in growing your own grapes': Miquel Hudin, 'Ancient Georgian winemaking loses one of its modern founders', *Harpers*, 13 April 2018.

297 'dismantled by communism': In the years following the collapse of the Soviet Union, the quality of Georgia's conventionial wine has gone from strength to strength. Around 50 per cent is exported to Russia. This has resulted in the drink being used as a political weapon, such as in 2006–2013, when Russia placed a ban on Georgian wine imports.

297 'out-producing Italy, Spain and Portugal': Stephen Buranyi, 'Has wine gone bad?', *Guardian*, 14 August 2018.

297 'father of modern winemaking': Mike Steinberger, 'The Tastemaker: Émile Peynaud invented modern winemaking, but don't blame him for what's wrong with modern wine', *Slate*, 30 July 2004.

298 'world's most sought-after wine consultant': Eric Asimov, 'Satan or Savior: Setting the Grape Standard', *New York Times*, 11 October 2006.

300 'The standard states': Among the criteria for natural wines is that 'additions' such as acid, sugar, tannin, water and colouring are forbidden. See

Jancis Robinson, 'The Definition of Natural Wine', *Financial Times*, 10 April 2020.

301 'John Steinbeck portrays Georgians': John Steinbeck, *A Russian Journal* (Penguin, 1948).

303 'tasted and looked like wine': See Michael Jackson, *The Beer Hunter*, Channel 4, 1990, for the most eloquent descriptions of Belgian beer diversity.

304 'changed so little': See also Michael Jackson, *Michael Jackson's Beer Companion* (Mitchell Beazley, 1997).

305 'add wheat to their grist': It is a significant proportion, around one-third of the mix, which is why lambics are often considered to be a subset of 'wheat beers'.

306 'old bookshop': Tim Webb and Joe Strange, *CAMRA's Good Beer Guide Belgium* (CAMRA Books, 2018).

307 'relatively young upstart': Louis Pasteur first discovered yeasts in the 1850s when he observed the single-celled fungi consuming sugars and converting them into ethanol and CO_2. In Copenhagen in the 1880s, Emil Hansen became the first person to isolate a pure yeast cell. The species was *Saccharomyces carlsbergensis*, named after the Carlsberg brewery laboratory in which it was isolated. This yeast works slowly at low temperatures and produces lager-style beers. Using different, faster-acting strains of yeast, which work at higher temperatures, results in the other main family of beer, ales. For centuries brewers saved their own yeast; strains that worked in one brew were added to the next. But from the 1880s onwards, following Pasteur's and Hansen's breakthroughs, it became possible to buy specific laboratory-produced yeast strains and so achieve consistent results in the brewhouse all year round. With greater consistency the era of mass-market beers arrived.

307 'lagers were dark in colour': Author interview with drinks writer Pete Brown, November 2020.

308 '95 per cent of all global beer': Garrett Oliver (ed.), *The Oxford Companion to Beer* (OUP, 2011), see entry for Pilsner.

313 'One of the best': Pete Brown and Bill Bradshaw, *World's Best Cider* (Sterling Publishing, 2013).

315 'Perry was a drink of kings': Ralph Austen, *A Treatise of Fruit Trees* (1676), quoted in Joan Morgan, *The Book of Pears* (Ebury Press, 2015).

316 'factory-sized production': An exception was Babycham, although the drink was eventually made with varieties other than perry pears.

PART NINE: STIMULANTS

321 'They have a very good drink ... ': Quoted in William Harrison Ukers, *All About Coffee* (The Tea and Coffee Trade Journal Company, 1922).

322 'the extraordinary thing happened': Marcel Proust, *In Search of Lost Time* (Vintage, 1996).

322 'a means of purifying the body': Ben Richmond, 'The Forgotten Drink That Caffeinated North America for Centuries', *Atlas Obscura*, March 2018.

323 'world's favourite drug': Tea also contains a chemical relative of caffeine that's even more potent, theophylline, although it's present in much smaller amounts.

324 'nearly $5 billion a year': Bruno Volsi et al., 'The dynamics of coffee production in Brazil', *PLoS ONE*, 14(7), 2019, DOI:10.1371/journal.pone.0219742.

326 'the tea plant *Camellia sinensis*': The other main variety, *Camellia sinensis-sinensis*, is more sensitive and has smaller leaves.

326 'in most of the world's vast plantations': The different types of loose-leaf tea (white, green, black, oolong or pu-erh) are determined by the way in which the leaves of the *Camellia sinensis* plant are processed (the amount of oxidation involved is crucial to deciding its flavour). White teas are the young and tender leaves; green tea is made when tea leaves are heated soon after picking, which fixes their colour; if leaves are withered and then bruised a little, causing oxidisation, this results in black tea. Oolong fits somewhere between green and black tea. And then there's pu-erh, arrived at after a longer, more complex process.

326 'the rarest pu-erh': There is an important distinction between raw pu-erh and a modern version, 'ripe' pu-erh. Raw cakes are those allowed to ferment naturally, in some cases over a period of decades (the focus of the story in this chapter). Ripe pu-erh goes through a process designed to speed up fermentation and replicate some of the characteristics of the ageing process for a mass-market version of the cakes. In a technique developed in the 1970s, leaves are piled up on concrete floors in warehouses, moistened with water and then left for two to three months in a batch fermentation (during which leaves will be moved around from top to bottom). This method produces much darker cakes. Because of this process it is highly unlikely the best-quality leaves (including the rarest leaves from ancient trees) will be used. Raw pu-erh can even be thought of as sun-dried green tea (i.e. minimal intervention). It should be added that you can still find great-tasting ripe pu-erh and disappointing (and expensive) raw pu-erh. This is why buying cakes from a source you can trust is essential.

326 'a quarter of all mammals found': Jia Qi Zhang et al., 'After the rubber boom: good news and bad news for biodiversity in Xishuangbanna, Yunnan, China', *Regional Environmental Change*, 19, 1713–24, May 2019.

326 'what scientists call "plant apparency"': A.M. Smilanich, R.M. Fincher, L.A. Dyer, 'Does plant apparency matter? Thirty years of data provide limited

support but reveal clear patterns of the effects of plant chemistry on herbi-vores', *New Phytologist*, 210 (3), May 2016, 1044–57, DOI: 10.1111/nph.13875.

330 'With their dirty fingers': A. Henry Savage Landor, *An explorer's adventures in Tibet* (Harper & Brothers, 1910).

330 'South-east of the Yangtze': Victor H. Mair and Erling Hoh, *The True History of Tea* (Thames & Hudson, 2009).

331 'global rubber prices tripled': Despite decades of research, synthetic materials can't match the natural product tapped from trees (it's tougher and more elastic).

334 'capacity of *la roya*': It thrives when there's plenty of moisture and where temperatures hover between 16°C and 28°C. See Stuart McCook, *Coffee Is Not Forever* (Ohio University Press, 2019).

334 'coffee harvests in Colombia': Jacques Avelino et al., 'The coffee rust crises in Colombia and Central America (2008–2013)', *Food Security*, 7. 303-321, 2015, DOI:10.1007/s12571-015-0446-9.

334 'cost of damaged crops': Maryn McKenna, 'Coffee Rust Is Going to Ruin Your Morning', *The Atlantic*, 16 September 2020.

334 'Migrant caravans travelling north': Oliver Milman, 'The unseen driver behind the migrant caravan: climate change', *Guardian*, 30 October 2018.

335 'the raw beans were chewed': Aaron Davis et al., *Coffee Atlas of Ethiopia* (Kew Publishing, 2018).

335 'the Oromo people of southern Ethiopia': Jonathan Morris, *Coffee: A Global History* (Reaktion Books, 2018).

336 'In the west are the Wellega': Aaron Davis et al., *Coffee Atlas of Ethiopia* (Kew Publishing, 2018).

336 'coffee may be sweet and subtle': Author interview with Aaron Davis, Kew's head of coffee research, January 2019.

337 'travel writer James Bruce': Jeff Koehler, *Where the Wild Coffee Grows* (Bloomsbury USA, 2018).

337 'presence of the volcanic glass obsidian': Author interview with Dorian Fuller, Professor of Archaeobotany at UCL, September 2018.

337 'became known as *qahwa*': It's from *qahwa*, some historians argue, that we get the word 'coffee', although others believe it comes from the name of the wild coffee zone, Kaffa.

337 'coffee drinking among dervishes': William Ukers, 'All About Coffee', *Trade Journal Company*, 1922.

338 'The Age of Enlightenment': For more on this idea see Steven Johnson, *The Invention of Air* (Riverhead Books, 2009).

338 'de Clieu kept it alive': Frederick L. Wellman, *Coffee (World Crop Series)*, (Leonard Hill Books Ltd, 1961).

339 'was called *bourbon*': James Hoffman, *The World Atlas of Coffee* (Mitchell Beazley, 2018).

340 'The most celebrated': Its proper name is Gesha, from the village. It was changed to Geisha by the Japanese, who were the first to pay high sums for it in auction. Although Geisha has some resistance to rust it has mostly been a success due to its exceptional taste.

340 'Scientists at the Royal Botanic Gardens': Aaron Davis et al., 'The Impact of Climate Change on Indigenous Arabica Coffee (*Coffea arabica*): Predicting Future Trends and Identifying Priorities', *PLoS ONE*, 7(11): DOI.org/10.1371/journal.pone.0047981.

343 '60 per cent are threatened': 'Kew scientists reveal that 60% of wild coffee species are threatened with extinction, causing concern for the future of coffee production', 16 January 2019, https://www.kew.org/about-us/press-media/kew-scientists-reveal-that-60-of-wild-coffee.

PART TEN: SWEET

345 'If the enemy is taking': Quoted from Lionel Giles, *Sun Tzu on the Art of War* (Luzac and Co., 1910).

349 'leading food exporters in the region': Basma Alloush, 'The importance of the agricultural sector for Syria's stability', Chatham House, August 2018, https://syria.chathamhouse.org/research/the-importance-of-the-agricultural-sector-for-syrias-stability.

349 'drought- and disease-resistant traits': Mark Schapiro, 'How Seeds from War-Torn Syria Could Help Save American Wheat', *Yale Environment 360*, Yale School of Environment, 14 May 2018, https://e360.yale.edu/features/how-seeds-from-war-torn-syria-could-help-save-american-wheat.

351 'The pistachio tree is the lung': Quoted in the *Bangkok Post*, 16 July 2020.

352 'across the border into Turkey': Shira Rubin, 'Syrian refugee chefs recreate the taste of home in Turkey', *Mashable*, 15 February 2016, https://mashable.com/2016/02/15/syrian-refugee-chefs-turkey/?europe=true.

352 'Like a fire': Lauren Bohn, 'Out of Syria', *Culinary Backstreets*, 16 March 2016, https://culinarybackstreets.com/cities-category/istanbul/2016/salloura-an-epic-of-sweets-chap-1-out-of-syria/. See also Lila Hasan, 'Legacy of Salloura Bakery continues in Istanbul via refugees', *Daily Sabah*, 5 August 2015.

355 'the control of water': Martin Asser, 'Obstacles to Arab-Israeli peace: Water', BBC News, 2 September 2010, https://www.bbc.co.uk/news/world-middle-east-11101797.

355 'the West Bank's water': *Amnesty International*, 'The Occupation of Water', 29 November 2017, https://www.amnesty.org/en/latest/campaigns/2017/11/the-occupation-of-water/.

355 'the World Bank highlighted': World Bank, 'Area C and the Future of the Palestinian Economy', 2014, http://documents1.worldbank.org/curated /en/257131468140639464/pdf/Area-C-and-the-future-of-the-Palestinian-economy .pdf.

355 'pitch-black qizha cake': Daniella Peled, 'A Taste of Nablus', *Roads & Kingdoms*, 24 September 2014, https://roadsandkingdoms.com/2014 /a-taste-of-nablus/.

358 'world's murder hotspots': William Finnegan, 'Venezuela, a Failing State', *New Yorker*, 14 November 2016.

360 'filled with "black gold"': Matthew Smith, 'The End of Venezuela's Oil Era', oilprice.com, 22 October 2020, https://oilprice.com/Energy/Energy -General/The-End-Of-Venezuelas-Oil-Era.html.

360 'cacao could do this again': As far back as the 1980s, Venezuelan governments had been advised to diversify the economy and reduce the reliance on the oil industry (at the time 80 per cent of export income). When oil prices started to fluctuate in the late 1980s, Caracas turned to the International Monetary Fund for help. The IMF recommended severe cuts in public spending. When these reforms were implemented, high levels of inflation and civil unrest followed. This led Venezuela on a path towards the more radical and socialist governments of Hugo Chavez and Nicolás Maduro.

361 'to settle unpaid taxes': Luc Cohen, 'Venezuela cocoa growers fear new pest: the government', *Reuters*, 27 December 2018.

361 'oil exports unsteady': By July 2020, Venezuela was pumping an average of 345,000 barrels of crude daily, the lowest level in nearly a century. See Smith, oilprice.com.

362 'even Coca-Cola's factories': 'Sugar shortage cuts Coca-Cola production in Venezuela', BBC News, 24 May 2016.

363 'chocolate sipped by Europeans': Sophie D. Coe and Michael D. Coe, *The True History of Chocolate* (Thames & Hudson, 1996).

363 'The Spanish Crown': H. Michael Tarver and Julia C. Frederick, *The History of Venezuela* (Greenwood Press, 2005).

364 'the fruits have a flavour': François Joseph Pons: *A Voyage to the Eastern Part of Terra Firma, Or the Spanish Main, in South-America, During the Years 1801, 1802, 1803 and 1804: Containing a Description of the Territory Under the Jurisdiction of the Captain-General of Caraccas, Composed of the Provinces* (Ulan Press, 2012).

366 'temperatures within the box': Harold McGee, *McGee on Food and Cooking: An Encyclopedia of Kitchen Science* (Hodder & Stoughton, 2004).

368 'She collected a thousand': Elena Molokhovets, *Classic Russian Cooking: Elena Molokhovets' A Gift to Young Housewives* (Indiana University Press, 1998).

368 'it was called Ni-Kola': Natasha Frost, 'Russia's Patriotic Alternative to Coca-Cola Is Made Out of Bread', *Atlas Obscura*, 18 April 2018.

369 'Until it's ready': Grigory Tarasevich, 'White kvass: An old drink with a new taste', *Russia Beyond*, 15 September 2013.

EPILOGUE: THINK LIKE A HADZA

371 'Are we being ... ': Jonas Salk, 'Are We Being Good Ancestors?', *World Affairs*, 1, 16–18, 1992.

375 'every minute of every day': Food and Land Use Coalition, 'Growing Better Report 2019', https://www.foodandlandusecoalition.org/global-report/. Also the author's conversation with one of the contributors to the 'Growing Better Report', the economist Jeremy Oppenheim.

376 '30 per cent of food for school meals': 'Crop swap: Thousands of edible plants could feed us on a hotter planet', Reuters, September 2020.

376 'supplying apples to schools': Michael Allen, 'Brexit: an opportunity for local food systems?', *Youris*, 2 October 2019, https://www.youris.com/bioec onomy/food/brexit-an-opportunity-for-local-food-systems-.kl

Acknowledgements

Eating to Extinction exists because of three people. One is Claire Conrad, my literary agent, who listened to me tell stories on radio and was convinced she was listening to a potential writer as well as a broadcaster. The second is my editor, Bea Hemming of Jonathan Cape, who patiently listened to my ideas, saw the bigger picture and imagined a more ambitious book than I believed was possible. A huge thank you to them both. The third person I'll mention at the end.

It wasn't hard to choose the endangered foods featured in this book. But telling these stories – and weaving them together – has involved the help of many kind and clever people, including several academic advisers. I would especially like to thank: Professor Dorian Fuller, who introduced me not only to the seed library at University College London back in 2018 when I started to write this book, but also to the wonders and mysteries of the world's earliest farmers; Professor Tim Benton of Chatham House, whose expertise in global food systems and the urgency of the challenges we now face has been invaluable; Dr Joan Morgan, whose feedback and encouragement has been a source of inspiration; Professor John Dickie, who provided much-needed support and advice as I started to write my first draft; Professor Harry West, who reminded me that the cultural dimension of endangered foods really matters; and Professor Jules Pretty, who shared his exceptional insights into wild foods and indigenous societies.

Finding many of these stories and the people in a position to tell them would have been impossible without the help of the Slow Food team in Bra. My heartfelt gratitude goes to Paola Nano, Giulia Capaldi, Paolo di Croce, Serena Milano, Michele Rumiz, Nazarena Lanza, Charles Barstow and, of course, Carlo Petrini. Many experts all over the world, working in various fields, have been unbelievably generous with their time and their knowledge, helping me to shape my ideas. Any remaining misunderstandings or mistakes are of course down to me.

For 'Wild': my thanks to Professor Alyssa Crittenden, an expert on the Hadza, who deepened my respect for these hunter-gatherers long after I had a chance to visit them. In Australia, thanks to Ben Shewry, Bruce Pascoe, Professor John Morgan at La Trobe University and Dave Wandin. Professor Monique Simmonds at the Royal Botanic Gardens, Kew, was my brilliant guide to all things medicinal in the wild food stories, while Phrang Roy taught me about the food and people of Megahalaya.

For 'Cereals': I'm indebted to: Claire Kanja, who was always prepared to break away from her PhD research at Rothamsted Research to explain the intricacies of sneaky crop diseases; Alptekin Karagöz in Turkey, for introducing me to the story of Mirza Gökgöl; Jeremy Churfass, along with Luigi Guarino and his colleagues at the Crop Trust, for sharing their passion for plant diversity. Thanks also to John Letts and Mark Nesbitt for invaluable help with all things einkorn and emmer. My rice advisers included Ruaraidh Sackville Hamilton and Debal Deb, who really helped me appreciate how beautifully diverse rice can be. Logan Kistler at the Smithsonian Institution was a great help with maize. Thanks also to Cary Fowler and Colin Khoury for conversations about Svalbard and Vavilov.

For 'Vegetables': my thanks to Alys Fowler, Phil H. Howard at Michigan State University, Colin Tudge, Geoff Tansey, Jessica Harris and Eve Emshwiller. Also thanks to Nik Heynen for bringing the story of the Geechee red pea up to date for me. Many thanks too to Josiah Meldrum and the team at Hodmedods and Tomas Erlandsson in Sweden for everything I needed to know about lentils.

For 'Meat': my thanks to Professor Greger Larson at Oxford for guidance on animal domestication, Simon Fairlie for many discussions on farming and livestock and to Bob Kennard for his excellent insights into sheep history and mutton. In the USA, my thanks to Jack Rhyan for helping me with bison history, to Jennifer Bartlett in Colorado for guiding me to bison (and maize).

For 'From the Sea': I was blessed to have the assistance of Callum Roberts and Chris Williams, whose years of research on fish and fisheries was crucial in writing this part of the book. Thanks also to Daniel

Pauly at the Sea Around Us, Ian Roberts at Mowi, and Mark Bilsby and Professor Ken Whelan at the Atlantic Salmon Trust.

For 'Fruit': thank you to fellow journalist Mike Knowles for his unique grasp of the fruit industry and Cindy Rijswick at Rabobank; to Fred Gmitter, Marco Caruso and Giuseppe Reforgiato for citrus wisdom; Fernando A. García for banana science; Vladimir Levin for apple history in the forests of the Tian Shan; and Barrie Juniper for a memorable day picking apples in Oxford.

For 'Cheese': my thanks to Andy Swinscoe at the Courtyard Dairy, Bronwyn Percival at Neal's Yard, Joe Schneider at Stichelton Dairy and Professor Michael Woods at Aberystwyth University.

For 'Alcohol': thanks to Jancis Robinson, Sarah Abbott, Jamie Goode, Tim Webb, Pete Brown, Carla Capalbo and Patrick Boettcher, Tom Oliver and Charles Martell, who were all so helpful in sharing their love and understanding of beer, wine and perry.

For 'Stimulants': thanks to Aaron Davis at Kew, the world's foremost expert on coffee and endangered varieties; and Don Mei at Mei Leaf tea for opening up the world of pu-erh for me.

For 'Sweet': thanks to chocolate experts Chantal Coady, Chloé Doutre-Roussel and Juan C. Motamayor.

For the Epilogue: thank you to Miles Irving, economist Jeremy Oppenheim and, again, Professor Tim Benton, for their ideas and suggestions.

Thank you to all my different travelling companions for helping me reach some remote places and explaining so much when we arrived. These are too many to mention but include Fatih Tatari in Turkey, Stephen Harr in the Faroe Islands, Rob Wallace and the Wildlife Conservation Society in Bolivia, and Remi Ie in Okinawa.

I also need to thank many people at the BBC, including the reporters, producers and contributors I've worked with over the years on *The Food Programme*. Particular thanks go to my editors Clare McGinn and Dimitri Houtart, and Controller of Production Graham Ellis for supporting my work over the years and for making it possible for me to take a career break from the BBC to write this book. My warm thanks to Sheila Dillon for being a great mentor, dear friend and inspirational colleague. Also, to my parents Elaine and Liborio Saladino for all their encouragement.

A special thank you goes to my wife, Annabel, who is the third person who made *Eating to Extinction* possible. She has been my closest collaborator in writing this book. To my sons, Harry and Charlie, I hope I've done you proud, and that one day you will love this book a fraction of the amount that I love you both. And finally, to Scout the dog, for all the walks in Lineover Woods in the autumn and winter of 2018, where many of my ideas began to take shape.

Index